REJECTION AND TOLERANCE

Transplantation and Clinical Immunology

Symposia Fondation Marcel Mérieux

VOLUME 25

Rejection and Tolerance

Proceedings of the 25th Conference on
Transplantation and Clinical Immunology,
24–26 May 1993

organized by
Fondation Marcel Mérieux and Université Claude Bernard-Lyon I

Edited by

J.L. Touraine
J. Traeger
H. Bétuel
J.M. Dubernard
J.P. Revillard
C. Dupuy

Springer-Science+Business Media, B.V.

A C.I.P. Catalogue record for this book is available from the Library of Congress

ISBN 978-94-010-4345-8   ISBN 978-94-011-0802-7 (eBook)
DOI 10.1007/978-94-011-0802-7

Printed on acid-free paper

Table of Contents

vi

Authors Part B: Follow-up of transplant patients and immunological monitoring

ETHICS AND ORGAN TRANSPLANTATION

Jean Bernard

From the outset, the pioneers of the new methods of transplantation were acutely aware of the importance of the ethical problems that organ transplantation involves.

In connection, for instance, with the kidney, Jean Hamburger, Jean Crosnier and Jean Dormont wrote a report as early as 1965 on the moral issues raised by organ substitution and transplantation. For the skin and bone marrow, Jean Dausset analysed the conditions of experimentation on man and suggested possible solutions to the difficulties experienced.

Transplantation has in fact its own history and geography, and over the past twenty-five years, two distinct trends have emerged :
- one of them inclines towards diversity : it concerns the diversity of the organs (even or uneven numbers, dead or living, regenerable or unregenerable), of the practices in different countries (from the huge publicity in South Africa to the discretion that reigns in California, and from French orthodoxy to the sale of organs in Brazil), and of the present laws, which range from anachronistic to very advanced.
- the second trend is towards unity, and is based on scientific and technical progress and on the closer relations and exchanges of knowledge among the teams concerned all over the world.

It is important to stress that the ethical model for transplantation can be extended to bioethics as a whole. This makes it possible to tackle and discuss the essential moral problems of biology and medicine, including experimentation on man, artificial life support, the definition of a person, profit-making and disinterestedness.

The present review will consider each of the moral problems that concern the donors and hosts respectively. The donor may be dead or living, and the deceased donor may be an adult or a foetus.

Deceased adult donors

The very principle of organ removal is controversial : is it lawful to violate death and dissect a corpse ? The idea that this is forbidden goes back to the dawn of history and primitive societies. The French writer Vercors described this worship of the dead in a beautiful novel called "Les animaux dénaturés" (denatured animals).

Attitudes to organ removal were surveyed in two studies by American authors : one of them, published in 1980, recorded a neutral attitude, or

1

J. L. Touraine et al. (eds.), Rejection and Tolerance, 1–9.
© 1994 Kluwer Academic Publishers.

grudging approval, by sixty-nine religious groups, and in the other more recent survey, twenty religious families expressed more varied reactions.

These attitudes, especially those of Buddhists and Moslems, were motivated by three wishes : not to go against the basic tenets in the fundamental scriptures, the hope of finding elements in these scriptures that would justify current practices, and love of one's neighbour and the desire to help him.

Pope Pious XI was the first to lift the ban on removing the cornea. After that, there was fairly general agreement on the right to organ removal, with some geographical variations. Thus, as certain eastern religious consider that the soul remains in the body for a week after death, it is forbidden, in Japan, to touch a corpse during that week. And as Dominique Lapierre recounts in The City of Joy, extreme poverty may reduce an Indian father to selling his body in advance, to provide his daughter with a dowry.

Acknowledgement of the right to remove organs from the dead implies that two conditions have been fulfilled : firstly, that death is certain and secondly, consent to such removal.

One of the most remarkable events of our time has been the need for human societies to define death. This definition may not have been very clear in the 1930s, when blood from corpses was used for transfusion (Judine, URSS, 1935) ; this was the first time that human tissue from the dead was used for therapeutic purposes. The definition necessarily became stricter when the removal of organs like the kidney became urgent. A moving report by Jean Hamburger had shown that a young girl whose heart was beating and whose lungs were breathing could nevertheless be dead. In many countries, the law defines death as the presence of several symptoms which are evidence of brain death, and requires two successive flat electro-encephalograms as well as the agreement of several physicians.

Further progress in biology may change this situation in the future. This would be the case if the results of experiments by Etienne Wolff on lower crustaceans, showing that indifferentiated cells can be differentiated into nerve cells, were first confirmed and then extended to mammals and man. It may be that every 50 or 100 years, human societies will have to find new definitions of death.

Consent may have been given either long before death or just before it (for instance by a person undergoing an operation, or someone condemned to death). It can also be given by the family of someone who has just died.

The right to remove an organ without consent or agreement may be a consequence of certain laws. This, for instance is the case in France for the Caillavet Law of December 22nd, 1976, whose provisions were completed by the decree of March 31st 1978 for its enforcement. The Americans have called this law courageous, but no law, however good, can solve all the moral problems with which physicians have to contend. What is more, there are great differences between countries and sometimes, as in the United States, differences between the States of a single country.

Two solutions to the problem of consent can be envisaged. The presence of a competent trained person capable of having the long explanatory talk with the bereaved familiy necessary to obtain its consent, prompted by human solidarity ; or else to advise persons at risk to carry with them a document allowing or forbidding organ removal in case of sudden death.

The second solution is the best, and is strongly recommended in Belgium and Austria. In Turkey, the agreement of 100 000 subjects to organ removal in case of accidental death was obtained in 1992 as a result of a vigorous campaign in favour of consent.

However, most healthy people do not think about their death, or dislike thinking about it and an energetic campaign to educate them to do so is undoubtedly necessary.

There is a definite relationship, which may be obvious, flaunted, hypocritical or dissembled, between the wealth of the host and the speed with which the desired organ becomes available. The resolutions passed by various American associations like the Transplantation Association are extremely instructive for their explanations of the different methods of buying and selling organs, methods which they condemn wholeheartedly or feebly.

In France, the Ministry of Health has issued instructions recommending that transplantations should only be performed in the public wards of the hospitals.

Deceased donors : the foetus

Foetal tissue grafting is not a new development, but has been done since the beginning of the century, under very diverse conditions. The failure of such grafts in diabetes was already reported in 1928. The effectiveness of foetal thymus transplantation in treating congenital thymus hypoplasia or DiGeorge syndrome was recognized in 1960. From Australia to France, and from the United States to Mexico, more than 1 000 foetal tissue transplantations have been performed during the past 30 years - the largest numbers in the former Soviet Union and China.

These foetal tissue or organ grafts have given rise to sharp controversy between physicians anxious to save their patients and representatives of moral and spiritual groups who, perhaps rightly, fear that in all good faith, this type of graft may lead to an increase in the number of voluntary abortions. Legal proceedings have even been instituted against certain very eminent physicians. When these matters were referred to the French National Ethics Consultative Committee by a very embarrassed court, the Committee stated that the foetus should be considered as a potential person, and listed three distinct cases : 1) hematopoietic grafting of the foetal liver should be permitted when it can save the life of a child with severe immune deficiency and when no HLA-compatible sibling donor is available ; 2) such grafts should not be permitted when the foetal tissue is to be used to manufacture cosmetics and beauty products and 3) cases involving new or recurring problems concerning, for example, the pancreas, the foetus or diabetes should be referred to an ethics committee.

Since this opinion was formulated, the situation has become at once simpler and more complex.

Simpler, because the number of indications for liver grafts has been reduced, to the benefit of the number for bone marrow graft. More complex, because of the use of foetal nerve cells for grafts in Parkinson's disease, which may involve the need literally to programme abortion as a function of the chronological development of the necessary foetal nerve cells.

Living donors

At present, the organs taken from living donors are the kidney, bone marrow and liver, although many more kidneys from corpses than from living persons are used for grafting.

The removal of an organ from a living person is an amputation. The donor is usually an adult, but in the case of bone marrow, a self-regenerating tissue, the donor is fairly often a child.

Adults   Two vital questions are at issue : is the sacrifice acceptable ? and is refusal acceptable ? The conditions of the sacrifice have been defined and the donor may either be a member of the patient's family or a volunteer. Most studies of donors have dealt with the volunteers. For a long time the attitude of transplantation centres towards them was very reserved. However, the authors of an American study recently stressed the importance and moral value of such altruism, by recalling that in June 1992, 27 000 patients in the United States ware awaiting an organ. The donor must be fully aware of the risks involved in organ donation, and pressure must not be brought to bear on him or her. A psychological examination is desirable. On no account must the donor be remunerated. The sale of kidneys, and in some cases advertisements in the press and bargaining over prices, are not part of our civilization's moral code.

Acceptance of generous sacrifices is frequent and refusals are rare and extremely varied. They may involve the refusal by a wanted habitual criminal to help a brother whom his bone marrow could have saved, or the refusal of a mother who had agreed to give her bone marrow to her own child, to give it to save another dying child. In Britain, a man on the list of volunteer bone marrow donors was persuaded by his wife to change his mind at the last minute, thus causing the death of another man whom his bone marrow could have saved.

A number of studies have dealt with the state of mind of the volunteer donor during the years after organ donation. Two kinds of feeling appear to predominate : discreet satisfaction at the thought of his courage, combined with anxiety about a possible deterioration in his health ; much later the donation is forgotten altogether.

Liver grafts involve particular problems. Like the bone marrow, the liver is a self-regenerating organ. However, the risk of peroperative death of the donor, which is very slight for bone marrow removal, must in the case of liver donation be taken into account. As such method has already be used for donors of other organs, certain bold innovators made the first attempts at liver lobe removal in Japan, the United States and in the French city of Lyons, even before ascertaining the views of the various national ethics committees which were subsequently consulted.

In Turkey, eight liver lobe transplantations from living persons were performed between 1990 and 1992. American specialists in ethics considered that the donation of a living organ could be accepted when the risk for the donor was less than 1/1000. The exact degree of risk in the case of the liver is not known, but it is certain that parents whose children's lives are in danger are prepared to accept a higher risk than that.

The present ethical attitude to grafting liver from living persons can be summed up as follows : 1) the only acceptable indication is the one concerning the grafting of a fragment of liver from a parent to a child suffering from a liver disease with a fatal outcome ; 2) the dangers involved in a long wait for a volunteer's liver may justify this indication ; 3) the only teams which should be allowed to practice such liver grafts are those that combine great technical skill with a sense of responsability, and 4) after a reasonable number of such grafts, say ten, a report should be made to the national ethics committee.

Child donors   The diseases that can be cured by a bone marrow graft often concern children. At the present time, HLA-compatible donors are brothers and sisters, and therefore also children. Should such children, who are not really able to give informed consent, be exposed to the slight but non-negligible risk involved in a general anaesthetic ? The reply to this question varies in different countries.

In many of them, parental consent has often been sufficient.

In various States of the USA, an independent Child Advocate is designated, who may be a jurist or a philosopher. The Advocate studies all the aspects of the case and gives or withholds the required permission.

In France, the law on bioethics, which has now passed its first reading in the National Assembly, provides for the designation of a magistrate to give or withhold such permission. This provision is reasonable, on condition that the decision is made within a very short period, as in many cases the patient's condition does not allow a long wait.

Here again, a new problem arose a few years ago. In Italy, the only child of a couple in Lombardy had very serious leukaemia and no compatible bone marrow donor was available, so that the child was condemned to die. His parents envisaged having another child, in the hope that its bone marrow would be compatible. They consulted an Italian doctor, who, in a quandary, asked for my advice. However, the parents conceived the second child without waiting for their doctor's reply. The younger child's bone marrow was compatible with that of the older child, and a few months later, the graft was performed and proved successful. Today, the parents and both children are healthy and happy.

In other countries, several families who learnt what had happened in Italy and were confronted with a similar dilemma also conceived a second child, but the results were less fortunate. Determination of the HLA group of a foetus leads to abortion when there is incompatibility. In at least two families, several successive pregnancies were terminated for such incompatiblity, until in one family, attempts to conceive an HLA-compatible child were given up, and in the other, an HLA compatible child was at last born. Are such procedures really acceptable ?

As is often the case in bioethics, progress in research can provide a solution to a problem created by previous progress. Thus, the use of umbilical cord blood, first attempted by Eliane Gluckman, and the creation of a European Cord Blood Bank, might in the near future reduce the gravity and frequency of the moral questions involved in bone marrow grafting.

The host   Other ethical problems concern the host, the first being his consent to the graft. Here, he must be very fully informed : the surgeon or physician must explain to the patient the conditions under which the graft will be performed, and the possible complications and subsequent developments. These developments should be compared to those expected, i.e. the prognosis, for other forms of treatment. One such patient, a farmer from the Poitou district with chronic myeloid leukaemia, was fully informed of the risks of a bone marrow graft, which might have shortened his life, as occurs in 25% of cases, or saved it (50% of cases). As a result, he refused the graft. However, in most cases, the hope that the graft will succeed predominates. One patient given a transplant put it this way : "Moral problems only exist for those who have never had an organ transplant".

"If I had understood correctly, my heart pumps my brother's blood through my arteries", a young girl, Marie, with severe medullary deficiency, told me last year. She had just been grafted with the bone marrow of her brother, Jacques, which fortunately was compatible with hers. And it was true ; Marie had become a chimera ; not the chimera of Greek mythology, with the body of a lion, the head of a unicorn and the tail of a serpent, but a chimera none the less, since her body contained her brother's bone marrow together with her own organs.

The grafting of nerve cells will, if it develops satisfactorily, open up new possibilities. Here is a story about its implications. Pierre loves Jeanne. After an accident, Jeanne has to have an arm amputated, and another arm is grafted in its place. Pierre continues to love Jeanne. Later, Jeanne develops a serious kidney disease, and undergoes a kidney transplant which proves successful. Pierre is still in love with her. After a while, a heart transplant is envisaged. How many of Jeanne's organs and tissues can be changed without changing Pierre's love ? The usual reply is that this depends on the brain. As long as it is unchanged, love persists. But if nerve cells are grafted, what is the limit ? How many billions of neurons can be grafted without Pierre's love being affected ? A great French poet refused to consider the question ; Pierre, he said, was in love with his image of Jeanne, which could not be changed by all the grafts in the world.

Morals and economics

Other problems, less spiritual but nevertheless very important, arise from the relations between morals and economics in the field of transplantation.

According to French law, organs and tissues must be given and not sold. In some countries, however, there has been a dangerous evolution in this respect. In India, for instance, the buying and selling of organs is an accepted practice which may even be recommended. In South Africa, the personal advertisements of an evening newspaper sometimes advertise the sale of a kidney. A French missionary priest in Africa did not know what advice to give a poor farmer in Zaire, whose five children were dying of hunger and who was thinking of selling one of his kidneys, because this would bring in enough money to feed the children well for several years.

From Bombay to Sydney, Ottawa and Munich, meetings have been devoted to these questions.
The following classification of donors has been suggested :
- Living member of the family
- Donor deeply moved by misfortune
- Altruist donor outside the family
- Officially remunerated donor
- Unofficiallly remunerated donor (surreptitious trading)
- Donation obtained by criminal threats

A fluctuating moral code is developing, which is temporarily founded on the following rules :
1. Banning of go betweens
2. Banning of advertising and publicity
3. Donors must be in good health

4. Separate medical examinations of donor and host

5. Independance of the surgical team operating on the donor

6. Long-term sound insurance policy for the donor

7. Moderate remuneration for the team performing the transplantation

8. Subsidy to be requested from charities to help poor patients in countries without a social security system.

9. Regular publication of the results obtained by the transplantation team

10. Grafts confined to a country's inhabitants only.

The conclusions reached in the studies conducted by American transplantation teams are not all acceptable, and imply the existence of some regrettable moral deviations. There is reason to fear the advent of a difficult period dominatated by money, but there are also grounds for hoping for a return to more satisfactory ethics, dominated by the absence of trading in parts of the human body.

The expenses connected with transplantation techniques, hospital expenses and medical and nursing staff salaries are often considerable. In many countries such as France, they are entirely met by the social security system. In various centres in the United States, they have to be paid by the patient and his family before the grafting, thus giving rise to selection based on means, which is morally unacceptable.

Even in countries like France, which refuse to give priority to the rich, very serious problems arise when - as frequently happens - patients whom a graft could save are on a waiting list.

In such cases, an ethical choice is hard to make, and must take three kinds of factor into account (but in what order and to what extent ?) : 1) the need to save the patients most and the degree of urgency at risk 2) the prospects of success, which imply that the graft should go to the patient whom it is most likely to save, and 3) the heartless justice of the " first come first served" principle ; can organs be assigned to persons not residing in a country, and in what proportion of cases ? Where, in this respect, should one draw the line between total permissiveness and a total ban ? As the liver graft pioneer Starzl remarked, "Would Mozart have been given priority ?".

The economic problems of organ transplantation may affect all of society. Thus, in certain cases, organ grafting may save money, as is the case for the kidney, because kidney dialysis places a heavy burden on the budgets of modern societies. By limiting the number of patients dialysed, kidney grafts save money.

For bone marrow grafts, however, the situation is quite different, as shown by the following two examples.

A bone marrow graft is a good treatment for thalassemia major (ß-thalassemia), but it is too costly for the budgets of Mediterranean islands. Hence the decision to recommend in utero diagnosis and systematic abortion in the case of thalassemia major, i.e. the death of the foetuses concerned, for purely financial reasons.

The second example comes from France. In a large provincial town, a bone marrow graft, the only chance of survival for a leukaemic child, had been planned for December 10th. However, the hospital's manager informed the doctors that he could not agree to the graft, as the year's overall spending had already exceeded the budget, and so the graft would have to be done the following year, i.e. too late. Only when strong pressure was exerted on the town's mayor was the necessary money forthcoming.

It is quite deliberately that I have not so far mentioned xenografts. Research in this field is in full swing, but not convincing results have so far been obtained. However, in the near future, important progress may be expected, either in grafting proper, or in xenoperfusion, with pig liver being used for a few days as an artificial organ until human liver becomes obtainable for grafting.

Here again, important strides will create new ethical problems.

One of these concerns the donors. The monkey, in particular, is receiving a great deal of attention from animal lovers, who are less sensitive to the fate of the pig. Nevertheless, defenders of animals' rights are prepared to ban all xenotransplantation.

Other problems concern the hosts. For instance, in a recent interview, I was asked whether I would personnally agree to being grafted with the organ of a baboon. My answer was "yes" for the liver or kidney, but "no" for the brain.

THE CRISIS OF ADOLESCENCE IN ORGAN TRANSPLANTATION

Pr. J. TRAEGER - Professeur Emérite de Néphrologie - Université Claude Bernard. - AURAL - 10 Impasse Lindbergh - 69003 LYON
Tél. : 78.54.81.92 - Fax : 72.33.82.96

The acceleration of knowledge in biological and medical sciences is one of the remarkable features of our times and in particular the development of organ and tissue transplantation has been incredibly rapid ; in the last 30 years we have passed from the first attempts on humans during the 50's to multiple organ transplantation including heart, liver, lung and pancreas. There has also been an extraordinary increase in the number of transplants performed so that now 150,000 kidney transplants have been carried out in the last 20 years. In fact every year more than 3,500 transplants are carried out in France alone.

Have we now reached the summit in the development of organ transplantation ? One can not be certain of this : if the technique of renal transplantation has been well established, it is probably not in the case of

11

J. L. Touraine et al. (eds.), Rejection and Tolerance, 11–26.
© 1994 *Kluwer Academic Publishers.*

transplantations of the other organs such as pancreas, lung, intestine and liver, and the day is still a long way off when all the technical factors and indications for transplantation of these organs becomes firmly established. One would rather say that we are at a state of "adolescence" in organ transplantation and that is why "Crisis of Adolescence" seems appropriate as title of this paper.

This crisis was predictable with a rapidly expanding speciality and with constantly changing techniques. Developments are frequently dramatic and surgically spectacular and attention from the media, which is often produced by organ retrieval from brain dead subjects, and concern as to definition of the time of death, have added to complexity of the problems involved. So the causes of the crisis were predictable. One could say that this is a usual development and that one could predict ethical and psychological problems in addition to administrative and organizational ones. It is necessary to analyze the factors to predict what should be done because adolescence is a turbulent period in which the future stability of the adult period depends.

This crisis in organ transplantation is characterized above all by a diminution in the total number of cases carried out each year. We already reached a plateau in the years 89 and 90 with an actual reduction in the total numbers of 10 % in 92. This reduction is found in all Western countries as indicated by Eurotransplant as well as by France Transplant. UNOS, which is the U.S. organization shows no reduction, but this is associated with an increase in the number of living donors, the total of whom are responsible for 30 % of transplantation in the U.S. compared to 10 % in France. The diminution in the number of transplants applies to all organs amounting to more than 10 % for cardiac transplants, the statistics of France Transplant indicate a drop of 5 % in liver transplants and a drop of 15 % in kidney transplants for 1992.

This reduction has not been caused by a lessening of demand since the waiting lists in France indicate, particularly for a kidney transplant patient, an increase to more than 5,400 in 1992, and the average waiting period is 23 months. The number of cardiac and liver patients , waiting transplantation remains constant (between 300 to 500) but this is due to the high mortality as compared to renal patients, who are able to survive a long time with dialysis.

The real cause of the diminution of the transplants is linked to a 20 % reduction in the availability of subjects who have suffered cerebral death between 1991 an 1992. This has been primarily due to the success of the campaign to reduce automobile accidents, but is also due to the improvement in the treatment of cerebral injuries. One might expect that in the coming years there will be further improvement, and a further reduction of the order of 25 % in cerebral death might be anticipated.

The diminution of availability of organs for transplantation has also been contributed to by an *obvious increase in the opposition of family members in giving permission for organ removal.* The statistics of France Transplant show an increase in this opposition from 47 % in 1991 to 62 % in 1992, which is a striking increase of 15 %. The increased opposition to providing permission for organ retrieval on the part of the public is the cause for considerable concern, and is inexplicable, in view of the fact that the results obtained in heart, kidney and liver transplantation show constant improvement.

In our attempts to analyze the psychological factors in the change of attitudes to transplantation one can refer to the poll carried out recently on a relatively modest number of 500 persons by "SOFRES" ("Les Français et le don d'organes"). Eighty-nine percent of those polled were in favour of organ donation but the percentage diminished to 81 % when they considered organ donation for themselves. When they made a decision as to donation when their wife, husband or children were involved the percentage of approval showed a further drop to 65 %. The difference between a decision for oneself compared to a decision for others is important -this disparity would presumably not be present if everybody indicated their approval during life.

The cause of refusal to donate is variable : moral or religious grounds are given as the reason in 37 % of cases. Twenty-five percent stated that they were concerned that their body would not be respected after death and 25 % could not give a reason why they refused. Lastly 10 % gave fear of the unknown nature of the procedure as their reason. One might speculate that the desire to maintain the integrity of the body after death has a religious basis associated with the desire for continuing existence in an "after life". It is interesting to note that the donation of organs is allowed by the religious authorities of all religions although this message is not fully appreciated by their congregations.

This raises the question whether the public has been properly informed ? The results of the french poll are extremely striking in that 98 % questioned could not give the name of the law concerning organ donation (Caillavet Law) and only 20 % realized that the law had the effect of presuming consent to organ donation in the absence of any expressed wish to the contrary. When the public is questioned as to who they consider best able to provide direction, 44 % thought that transplant recipients would be, 33% thought their family doctors, and only 25 % thought that members of the transplant team would be most effective. This suggests that *there has developed a certain questioning by the public of the infallibility of medical and surgical teams.*

The information provided to the public by the media has changed over the course of the last few years. This has changed the public perception of transplantation and of the medical profession providing this service.

Firstly there has been a *plethora of information* which one has not the time to absorb. One is subjected to "background noise" with information about AIDS, HIV transmission by transfusion and transplants, and by sensational accounts of organ retrieval, causing a confusion on the subject of organ transplantation.

The second characteristic of the media presentation is its entire *concentration on sensational occurences* with a notable abscence of any reference to their infrequent occurrence.

Who is responsible for this state of affairs ? One can think of three possible groups.

Firstly the journalists. Although they are required to provide an increasing amount of information to satisfy the appetite for new in the modern world, they should be expected to be more responsible and consider the adverse effects of unbalanced reporting.

Doctors dealing with the media should not be too ready to claim personal success in their results. For instance, in renal transplantation one frequently hears of great success in results obtained over the course of the first year without reference to the less favourable survival over the long term. There is a great danger in producing incomplete information because the effects of deceiving the public is to diminish their faith in the medical profession. An addiditional and later effect of this incomplete presentation of the results is that it produces an unrealistic expectation of success which, if not realized, the public ascribes to the incompetence of the professionals providing the service.

Thirdly, *government officials* who in the course of their work obtaining information which may be provided to the press, should be aware of the dangers of misinterpretation or in emphasis of words and statements in their reports. A good example of this recently occured in the report of one French Inspector General of Health when the newspapers headlined "Anarchy in Organ Retrieval". The word "anarchy" did actually occur in the report but it was picked up by the journalists for sensational purposes. In the report the term was appropriate, but appearing as a headline the effect on the public was catastrophic and resulted in an increase in the frequency of refusals of permission for organ retrieval. A little foresight and moderation in the choice of words would have avoided these damaging effect.

Another aspect of the crisis concern the necessity of changes in the structure of the organisations who control the transplantation service. The regulations have became more complex because in the volume and variety of transplantations and also formulation of rules regarding immunological compatibility. This great increase in the data management requires more expenses and more money. An increase contribution of the state to this cost should not be accompanied by increased participation by governement in medical and scientific decision making.

Let us now consider the possibilities for dealing with the problems of finding organs for transplantation. One might consider the possibility of *providing some financial incentive* to donors which is a subject presently being discussed in the U.S.A. In France it is at present not possible as it is contrary to the laws of the country.

Some people might think it would be reasonable to provide an incentive in the form of pension or health benefits from the State.

The other incentive being considered in some circles is to reserve transplantation to those who have offered their organs for salvage in the past but this is obviously extremely difficult to apply.

One might pay greater attention to *encouraging donations on the part of close relatives* as is evident in the Minneapolis group where 60 % of the transplants are the result of donations of relatives, compared to 30 % overall in the U.S.A. and 10 % in France. When we consider the very favourable results (100 % survival of the kidney transplant taken from HLA identical siblings), one realizes that this is the most effective source of transplant material.

The possibility of *recovery of transplant from old subjects,* more than 60 should not be excluded. However, it remains to be proved that the graft survival remains of the same order as with younger transplant.

The possibility of recovery of organs of brain dead subjects after cessation of cardiac activity should be kept in mind. This would require the training of a teams in suitable hospitals who would be immediately available, and involve instituting aortic cooling of the organs. The experience in Maastricht has indicated that such a service would result in an increase of 20 % in organ retrieval.

Modelling the future of organ exchange (OPELZ) could lead to a lesser loss of transplants in combining good HLA-match with better allocation through more active exchange in a larger waiting list (10000) - though the problem of the detrimental effect of a longer cold ischemia time remains to be solved.

Finally, *xenografting* represents for many a means of counteracting to a certain degree the shortage of organs. This might well be a satisfactory solution to the problem in the future, perhaps in as little as ten years. But this would require considerable scientific research to overcome the difficulties now present. We must keep in mind that xeno grafting is unlikely to be a solution for all cases and one must guard against having the public believe that further organ donation was no longer necessary.

To conteract negative attitudes of the public to organ transplantation *more information and better information is required*. The Associations for the Promotion of Organ Donation have a very important role in this respect in furthering instruction in schools, colleges and also in the Armed Forces, to promote the notion of communal responsability and knowledge of the law concerning organ donation. This process of information should be a continuous activity since it has been shown that relaxing the process results in the message being soon forgotten. This is even the case among nurses and doctors working in transplant team.

The family doctors seldom have the time to attend meetings of these associations and an effort should be made to include information about advances in organ transplantation and organ retrieval in postgraduate courses.

Finally, it behooves the medical and governmental serves to ensure that the information provided to the media does not raise unrealistic expectations and also does not create anxiety in the population.

Turning to the question of whether the law should have a place in organ transplantation. The Caillavet Law is based on the presumed consent and one could expect that a modification of this statute would be severely detrimental to our service. Indeed, this Law appears to be the best available and is envied and copied by other countries. Recents studies on ethical problems in transplantation have clearly demonstrated that this Law is the most effective. If this Law became subject to restriction in response to ill-informed public opinion, a

15 % to 20 % increase in refusal is to be expected. The Caillavet Law is perhaps not perfect but does produce the greatest saving of human life. A possible acceptable modification of the Law could be the establishment of a complete computer registration of persons refusing which would be readily available to the medical team, as is presently in effect in Belgium.

On the question of *legislating the definition of brain death* one must consider that continuing development in technology such as angiography and isotope procedures would be incompatible with rigid legal definitions. It would seem preferable to continue the process established in 1964 by the Academy of Medicine when publishing rules regarding the definition of cerebral death.

CONCLUSIONS :

The general population should have a clear idea whether it whishes to benefit from having an organ transplantation service. If it does, *it must consider the negative effects of ill-considered regulations and information.* Although regulation is directed to prevent and diminish the risk of abuses of the service, these abuses are in fact infrequent and not a serious problem in the developed world. The effect of ill-considered regulation is exemplified by a recent direction concerning the retrieval of corneal material which produced in France a reduction to almost zero in the number of the operation which had allowed 3,000 to 5,000 people to recover their sight in France.

It is a simple calculation to calculate the effects of a 20 % reduction in organ donations. This would result in France in a loss of material to carry out life saving transplantation on 150 cardiac and 150 hepatic patients and more than 400 cases of renal failure would have to continue with dialysis.

One might speculate that it is the fear of the unknown which is responsible for the tendency to produce legislation to limit progress in organ transplantation. Although transplantation of kidneys is quite generally accepted nowadays, one remembers the sensation caused in 1967 when Barnard performed the first cardiac transplantation. Nowadays transplantation of liver, lungs, pancreas, and even of total abdominal viscera, is being performed, and perhaps the rapid progress is considered to be menacing because it raises the specter of transplantation of the brain... History shows us that rapid progress in science can produce a tendency by legislators to resort to restrictive law making.

Pr. Murray (who won the Nobel prize for his work in organ transplantation) at the Congress of Transplantation in Developing Countries held in Singapore in May 1992 stated "The very success of transplantations has created a scarcity of donors organs, that in turn has led to their unethical allocation. The solution of this unexpected and degrading situation, does not, in my opinion, lie in ethics, politics, law or even religions but in the professional standard of surgical and medical care".

I believe that one must place one's trust in the profession which has for the past 30 years been performing transplantations which have resulted in the saving of more than 100,000 lives.

This is not to say that those engaged in transplantation services do not require the advice, moral guidance and support of those who have given thought to the moral, ethical and legal consequences of advances in medical science, but one might have fear that if these concerns are manifest by restrictive laws the result would be an overall reduction in progress of life saving activities.

26

Acknowledgements

Pr. J.L. TOURAINE, Dr. BETUEL, Dr. COLPART (LYON) for their informations. Dr. John FRASER (VANCOUVER) for his great help in a precise translation.

FROM SEROLOGY TO MOLECULAR HISTOCOMPATIBILITY TESTING

E.D. Albert, Immunogenetics Laboratory, Children's Hospital, Ludwig-Maximilians-University, Pettenkoferstraße 8a, 8000 München 2, FRG.

Introduction

The past five years have introduced a vast technological change in the methodology for histocompatibility testing. The availability of gene probes for the various HLA loci has allowed to study the polymorphisms at these loci at the DNA level using the technique of restriction fragment length polymorphisms. The availability of first allelic sequences together with the new technique of polymerase chain reaction has very quickly lead to a wealth of information on polymorphic sequence of all the classical HLA loci (Marsh and Bodmer, Zemmour and Parham).

The first systematic application of DNA typing for histocompatibility testing has in a retrospective analysis of donor-recipient pairs of kidney transplantation documented a very high degree of reproducibility between different laboratories for the RFLP analysis used (Opelz et al.). In addition, it became apparent, that a surprisingly large percentage of the donor and recipient typings were incorrect. The use of the correct DNA typing results for retrospective matching resulted in an improved correlation between matching and clinical outcome. Although a number of investigators maintain, that at least in some centers the quality of serology is better than it appears from this multi-center study, it is clear that the advantages offered by the new DNA technology should be utilized in clinical histocompatibility testing.

Advantages of DNA Typing

The major advantages are both of practical and of theoretical nature. On the practical level, it is the fact that genomic DNA can be extracted from very small amounts of blood. Normally, DNA extracted from 5 ml of EDTA blood yields enough material to perform several thousand different tests. The DNA thus extracted may be stored in a simple refrigerator or a - 20°C freezer, thus providing the opportunity for repeated testing, extended testing, exchange of reagents and for standardization. The second practical advantage, which is in our opinion the most important one is, that reagents of defined quality can be produced by anyone in unlimited quantity. This is a very obvious improvement over the situation in serology, where the time consuming, expensive and frustrating screening for antisera is the most important cost-factor. It is unquestionable that a multitude of monoclonal

J. L. Touraine et al. (eds.), Rejection and Tolerance, 27–31.

antibodies are available, which - theoretically - can also be expanded in unlimited quantities. There are, however, not enough different monoclonal anti-HLA antibodies to cover the entire range of specificities now defined by alloantisera. There is no question at all that monoclonal antibodies are essential tools for the detection of expression or for the precipitation of HLA molecules.

The most important theoretical advantage of DNA typing is the increased power of resolution: Many more alleles can be recognised for the known loci (as for example DRB1, DQB1, HLA-A) and loci whose polymorphism has been only partially detected by serology (HLA-C, HLA-DP), and Polymorphisms which have so far not been detected at all by serology, can now be defined to give a more complete description of the biological variability of the MHC. Such polymorphisms include those of HLA-DQA1, -DPA1 and of the promotors which have been shown to be polymorphic for DRA, DRB1, DQA1 and DQB1. It is quite likely that further regulatory and structural polymorphisms of the MHC will be discovered, all of which can be defined on the DNA-sequence level (Sherman et al., Singal et al., Auffray et al., Kimura et al).

The Choice of DNA Typing Techniques

From the above, it becomes obvious, that todate, every sincere histocompatibility typing laboratory must include DNA typing techniques in order to benefit the patient. As the field is still in a phase of very rapid technological development, it is very difficult to predict which will be the final techniques. Presently it appears as if for different clinical needs different techniques will be employed. In the following, we shall give a brief presentation of the principle technologies available todate.

1. Restriction Fragment Length Polymorphism (RFLP) (Bidwell 1988):
This technique, which has been shown to be highly reproducible in multi-center studies is presently being phased out, because the technique is time consuming, offers a relatively low power of resolution at today's standards, requires relatively large amounts of genomic DNA and is generally performed with radioactive labeling of the gene probes. In spite of these negative aspects, it must be stressed, that this is the only DNA typing technique so far, for which there has been a large scale multi-center reproducibility study with very good results (Opelz et al.). In addition, it is a technique in which it can be very easily recognised, if there have been technical problems.

2. Oligonucleotide Typing of PCR Amplified DNA (Nevinny-Stickel et al. a & b)
This technique is presently most commonly used and utilises non-radioactively labeled oligonucleotides (for example digoxigenin or biotin labeling). With this technique, practically all allelic variants which are presently known, can be typed for except for a very small number of ambiguous heterozygote types. This technique is very well suited for large scale non-urgent typing, it is however not fast enough, to be used for prospective typing of organ donors. One major advantage is that most

steps of the procedure can be automated and that each oligonucleotide hybridisation of a given membrane can be controlled for specificity and sensitivity.

3. Reverse Oligotyping (Cros et al.):
In this technique, which is very convenient and can be applied for acute donor typing, a set of oligonucleotides is fixed into a microtiter plate and the amplified target DNA is hybridised to the primers in the plate. It appears very difficult with this technique to perform appropriate controls.

4. Specific Amplification (PCR-SSP) (Olerup et al., Bein et al.):
This technique, which relies on the specificity of amplification brought about at the 3' end of the primer is very fast, so that it can be employed in acute donor typing. Each typing requires a large number of pipetting steps and the transfer of a large number of amplificates into a gel. This makes it very cumbersome for large scale testing. The inclusion of a internal positive control does not rule out the occasional occurence of an undetected false negative reaction.

5. Sequencing:
Direct sequencing of PCR amplified exons has been shown to represent a feasable alternative to the other techniques, provided the availability of an automated sequencer. This method provides of course the highest possible power of resolution, but it is too slow for application in acute donor typing. Adequate controls can be included by sequencing in both directions and from repeated amplifications.

From the above, it can be seen that the choice of techniques depends on the clinical needs and it is becoming apparent, that a well equipped laboratory should be able to perform a fast technique for donor typing (PCR-SSP or reverse oligotyping) and one technique for large scale typing and control typing (oligonucleotide typing) as well as the facility for sequencing in order to clarify ambiguous results and questionable homozygosity.

Standardisation and Quality Control

It is one of the greatest advantages of the DNA technology, that the nucleotide sequence of a given gene can be used as a standard. The DNA which has been used for the determination of the sequence can be kept either as DNA or in form of a cell line and can be distributed for crossreferencing purposes. Since it is possible to ship large numbers of DNA samples at ambient temperatures, quality control exercises can be easily performed. There is now a number of different techniques that may lead to a DNA typing result and it must be expected that more new techniques will appear and present ones will diverge in the different laboratories. Since there is a common standard consisting of the DNA sequence, it can be left up to the individual laboratory to choose the particular technique which is most suited under the given circumstances. The quality control consists of a sizable number of coded DNA samples with blind duplicates and triplicates and negative controls for which a correct result must be reported regardless of the techniques which has led to this result. It has been our experience that the testing of coded samples and the open reporting of the results has a very strong educational effect.

Conclusion

Although it is very clear that classical HLA serology will remain the technique of choice for the performance of crossmatches and for the characterisation of preformed HLA antibodies in the sera of transplant recipients. In addition, it must be acknowledged that the typing for class I determinants is presently more efficient and less time consuming by classical serology than by DNA techniques. This may, however, change in the near future as more automated techniques are becoming available. In the field of bone marrow transplantation, it is widely accepted that subtypes of serologically defined HLA antigens are of major importance in unrelated bone marrow transplantation. The subtypes however, cannot be safely determined by serology, but must be defined in one-dimensional isoelectric focusing, a technique which is too time consuming and cumbersome to be used by all laboratories involved in donor searches. Also here, there is a rapid development in the direction of a recognition of these subtypes by DNA techniques. We will therefore strife to first define all these class I subtypes on the DNA level and will then switch to DNA typing of class I in general, when appropriate, simplified techniques become available.

From all this, it can be seen that it is the obligation of the histocompatibility testing community to accept the challenge of the technological change towards molecular biology. The unlimited supply of test reagents as well as the far improved possibilities for standardisation and quality control on the DNA level will make this change faster than most serologists today believe.

Acknowledgements:
Supported by the SFB 217.

References:

Andersen LC., Beaty JS., Nettles JW. et al.: Allelic polymorphism in transcriptional regulatory regions of HLA-DQB genes. J. Exp.Med., 1991, 173: 181-192.

Auffray C., Lillie JW., Korman AJ et al.: Structure and expression of HLA-DQα and -DXα genes: interallellic alternate splicing of the HLA-DQα gene and functional splicing of the HLA-DXα gene using a retroviral vector. Immunogenetics 1987, 26: 63-73.

Bein G., Gläser R., Kirchner H.: Rapid HLA-DRB1 genotyping by nested PCR amplification. Tissue Antigens 1992, 39: 68-73.

Bidwell J.: DNA-RFLP analysis and genotyping of HLA-DR and -DQ antigens. Immunology today, 1988, 9: 18-23.

Cros P., Allibert P., Mandrand B., Tiercy JM. and Mach B.: Oligonucleotide genotyping of HLA polymorphism on microtitre plates. Lancet 1992, 340: 870-873.

Kimura A., Sasazuki T.: Polymorphism in the 5ß-flanking region of the DQA1 gene and it's relation to DR-DQ haplotype. In: HLA 1991 (eds Tsuji K., Aizawa M., Sasazuki T.) Vol. II: 382-385, Oxford Sci. Publ. 1993.

Marsh SGE., Bodmer JG.: HLA class II nucleotide sequences 1991. Immunogenetics 1991, 33: 321-334.

Nevinny-Stickel C., Bettinotti MdIP., Andreas A. et al.: Nonradioactive HLA class II typing using polymerase chain reaction and digoxigenin 11-2'-3'-dideoxy-uridinetriphosphate labeled oligonucleotide probes. Hum.Immunol. 1991, 31: 7-13.

Nevinny-Stickel C., Hinzpeter M., Andreas A., Albert ED.: Nonradioactive oligotyping for HLA-DR1-DRw10 using polymerase chain reaction, digoxigenin-labeled oligonucleotides and chemiluminescence detection. Eur.J.Immunogenetics 1991, 18: 323-332.

Olerup O. and Zetterquist H.: HLA-DR typing by PCR amplification with sequence-specific primers (PCR-SSP) in 2 hours: An alternative to serological DR typing in clinical practice including donor-recipient matching in cadaveric transplantation.

Opelz G., Mytilineos J., Scherer S., Dunckley H., Trejaut J., Chapman J., Middleton D., Savage D., Fischer O., Bignon JD., Bensa JC., Albert E. and Noreen H.: Survival of DNA HLA-DR typed and matched cadaver kidney transplants.
The Lancet, 1991, pp. 461-463.

Sherman PA, Basta PV, Ting JPY: Upstream DNA sequences required for tissue specific expression of the HLA-DRα gene. Proc.Natl.Acad.Sci. 1987, 84: 4254-4258.

Singal DP, Qui X., D'Souza M., and Sood SK.: Polymorphism in the upstream regulatory regions of HLA-DRB genes. Immunogenetics 1993, 37:143-147.

Zemmour J. and Parham P.: HLA class I nucleotide sequences, 1992. Europ.J. Immunogenetics, 20:1: 29-45.

CONTINUING DEVELOPMENTS IN TRANSPLANTATION

Peter J. Morris

Nuffield Department of Surgery

University of Oxford, John Radcliffe Hospital

Headington, Oxford OX3 9DU, UK.

Tel: 0865 221297   Fax: 0865 68876

Introduction

We have come a long way in transplantation since the pioneering efforts of

David Hume in the late 40's and early 50's, when a series of cadaver kidneys

were implanted in the thigh with vascular anastomoses to the femoral vessels

and with the ureter draining onto the skin. No immunosuppression was used

but surprisingly some of these kidneys functioned for several weeks. Since

J. L. Touraine et al. (eds.), Rejection and Tolerance, 33–45.

that time we have seen major advances in transplantation so that now renal transplantation is the accepted therapy for most patients with end-stage renal failure, and liver and cardiac transplantation are the preferred treatment for many patients with end-stage failure of those organs. In addition, there have been important developments in lung and pancreatic transplantation amongst the other organs, such that they can almost be considered as acceptable therapies in certain situations. Apart from organ transplantation, there have been continuing advances in tissue transplantation, in particular bone marrow transplantation which provides the treatment of choice for many types of leukaemia, as well as certain immunodeficiency syndromes, provided a suitable matched donor (usually a family member) is available.

These enormous advances in the success of transplantation can be attributed to a number of developments such as the recognition of brain death and in particular brainstem death, ever improving techniques of organ preservation, the recognition of HLA as the major histocompatibility complex of man, as well as the recognition of the importance of the crossmatch between donor and recipient. However, it is the marked improvement in immunosuppression that has occurred over these years and which continues to occur, which has had the biggest impact on improved graft survival in the transplantation of all organs.

Table 1   Immunosuppression in organ transplantation, 1950-1980

Total body irradiation

Azathioprine and high dose steroids

Cyclophosphamide

Thoracic duct drainage

Thymectomy

Splenectomy

Graft irradiation

Azathioprine and low dose steroids

Antilymphocyte globulin

From 1950 to 1980 a variety of immunosuppressive regimens had been used (Table 1), commencing with total body irradiation in the early years of renal transplantation. But the advent of azathioprine in the early 60's and the recognition that the addition of steroids provided better prophylaxis against rejection led to an explosion in renal transplantation. Results continued to improve after the introduction of azathioprine, particularly as the morbidity associated with the steroids was found to be markedly decreased by the use of low dose steroids, but without sacrificing

Table 2   Immunosuppressive drugs in the 1990's

Drug	Mechanism of action
Cyclosporine	Inhibits T cell activation
FK506	Inhibits T cell activation
Mofetil Mycophenolate	Inhibits purine metabolism, antiproliferative
Rapamycin	Inhibits lymphokine generated signal, antiproliferative
15-deoxspergualin	Not known
Brequinar Sodium	Inhibits pyrimidine metabolism, antiproliferative
Leflunomide	Not known, antiproliferative

graft survival. The advent of cyclosporine in the early 80's represented a major advance in immunosuppression with graft survival in the case of kidney transplantation improving by 10% to 15%. This in turn resulted in a rapid expansion of cardiac and liver transplantation throughout the world. Cyclosporine has many side effects, nephrotoxicity being one of the more significant ones, and as a result a number of immunosuppressive protocols are used, all based on cyclosporine. However, there is no evidence that one protocol is better than another in terms of patient and graft survival. Triple therapy (low dose cyclosporine, azathioprine, prednisolone) is a very popular protocol, only because it is relatively simple to use and relatively free of side effects.

As cadaveric graft survival today is 80% and better at 1 year in the case of the kidneys, also of the heart, and not far behind in the case of the liver, one might be forgiven for feeling that most of the problems of transplantation have been resolved. This is far from the truth, and several major obstacles to longterm graft and patient survival remain. These are firstly rejection, and chronic rejection in particular. Although acute rejection leading to the loss of the transplanted organ is relatively uncommon, chronic rejection causing a steady attrition of grafts after the first year is a major problem which is not responsive to current therapy. Second, cardiovascular disease is an ever growing problem as patients survive longer, and indeed this is the major cause of mortality after renal transplantation in Europe at this time. Third, infection always remains a hazard in the immunosuppressed patient but with more effective treatments available for viral and fungal infections, this has become a far less common cause of mortality. Finally, as patients survive longer with a functioning graft, the spectre of cancer in the immunosuppressed patient becomes increasingly evident. For virtually all types of cancer show an increased incidence in the transplant population, but the cancers that might have a viral aetiology are those that show the highest incidence, e.g. squamous cell cancer of the skin, cervical cancer of the uterus, and non-Hodgkins lymphoma. As our current cohort of relatively young patients with long surviving grafts moves into the cancer age it may well be that we will see an epidemic of cancers occurring in these patients.

For all these reasons, although graft survival at one year is very satisfactory, long term graft survival is poor and the morbidity in many of these long surviving patients is considerable. There is no question that better, but less toxic and more specific, immunosuppression is required.

Newer approaches to immunosuppression

Immunosuppressive drugs

A large number of new drugs are undergoing clinical trials, or are about to. Different mechanisms of action and the possibility of synergistic actions may allow better immunosuppression with less side effects of the drugs themselves. Some of these newer agents are listed in Table 2, together with their mechanism of action.

FK506, a macrolide antibiotics, has undergone extensive trials in Pittsburgh in liver, kidney, small bowel, pancreatic and cardiac transplantation, and more recently two large multi-centre trials of FK506 in liver transplantation have been completed in North America and Europe. FK506 may be an improved immunosuppressive agent in comparison with cyclosporine in liver transplantation, but limited data so far does not suggest it is superior in renal transplantation. It is associated with a number of side effects, in particular nephrotoxicity, but it does not cause the facial brutalization seen with cyclosporine nor is it associated with hypertension to the same extent. In Pittsburgh, FK506 has produced exceptionally good results also in cardiac transplantation and has allowed a considerable number of successful combined liver and small bowel transplantation procedures to be performed, and more recently successful small bowel transplantation alone in a number of patients.

Rapamycin (a macrolide antibiotic) is another very interesting immunosuppressive agent which is an antiproliferative drug and is highly potent in experimental models of transplantation. It is about to undergo clinical trial.

Perhaps of greatest interest and generated by the discovery of these new immunosuppressive agents, is the increase in knowledge about their mechanism of action at the molecular level that has emerged in the last few years. Cyclosporine, FK506, and rapamycin all bind to a family of proteins in the cytoplasm known as immunophilins. Cyclosporine binds to an immunophilin known as cyclophilin, while FK506 and Rapamycin bind to FK binding protein (FKBP). It is this complex of the drug and its immunophilin which is the active agent. The complex of cyclosporin and cyclophilin, or

FK506 and FKBP, each bind to a protein phosphatase known as calcineurin. Calcineurin is thought to play a key role in the signal transduction which leads to activation of the IL2 gene and similar genes within the nucleus. The binding of the drug and its immunophilin complex inhibits this phosphatase activity of calcineurin, and therefore prevents the signal transduction which leads to activation of the enhancer region of the IL2 gene, thus blocking transcription of this cytokine gene. On the other hand, Rapamycin which binds to the same immunophilin as FK506, namely FKBP, (and indeed to the same epitope) inhibits proliferation of the activated T cell by blocking the signal generated by IL2 attaching to its IL2 receptors, and so proliferation of the activated T cell is prevented. What the complex of Rapamycin/FKBP attaches to is unknown, but it is obviously not calcineurin. As we unravel the action of these drugs at a molecular level, which will undoubtedly shed further light on signal transduction, the possibility of designing drugs with very specific sites of action seems likely.

Another interesting drug, RS61443 (mofetil mycophenolate) is an anti purine drug and it too prevents proliferation of activated cells. It is undergoing extensive clinical trials and in early phase I trials look very impressive both at preventing rejection and also for treating steroid resistant rejection. Another fascinating observation made in two different experimental models is that this drug prevents smooth muscle hypertrophy which is a feature of chronic rejection. That in itself, if found to occur in man, could represent a major advance in immunosuppression.

Monoclonal antibodies

Monoclonal antibodies provide an expectation that immunosuppression might be targeted very precisely to a cell surface molecule involved in cell activation or in cell interactions involved in the development of an immune response.

Monoclonal antibodies may act by deletion of the cell bearing the target, modulation of the target antigen or blinding of the target antigen. The only antibody in widespread clinical use is OKT3 directed against the CD3 molecule which is part of the T cell receptor complex. OKT3 is a potent immunosuppressive agent in preventing rejection or treating steroid resistant rejection. Whether it is superior to a good antilymphocyte or antithymocyte globulin is debatable, and probably the answer is that it is not. A number of other antibodies have been tested in phase I or in randomised trials. Some of these are an antibody to the IL2 receptor (anti CD45), an anti-T cell receptor antibody, an anti-CD4 antibody and an anti-LFA1 antibody. These trials have at least in their very early stages proved to be rather disappointing compared with the successful immunosuppression achieved by analogous antibodies in experimental models of allotransplantation.

Another more recent but very interesting approach to immunosuppression is to block the second signal which is required for T cell activation and which is mediated by the CD28 molecule and its interaction with B7 on the antigen presenting cell. Again in an experimental system this has produced impressive specific immunosuppression.

It must be admitted that the promise of monoclonal antibodies in the clinic has yet to be realised, but nevertheless they do allow immunosuppression to be targeted very precisely, and this in turn may allow specific forms of immunosuppression to be induced in due course. The more recent development of genetic engineering of chimaeric and humanised antibodies promises to decrease the likelihood of sensitisation against murine protein, almost inevitable with murine monoclonal antibodies.

Cell transplantation

Over this next decade we are likely to see many attempts to transplant cells as replacement therapy, in addition to the widely and very successful form of cell transplantation, namely bone marrow transplantation. In bone marrow transplantation the isolation and transplantation of haematopoietic stem cells is likely to represent a significant advance in this area. In other approaches to cell transplantation developments in the techniques of transplanting isolated pancreatic islets for type I diabetes in man and the transplantation of dopamine secreting neuronal tissue in patients with

Parkinson's disease may become relatively standard procedures. There are many problems associated with cell transplantation, all of which are illustrated in the development of pancreatic islet transplantation in type I diabetes. Thus, there are the problems associated with the preparation of a suitably pure islet cell suspension in sufficient numbers to allow correction of the diabetic state. Until these technical problems are resolved it is very difficult to evaluate what the extent of the immunological problems are, but suffice it to say they are likely to be no different than transplantation of other allogeneic tissues. Although progress has been slow, a considerable number of successful islet transplants in type I diabetics have been performed over the last two years as judged by normal levels of c-peptide secretion after transplantation in a substantial number of patients. However, the ultimate success of islet transplantation, namely the freedom of the patient from insulin therapy, has only been achieved in a handful of patients. Thus, for the moment, a vascularised whole organ pancreatic graft remains the only effective way of correcting type I diabetes, but this is a major procedure with considerable morbidity and can only be justified in patients who require a kidney transplant as a result of their diabetic nephropathy and who need immunosuppression in any case.

Immunoisolation

Following on from the potential developments in cell transplantation, an obvious solution to the problem of rejection of a cell transplant is to isolate the cellular transplant within a membrane capsule that would allow nutrients to pass into the capsule and allow the secretory products of the cellular transplant to pass out of the capsule. Thus, if the technology could be solved, islet transplantation and neuronal transplantation would be important areas for the application of this technique. Encouraging results are being produced in experimental allograft models and clinical application may not be too far away.

Xenotransplantation

The ever increasing shortfall between supply and demand means that over the last two or three years there has been an enormous growth of interest in the possible use of organs from animals for transplantation. Although transplantation from higher order primates, such as the chimpanzee, could probably be carried out successfully with modern immunosuppression, this is not likely to be ethically acceptable any longer. Thus donors that are more likely to be acceptable for the provision of tissues and organs are species that we eat, such as the pig. Unfortunately man has natural cytotoxic antibodies against most species including the pig, the antibodies being directed mostly against the sugar moiety of the target xenoantigen, gal 1,3 α galactose. Thus transplantation of an organ such as a pig kidney or a pig heart into a human would result in hyperacute rejection. If the problems presented by this natural cytotoxic antibody can be over come by deleting the recipient of the antibody before transplantation, or of complement, or indeed by using as organ donors transgenic animals that might express human complement inhibitors on their endothelium, for example this might allow successful transplantation from such disparate donors to humans. However, successful xenotransplantation probably still lies somewhere in the future.

Conclusions

Transplantation has made incredible advances over the past 40 years but without question the advances we will see over the next 10 to 15 years will outstrip even those previous, almost miraculous, events in the field of transplantation, so many of which we have heard described at these courses here in Lyon over the past 25 years. There are still many problems associated with transplantation which need to be resolved by better and more specific immunosuppression and hopefully it might even prove possible to induce tolerance to an organ allograft in a human patient in the not too distant future.

The "Burst" of Pulmonary Transplantation: Thirty Years of Progress

James H. Dauber, MD

University of Pittsburgh

Veterans Affairs Medical Center

Pittsburgh, PA, USA

Introduction

Compared to other major organs such as the kidney, liver, and heart, transplantation of the lung has not enjoyed widespread application until just recently. Despite the first attempts at both experimental and clinical pulmonary transplantation coinciding with those for other major organs, clinical success with the lung did not keep pace with that for these other organs. In fact, a long string of failures resulted in virtual abandonment of lung transplantation by 1978. This short review will recount the history of lung transplantation, the principal causes of the spectacular early failures, the advances which heralded in the modern era of pulmonary transplantation, and the refinements that permitted the burst of activity that has occurred over the last five years. Finally, the formidable challenges that now threaten to cause the "burst " to implode will be presented.

Experimental Pulmonary Transplantation

The first technically successful allograft of a canine lung is attributed to Carrel and Guthrie in the early twentieth century [1]. The techniques developed during a series of autographs and allografts of several organs represented ground breaking

47

J. L. Touraine et al. (eds.), Rejection and Tolerance, 47–64.
© 1994 Kluwer Academic Publishers.

work in vascular surgery. The achievements earned Dr. Carrel a Nobel Prize in 1912. Because of a lack of understanding about rejection and technical obstacles, the field remained dormant until the late 1940's. Improvements in thoracic surgery and advances in transplantation immunology stimulated renewed efforts, culminating in the report of Hardin and Kittle in 1954 of prolonged survival of canine lung allograft recipients which had been immunosuppressed with corticosteroids and azathioprine [2]. Continued refinements with this model paved the way for the first human lung allograft in 1963.

Clinical Pulmonary Transplantation

The Beginnings

In the summer of 1963, two human single lung transplants were performed three weeks apart at Jackson, Mississippi [3] and Pittsburgh, Pennsylvania [4]. In each instant the recipient had far advanced lung disease but showed remarkable improvement in ventilation within hours of receiving a new lung. Both were taken off mechanical ventilation within 24 hours after engraftment and maintained adequate lung function for the first postoperative week. Immunosuppression consisted of cortisone and azathioprine. The recipient from Jackson, Mississippi, who had pre-existing renal insufficiency, succumbed to renal failure and malnutrition on the 17th postoperative day. The grafted lung, however, appeared normal on both gross and microscopic evaluation at autopsy. In contrast, the recipient from Pittsburgh succumbed from overwhelming staphylococcal infection of the engrafted lung which, in retrospect, may have been present at the time of harvest. These two reports provide a fascinating account of the problems and challenges that had to be conquered before pulmonary transplantation came of age. They also spawned a number of attempts at other centers where the results provided no cause for optimism

The Promise Not Fulfilled

A total of 38 attempts in the next 15 years produced no long-term survivors! The longest lived recipient died less than one year following a single lung transplant and the majority succumbed much more quickly [5]. Breakdown of the bronchial anastomosis was one of the leading causes of mortality in this era. The other was infection. Both were believed to stem mainly from reliance on high doses of corticosteroids to prevent rejection. In the doses required to prevent rejection, these agents profoundly slowed wound healing and impaired host defense against infection.

The Resurrection

Fortunately, an effective alternative to corticosteroids and azathioprine for immunosuppression appeared in the form of cyclosporine in 1976. By 1979 it was being employed successfully in human kidney transplantation and promised considerable benefits for liver, heart, and lung transplantation. When cyclosporine was used in conjunction with antilymphocyte globulin to prevent rejection, corticosteroids could be entirely avoided in the early postoperative period. This approach toward immunosuppression permitted more rapid and complete healing of surgical wounds than where high doses of steroids were used immediately following surgery to achieve the same end. After the group at Stanford demonstrated the efficacy of cyclosporine-based immunosuppression in a primate model of heart-lung transplantation, they next applied it to humans. Their report of long-term survival in three human heart-lung recipients ushered in the modern era of pulmonary transplantation in 1982 [6]. In the same year, programs were initiated at Harefield Hospital in England and in Pittsburgh, Pennsylvania for heart-lung transplantation, and in Toronto where the focus was on single lung transplantation. Many additional programs followed in the next five years.

<u>Successes and Limitations</u>

In the ensuing five years, the number of procedures gradually increased. By early 1987, the total amounted to about 450 cases worldwide. The emphasis was on heart-lung allografting and the majority of procedures were performed for pulmonary

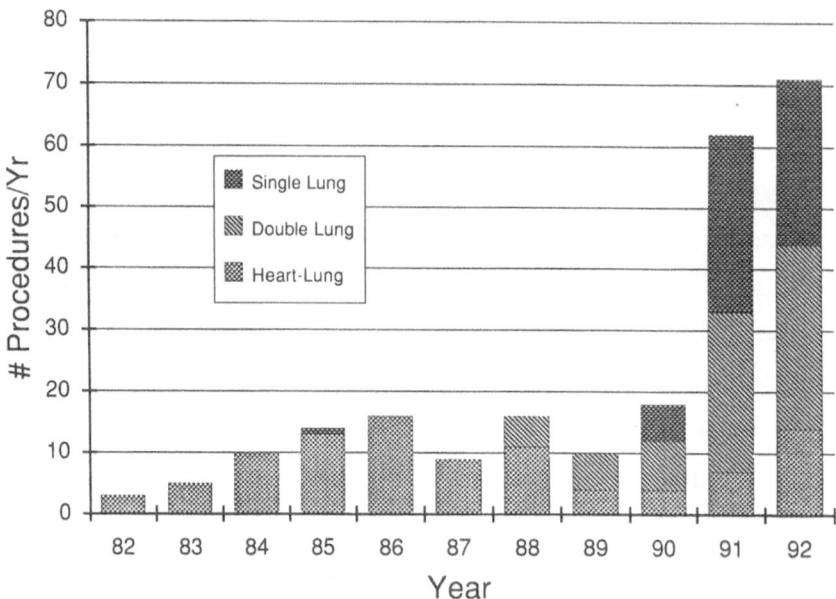

Figure 1. The yearly rate of pulmonary transplantation at the University of Pittsburgh from the inception of the program in 1982 until the end of 1992. During this period a total of 233 procedures were performed. All but one of the procedures between 1982 and 1987 were heart-lung transplants. The rate of heart-lung transplantation actually declined after 1986. The growth in pulmonary transplantation has been with single and double lung transplants which currently account for 85% of all procedures.

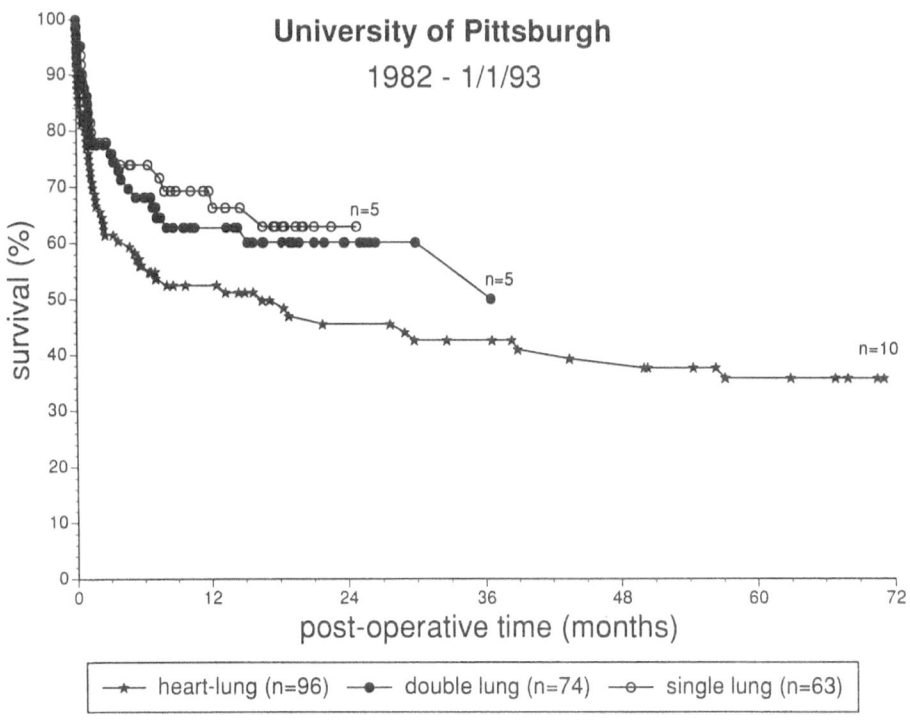

Figure 2. Actuarial survival rates for recipients of a lung or heart-lung transplant at the University of Pittsburgh from 1982 to the end of 1992. The mortality rate in the early postoperative period was higher for heart-lung recipients than for single or double lung recipients. This reflects a steep rate of loss in the first 4 years of the program when only heart-lung transplantation was being performed. None-the-less the proportion of recipients with a heart-lung allograft who were alive after 5 years is nearly 50%, a survival rate far exceeding that expected of the underlying disease for which transplantation was performed.

vascular disease, either primary pulmonary hypertension or pulmonary hypertension secondary to congenital heart disease. Concern over the irreversibility of right ventricular failure prompted transplant surgeons to graft a new heart as well as new lungs in recipients with cor pulmonale [7,8]. Single lung allografts were implanted in

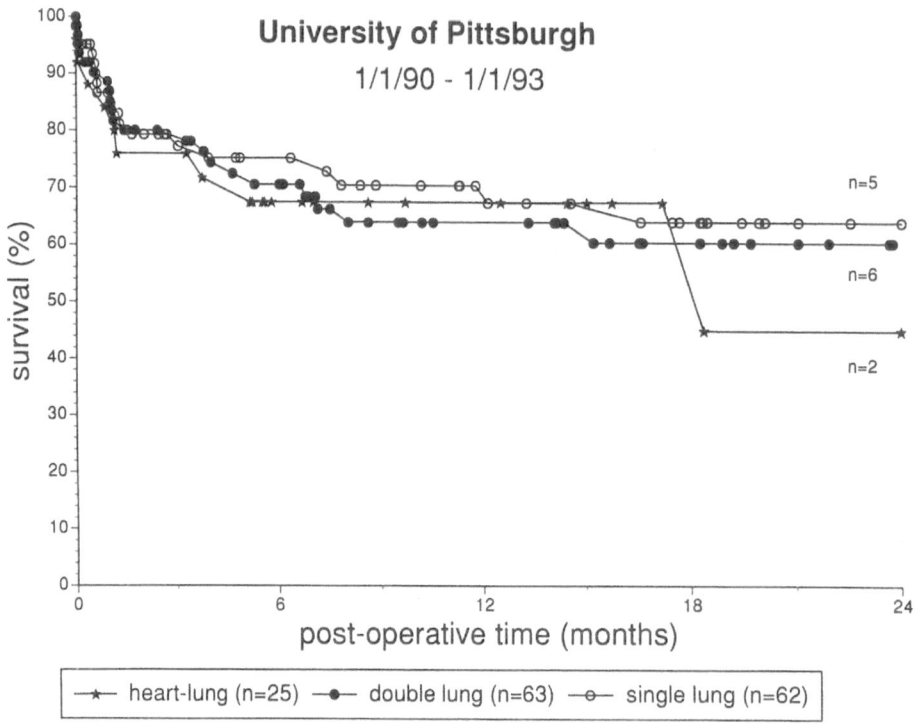

Figure 3. Actuarial survival rates for recipients of lung or heart-lung allografts at the University of Pittsburgh from 1990 through 1992. Compared to the previous analysis in Figure 2, survival for the three major forms of pulmonary transplantation are comparable.

patients with endstage pulmonary fibrosis but preserved right ventricular function at Toronto [9].

One year survival during this period ranged from 40 to 50%. The major cause of death in the early postoperative period was infection. Although dehiscence of airway anastomoses was encountered, the toll this complication extracted was much less than in the pre-cyclosporine era. The leading causes of infection in the early postoperative period were bacteria, cytomegalovirus, and fungi, particularly Candida species [10]. Perioperative bleeding related to coagulopathies and primary graft dysfunction related to inadequate graft preservation posed additional major challenges. Rejection of the lung allograft in the early postoperative period proved to be quite frequent and discordant with cardiac rejection [7]. Although rarely fatal because it usually responded to pulsed doses of corticosteroids, acute rejection posed a substantial diagnostic challenge. Tissue confirmation was considered desirable prior to therapy, since augmented immunosuppression greatly enhanced the risk for opportunistic infection. During this era transbronchial biopsy via the fiberoptic bronchoscope was considered hazardous and the tissue obtained inadequate for diagnosis. A larger specimen of tissue could be obtained by the transthoracic route, but only at the expense of considerable morbidity. This situation resulted in many cases of rejection being diagnosed on clinical grounds alone. Not uncommonly, high doses of corticosteroids were given to recipients with infection or preservation injury, often with a dire outcome.

Other limitations slowed the application of pulmonary transplantation during this period. Procurement of lungs was not centralized and the need for organs not widely appreciated. Thus, many potential donor lungs went unused. Concern over preservation of the lung led to elaborate techniques for harvesting and transporting organs. For example, the donor was brought to the recipient before harvest [6], or the heart-lung bloc was preserved with an autoperfusion system employing warmed donor blood [7]. Such systems often made procurement a logistical nightmare. Probably the most critical limitation was the growing demand for donor hearts for lone cardiac transplantation. This reduced the availability of heart-lung blocs, which eventually resulted in a decline in the rate of pulmonary transplantation at many centers by 1987 (Figure 1).

Advances Leading to the Burst in Pulmonary Transplantation

Fortunately, a series of advances converged at this juncture which greatly propelled activity in pulmonary transplantation. Arguably the most crucial was the understanding that the failing right ventricle could regain normal function once the burden of pulmonary hypertension was lifted. This revelation derived from successful efforts to relieve thrombogenic pulmonary hypertension complicated by cor pulmonale by thrombectomy [11]. Eliminating the need for a new heart for the majority of potential lung recipients awaiting heart-lung transplantation stimulated rapid growth of single and double lung transplantation.

Simplified procurement techniques and a growing awareness of the need for donor lungs helped to expand the supply. Perfusion of the donor lung with vasodilators followed by special electrolyte infusions and cryopreservation permitted ischemic times of up to six hours, resulting in more organs being available through distant procurement [12].

Up to this time, conventional thinking dictated that single lung transplantation would be ineffective for treating endstage pulmonary emphysema [13]. Despite experimental results to the contrary [14], most pulmonary physiologists reasoned that ventilation perfusion mismatch would worsen following single lung transplantation from increased perfusion and diminished ventilation to the allograft. Reports of successful lung transplantation for emphysema in 1989 finally dispelled this mistaken belief [15]. Consequently, emphysema has become the leading indication for single lung transplantation due to the large reservoir of potential candidates who have prolonged survival despite severe limitations from their underlying disease.

Bleeding in recipients who required cardiopulmonary bypass had long been one of the feared complications of pulmonary transplantation since unanticipated pleural and mediastinal adhesions and abnormal bronchial arterial circulation usually led to serious hemorrhage in these anticoagulated subjects. The technique of sequential bilateral single lung transplantation avoided the need for cardiopulmonary bypass in many recipients who required double lung transplantation [16]. Recipients with cystic fibrosis probably benefitted the most from this advance because prior to this significant pleural adhesions often eliminated them from consideration for transplantation.

Control of the infectious complications has been a challenge since the inception of pulmonary transplantation. Although the situation improved when cyclosporine became available, infection still remained the leading cause of death. The aggressive application of fiberoptic bronchoscopy with bronchoalveolar lavage (BAL) dramatically improved the accuracy and timeliness of diagnosis of infection in the allograft [10]. It also provided useful information about the course of opportunistic infections in these recipients. This, along with better monitoring of infection in the donor lung at the time of harvest, led to more effective specific therapy and regimens for prophylaxis against most forms of opportunistic pathogens. Broad spectrum antibacterial coverage for the first three to five postoperative days, based on results of cultures of the donor trachea and knowledge of the recipient's flora preoperatively, markedly reduced morbidity and mortality from early bacterial pneumonia [12]. Low dose Amphotericin in recipients whose donor lung harbored Candida species nearly eliminated life threatening infection from these agents [10]. Prophylactic treatment of recipients at risk for primary or secondary infection from cytomegalovirus with ganciclovir, in particular, has dramatically reduced morbidity and mortality from this all too common and potentially lethal infection [17]. Pneumonia from Pneumocystis carinii has all but been eliminated by the prolonged administration of regimens of oral sulfa drugs such as trimethoprim/sulfamethoxazole or dapsone [10]. Despite these encouraging advances, the vigil for infection must be maintained to maintain control of infection from well recognized agents and to discover new types of infection from heretofore unrecognized pathogens.

The recognition that transbronchial lung biopsy was a relatively non-invasive but highly effective approach for the diagnosis of allograft rejection revolutionized the management of this complication [8]. Prior to this realization in the late 1980's, detection of acute cellular rejection was a major diagnostic challenge. Because morbidity from a transthoracic lung biopsy was often unacceptable, diagnosis was frequently made without benefit of tissue. The relative ease and safety with which transbronchial lung biopsy may be performed repeatedly in these patients has greatly facilitated detection and management of acute allograft rejection. It has also contributed to our understanding of the syndrome of chronic rejection, which will be described later, as well [18].

The "Burst" of Pulmonary Transplantation

The convergence of these advances and their concerted application by transplant teams throughout the world have greatly improved survival following all forms of pulmonary transplantation. These results have engendered tremendous enthusiasm for the procedure on the part of physicians and patients. Consequently, the growth of pulmonary transplantation accelerated dramatically between 1987 and the present. Extrapolation of results from the Registry of the International Society for Heart and Lung Transplantation [19] and the St. Louis International Lung Transplant Registry (E.P. Trulock, personal communication) suggests that the total number of procedures performed worldwide in 1987 probably did not exceed 200, but by 1993 the yearly rate was approaching 900. Virtually all of this growth can be attributed to single and double lung transplantation, as the number of combined heart-lung allografts during this interval has remained relatively stable at around 200 per year. Figure 1 depicts activity at the University of Pittsburgh from 1982 through 1992. It is an accurate reflection of the large trends described above. Whether or not the "burst" will persist and expansion of activity continue at is present rate is unknown. This will depend principally on the supply of donor organs. The more the success rate for pulmonary transplantation improves, however, the greater the disparity between supply and demand.

Indications for the Various Forms of Pulmonary Transplantation and Related Survival

Although controversy still exists, there is a growing consensus about indications for the three principal approaches: single lung, double lung, and combined heart-lung transplantation. The major indications are listed in Table 1. More experience must accrue with the use of single and double lung transplantation for pulmonary vascular disease and the quality of long-term survival following single lung transplantation for endstage parenchymal lung disease must be better defined before these guidelines become firm. But at the present rate of activity in the field of pulmonary transplantation, these issues should be settled soon.

Long-term survival of recipients worldwide has progressively improved during the last ten years. Figure 2 depicts survival results at the University of Pittsburgh during this period. The combined five year survival rate now appears to exceed 50% whereas in the early days of this program only 50% of newly transplanted recipients lived to be discharged from hospital! In this analysis the two year survival rate for

Table 1. Indications for the Major Forms of Pulmonary Transplantation

I.   Single Lung Transplantation

     A.   Emphysema

     B.   Diffuse Pulmonary Fibrosis

     C.   Lymphangiomyomatosis

     D.   Pulmonary Hypertension?

II.   Double Lung Transplantation

     A.   Pulmonary Hypertension

          1.   Primary Pulmonary Hypertension
          2.   Collagen Vascular Disease
          3.   Eisenmenger's Syndrome from Repairable Congenital Heart Defect

     B.   Septic Lung Disease

          1.   Cystic Fibrosis
          2.   Bronchiectasis
              a. Idiopathic
              b. Immune deficiency?

     C.   Emphysema

          1.   Complicated by recurrent infection or evidence of bronchiectasis
          2.   Alpha-1-Antitrypsin Deficiency
          3.   Bullous Lung Disease

III.   Heart-Lung Transplantation

     A.   Pulmonary hypertension from uncorrectable congenital heart disease

     b.   Pulmonary vascular disease with irreversible left ventricular failure

recipients of a heart-lung allograft is lower than that for single and double lung allografts, but the former value is heavily weighted by high initial mortality rates in the early years of the program. Figure 3 compares survival rates for the three procedures since 1990. Clearly, survival rates at all times during the postoperative period are comparable for heart-lung versus lung transplantation. The proportion of recipients alive after two years is now about 60% for all procedures. In the absence of transplantation, the expected mortality rate approaches or is 100% for all patients being considered for transplantation in our program (I.L. Paradis, University of Pittsburgh, personal communication). Quality of life is also much improved for these recipients. Although results from formal assessments are still pending, it is clear to anyone intimately involved with these recipients that they are able to participate in most of the activities pursued by normal individuals. These achievements have established a role for pulmonary transplantation in the treatment of endstage cardiopulmonary diseases, but considerable challenges remain which must be met before the procedure can be considered highly successful.

The Future of Pulmonary Transplantation - Will the "Burst" Implode?

One of the problems which will retard the widespread application and success of this promising treatment is common to the entire field of solid organ transplantation. Although a dire shortage of organs plagues virtually all forms of transplantation, it is relatively more acute for lung transplantation since many donors who provide suitable hearts, livers, and kidneys do not provide suitable lungs. The reason for this is that the lung is more commonly injured and/or infected than other donated organs. Such a discrepancy is likely to persist despite the advent of better methods for harvesting and preserving the lung. The recent expansion in the number of lung transplantation programs throughout the world only aggravates this shortage since it diminishes the number of organs available to established centers who have contributed heavily to the advancements in this field and are best positioned to do so in the future.

Despite encouraging progress in the control of infection, this complication continues to pose a major challenge. The lung allograft seems to have a unique vulnerability to infection because of its intimate contact with the external environment and the fact that current surgical implantation techniques, the relatively non-selective immunosuppression regimens, and injury from poor preservation and rejection all combine to impair the mechanisms for lung defense both acutely and chronically. Consequently, as the prevalence of pneumonitis from bacteria, CMV and P. carinii declines, other pathogens assume greater importance. For example, infection with Aspergillus species now represents a major diagnostic and therapeutic dilemma. Primary infection with Epstein-Barr virus causes minimal direct morbidity, but strongly predisposes the recipient to lymphoproliferative disease. This transplant-related neoplasm is particularly common in the pediatric lung recipient and often afflicts the allograft [20]. Reduction in the level of immunosuppression has proven highly successful in controlling progression of the neoplasm, but it predisposes the recipient to allograft rejection. The resurgence of pulmonary tuberculosis in the United States may eventually create substantial risks for recipients due to contamination of the donor supply and increased rate of airborne transmission of the disease.

The final problem to be discussed which looms larger than all the others is chronic allograft rejection. All solid organs appear susceptible to a progressive decline in function due to a process that has been given the name chronic rejection. The lung allograft is no exception. By 1985, a syndrome characterized by progressive obstruction to airflow and the presence of histologic bronchiolitis obliterans was recognized as a late complication of pulmonary transplantation [21]. In the last five years the prevalence of this syndrome has been more accurately established as the number of long term survivors has grown. Depending on how the syndrome is defined, the prevalence ranges from 30 to 50% of recipients who live more than six months. Mechanisms of injury remain poorly defined but likely involve immunologic responses to donor antigens that are initiated and/or amplified by infection and probably other still poorly understood factors. For these reasons, the syndrome has come to be known as chronic lung rejection.

Conditions which are strongly associated with the emergence of chronic rejection include clinically significant ischemic injury to the donor airway in the immediate postoperative period, recurrent severe acute rejection episodes and infection with CMV, P. carinii in the early postoperative period, and bacteria in the late postoperative period [22] (I.L. Paradis, University of Pittsburgh, personal communication). Most centers have elected to treat this condition by augmenting immunosuppression, either acutely with pulsed doses of corticosteroids or anti-lymphocyte globulin, or chronically by pushing maintenance immunosuppression to tolerance. Response to therapy has generally been disappointing with the majority of recipients experiencing only a short-term remission or none at all [22]. This group suffers from a progressive decline in flow rates leading to severe disability and eventually death. The true rate of mortality has not been established, but probably approaches 50%. Even when there is a response to therapy, the recipient rarely regains premorbid levels of lung function. The role of retransplantation in the treatment of chronic rejection has not been well defined. Although it has been effective in a handful of recipients [19], it is often a technically challenging procedure which raises concerns about the ethics of organ utilization. The experimental immunosuppressive agent, FK-506, has also been employed in the treatment of these recipients at the University of Pittsburgh. Although it seems to reduce the frequency of acute allograft rejection when compared to Cyclosporin A [23], it has not had an appreciable effect on the chronic lung rejection in our hands. As might be expected, the magnitude of the problem posed by chronic lung rejection has engendered considerable pessimism regarding the overall efficacy of pulmonary transplantation in some transplant physicians. Although this author does not share this degree of pessimism, he appreciates that better means of prevention and treatment of chronic rejection are badly needed.

Summary

After thirty years of experience, the field of pulmonary transplantation appears finally to have achieved the same level of success as cardiac and hepatic transplantation. Along with prolonging life for patients with endstage lung and heart disease, pulmonary transplantation has also definitely improved the quality of their existence. The situation remains far from optimal, however. Shortage of donor lungs, inadequate control of opportunistic infection, and prevention of chronic allograft rejection must all be successfully addressed for this promising treatment to benefit all of the potential candidates who look to it for salvation.

Acknowledgements

The author would like to thank Ms. Alice Lawson for her excellent clerical assistance and Mr. Wayne Grgurich for preparation of the graphics.

References

1. Carrel A. The surgery of blood vessels, etc. Johns Hopkins Hosp Bull 1967; 18:18-28.

2. Hardin CA, Kittle CF. Experience with transplantation of lung. Science 1954; 119:97-100.

3. Hardy JD, Webb WR, Dalton MLJ. Lung homotransplantation in man. JAMA 1963;186(No.12):1065-1075.

4. Magovern GJ, Yates AJ. Human homotransplantation of left lung: report of a case. Ann NY Acad Sci 1964;120(1):710-718.

5. Veith FJ. Lung transplantation. Surg Clin NA 1978;58(2):357-364.

6. Reitz BA, Wallwork JL, Hunt SA, et al. Heart-lung transplantation: Successful therapy for patients with pulmonary vascular disease. N Engl J Med 1982; 306:557-564.

7. Griffith BP, Hardesty RL, Trento A, et al. Heart-lung transplantation: Lessons learned and future hopes. Ann Thorac Surg 1987;43:6-16.

8. Hutter JA, Despins P, Higenbottam T, Stuart S, Wallwork J. Heart-lung transplantation: Better use of resources. Am J Med 1988;85(1):4-11.

9. Pearson FG. Lung transplantation. Arch Surg 1989;124:535-538.

10. Dauber JH, Paradis IL, Dummer JS. Infectious complications in pulmonary allograft recipients. Clin Chest Med 1990;11(2):291-308.

11. Dittrich HC, Nicod PH, Chow LC, Chappuis FP, Moser KM, Peterson KL. Early changes of right heart geometry after pulmonary thromboendarterectomy. J Am Coll Cardiol 1988;11(5):937-943.

12. Zenati M, Dowling RD, Armitage JM, et al. Organ procurement for pulmonary transplantation. Ann Thorac Surg 1989;48:882-886.

13. Bates DV. The other lung. N Engl J Med 1970;282:277-279.

14. Veith FJ, Koerner SK, Siegelman SS, et al. Single lung transplantation in experimental and human emphysema. Ann Surg 1973;178(4):463-476.

15. Mal H, Andreassian B, Fabrice P, et al. Unilateral lung transplantation in end-stage pulmonary emphysema. Am Rev Respir Dis 1989;140:797-802.

16. Pasque MK, Cooper JD, Kaiser LR, Haydock DA, Triantafillou A, Trulock EP. Improved technique for bilateral lung transplantation. Ann Thorac Surg 1990; 49:785-791.

17. Duncan SR, Paradis IL, Dauber JH, et al. Ganciclovir prophylaxis for cytomegalovirus infections in pulmonary allograft recipients. Am Rev Respir Dis 1992;146:1213-1215.

18. Yousem SA, Paradis IL, Dauber JH, Griffith BP. Efficacy of transbronchial lung biopsy in the diagnosis of bronchiolitis obliterans in heart-lung transplant recipients. Transplantation 1989;47(5):893-895.

19. Kreitt JM, Kaye MP. The registry of the International Society for Heart and Lung Transplantation: Eighth official report-1991. J Heart Lung Transplant 1991; 10:491-498.

20. Armitage JM, Kormos RL, Stuart RS, et al. Posttransplant lymphoproliferative disease in thoracic organ transplant patients: Ten years of cyclosporine-based immunosuppression. J Heart Lung Transplant 1991;10(6):877-887.

21. Yousem SA, Burke CM, Billingham M. Pathologic pulmonary alterations in long term human heart-lung transplantation. Human Pathol 1985;16:911-923.

22. Scott JP, Higenbottam TW, Clelland CA, et al. Natural history of chronic rejection in heart-lung transplant recipients. J Heart Transplant 1990; 9:510-515.

23. Griffith BP, Hardesty RL, Armitage JM. Acute rejection of lung allografts with various immunosuppressive protocols. Ann Thorac Surg 1992;54:846-851.

Xenotransplantation: The Current Status of Understanding

Fritz H. Bach, MD, Willem J. Van der Werf, MD, Martin L. Blakely, MD, Bernard Vanhove, PhD, Rainer de Martin, PhD, and Hans Winkler, PhD. Sandoz Center for Immunobiology, Harvard Medical School, 185 Pilgrim Road, Boston, MA 02215. Tel. 617-732-1199 Fax 617-732-1198

Introduction

Xenoreactive natural antibodies (XNA) present in the blood of all individuals and reactive with antigens on cells of phylogenetically widely-separated species, as well as complement (C) play major roles in initiating hyperacute rejection (HAR) of a discordant xenograft. Depletion of either of these entities appears to result in prolongation of graft survival [1-4].

Several years ago, one of us (FHB) suggested that HAR initiated by XNA + C might be caused by the deposition of recipient XNA on donor organ endothelial cells (EC), and that the XNA and activated recipient C would result in EC activation, the consequences of which would lead to HAR. It is well known from a series of studies in other systems, that hemorrhage and thrombosis are the consequences of EC activation by IL-1, TNF, lipopolysaccharide, or other stimuli. These phenomena appear to be in the final common pathway leading to rejection of a transplanted discordant organ no matter whether the rejection episode occurs after 12 to 15 minutes, as with transplantation of an immediately-vascularized organ from guinea pig to rat, in 1 to 2 hours, as with transplantation from pig to primate, or after several days, as occurs if XNA and complement are temporarily lowered, or their actions abrogated, in the primate recipient. We review below, very briefly, the involvement of XNA, complement, and EC activation in discordant xenograft rejection.

This is paper #605 from our laboritories.

J. L. Touraine et al. (eds.), Rejection and Tolerance, 65–70.

Xenoreactive Natural Antibodies

The evidence that XNA are primarily of the IgM isotype is strong, although one should not at this point rule out a role for IgG. Studies by immunopathology of rejecting pig hearts in rhesus monkeys show primarily, if not solely, IgM depositing on the endothelium of the donor organ. IgG, when found, appears to have the same distribution as albumin, and is thus likely present secondary to loss of vascular integrity and diffusion of solutes from the intravascular space into the sub-endothelial tissues [5].

The titers of IgM XNA in different humans vary widely. In recent studies by Vanhove in our laboratories, studying 50 individuals picked at random, the titer of XNA varied more than 400 fold between the individual with the highest titer as compared with the one with the lowest [6]. In our previous studies of a smaller panel of sera, we found that this variation in titer did not correlate with either the amount of IgM in the serum nor the titers of the ABO isohemagglutinins [7].

One obvious goal is to remove the XNA, or lower titers *in vivo* to levels at which HAR will not occur. Previously, the two major methods that have been used were plasmapheresis and absorption of the XNA on donor species organs, such as the kidney, by passaging blood of the potential recipient through one or more donor organs before transplantation. Both of these approaches are effective, however, the XNA rapidly return to the circulation [1]. Thus, in the last few years, other approaches have been evaluated.

A number of new immunosuppressive agents have become available that suppress elicited antibody formation. Such agents include mycophenolate mofetil (RS 61443) [8], 15-deoxyspergualin [9], rapamycin and brequinar [10]. We have shown, primarily in rats, that several of these including RS 61443 as well as rapamycin and brequinar are able to suppress XNA titers, and if XNA are depleted by physical methods, to maintain the lowered levels achieved [10]. In addition, Soares, Bazin, one of us (FHB) and our colleagues have used a mouse anti-rat μ chain monoclonal antibody to suppress XNA to undetectable levels, which can be maintained for a few days after cessation of antibody therapy [11]. These approaches will hopefully not only be of use for clinically-relevant therapies, but will allow testing of important questions regarding the role of XNA in the rejection process.

One aspect of the XNA problem deals with the target antigens on pig EC that are recognized by the XNA. We and others, using various methods to isolate potential candidate targets, have shown that in addition to the triad (gp115, gp125, and gp135) we previously identified [12], there are other prominent target molecules, including ones with molecular weights ranging from 40 kD to 200 kD [13]. Once identified and isolated, the targets of the XNA could be administered *in vivo* in an attempt to block XNA binding to EC, or used on columns to deplete XNA before transplantation.

Complement

Inhibition of complement has represented a formidable barrier in the past, however, techniques have recently been introduced that show promise in this regard. Fearon and colleagues genetically engineered a soluble form of complement receptor type 1 (sCR1) which has been shown to inhibit complement and allow prolonged survival of discordant xenografts in both rats and primates [14]. A highly purified preparation of cobra venom factor has also yielded encouraging results with minimal toxicity to the recipient.

Dalmasso, working with us in Minnesota, had the idea of introducing human forms of membrane-associated inhibitors of complement, such as decay accelerating factor (DAF) [15], into pig EC to inhibit complement. Dalmasso and we [16], as well as David White and colleagues [17], have shown that there is potential validity to this idea. A major goal is to derive a transgenic pig that expresses high levels of human inhibitors of complement.

EC Activation

Addition of human serum to monolayers of pig EC *in vitro* results in various changes that are characteristic of EC activation. (We do not review in this paper, the loss of heparan sulfate from EC treated in this manner, which we have discussed [18].) Perhaps of greatest interest in this regard is that the EC stimulated with human serum promote coagulation as compared with quiescent EC. Consistent with these procoagulant changes, that presumably reflect the up-regulation of the gene for tissue factor and expression of that product on the cell surface [19], is the observation that a number of different genes are up-regulated (as measured by accumulation of mRNA) with the addition of human serum to the EC. Present studies in our laboratories suggest that XNA without complement do provide a stimulus to the EC [20].

We believe that these changes may well reflect what takes place *in vivo* as well. Guinea pig hearts transplanted to rats that have been treated with cobra venom factor survive between 2 and 5 days, depending on the addition of other therapies. Examination of the heart at the time of rejection by immunopathology shows evidence of IL-1, tissue factor, as well as expression of P-selectin and E-selectin, all markers of EC activation. Further experiments will be needed to evaluate to which extent the consequences of EC activation are the cause of rejection; we regard it as very likely that they play such a role.

Accommodation: a working model for xenograft survival

We have suggested [16] that it may not be necessary to remove XNA and compromise the complement system, and perhaps manipulate other factors, for the life-time of the graft, to prevent vascular rejection. (It is important to emphasize in this context that there will surely be a cell-mediated immune rejection response in the pig to primate situation if the vascular problem is averted; we are not dealing with that here, nor discussing the therapy of such rejection.) Based on findings in allotransplantation across the ABO barrier [21], we proposed as a working model that if XNA and complement, and perhaps other factors, are compromised for some time after the transplant is in place, that at a later time, when the transplanted organ and the EC of that organ have had time to "heal in", it may be possible to let XNA, C and other factors return to normal without evoking EC activation to the extent that vascular rejection occurs. We have referred to such a situation as "accommodation" and have discussed possible reasons why accommodation may be achieved. Whether accommodation, which we believe we did achieve in one rhesus recipient of a pig heart [18], can be reproducibly achieved must be the subject of future experiments.

References

1. Bach FH, Platt JL, Cooper D. Accommodation: the role of natural antibody and complement in discordant xenograft rejection. In: Cooper D, Kemp E, Reemtsma K, White DJG, editors. Xenotransplantation- the transplantation of organs and tissues between species. Heidelberg, Germany: Springer-Verlag. 1991: 81-100.

2. Blakely ML, Van der Werf WJ, Hancock WW, Bach FH. Prolonged suppression of xenoreactive natural antibodies and elimination of hyperacute rejection in a discordant xenotransplant model. Transplantation, submitted.

3. Pruitt SK, Baldwin WM, Marsh HC, Lin SS, Yeh CG, Bollinger RR. The Effect of soluble complement receptor type 1 on hyperacute xenograft rejection. Transplantation 1991;52:868-873.

4. Bach FH, Van der Werf WJ, Blakely ML, Vanhove B, de Martin R, Winkler H. Discordant Xenografting: A Working model of problems and issues. Xeno, in press.

5. Platt JL, Bach FH. Mechanisms of tissue injury in hyperacute xenograft rejection. In: Cooper DKC, Kemp E, Reemtsma K, and White DJG, editors. Xenotransplantation, 1990.

6. Vanhove B, Bach FH. Human xenoreactive natural antibodies: avidity and targets on porcine endothelial cells. Transplantation, in press.

7. Platt JL, Lindman BJ, Geller RL, et al. The role of natural antibodies in the activation of xenogeneic endothelial cells. Transplantation 1991;52:1037-1043.

8. Figueroa J, Fuad SA, Kunjummen BD, Platt JL, Bach FH. Suppression of synthesis of natural antibodies by mycophenolate mofetil (RS-61443). Transplantation 1993;55:1371-1374.

9. Leventhal J, Flores H, Gruber S, et al. III: Natural antibody production can be inhibited by 15-Deoxyspergualin in a discordant xenograft model. Transplantation Proc 1992;24:714.

10. Blakely ML, Van der Werf WJ, Hancock WW, Bach FH. Prolonged suppression of xenoreactive natural antibodies and elimination of hyperacute rejection in a discordant xenotransplantation model. (Submitted)

11. Soares MP, Latinne D, Elsen M, Figueroa J, Bach FH, Bazin H. In vivo depletion of xenoreactive natural antibodies with an anti-μ monoclonal antibody. Transplantation, in press.

12. Platt JL, Lindman BJ, Chen H, Spitalnik SL, Bach FH. Endothelial cell antigens recognized by xenoreactive human natural antibodies. Transplantation 1990;50:817-822.

13. Hofer -Warbinek R, et al. Unpublished observations.

14. Hebell T, Ahearn JM, Fearon DT. Suppression of the immune response by a soluble complement receptor of B lymphocytes. Science 1991;254(5028):102.

15. Dalmasso AP, Vercellotti GM, Platt JL, Bach FH. Inhibition of complement-mediated endothelial cell cytotoxicity by decay accelerating factor: Potential for prevention of xenograft hyperacute rejection. Transplantation 1991;52:530.

16. Bach FH, Turman MA, Vercellotti GM, Platt JL, Dalmasso AP. Accommodation: A working paradigm for progressing toward clinical discordant xenografting. Transpl Proc 1991;23:205.

17. White DJ, Oglesby T, Liszewski MK, et al. Expression of human decay accelerating factor or membrane cofactor protein genes on mouse cells inhibits lysis by human complement. Transpl Proc 1992;24(2):474.

18. Bach FH, Dalmasso G, Platt JL. Xenotransplantation: A current perspective. Transplantation Reviews 1992;6:1-7.

19. Hofer E, et al. Unpublished observations.

20. Vanhove B, Lipp J, de Martin R, Bach FH. Affinity purified human xenoreactive natural antibodies deliver an activating signal to pig endothelial cells. In preparation.

21. Alexandre GPJ, Latinne D, Gianello P, Squifflet JP. Preformed cytotoxic antibodies and ABO-incompatible grafts. Clin Transplantation 1991;(Spec . issue) 5: 583-594.

XENOTRANSPLANTATION: THE PRESENT AND THE FUTURE

BERNARD WEILL and DIDIER HOUSSIN
Faculté Cochin, 75674 Paris cedex 14 France
Tel (33)(1) 42 34 18 10 FACS (33)(1) 40 51 73 30

The first xenotransplantations were performed at the beginning of the twentieth century. Actually, only 46 xenotransplantations were published between 1906 and 1970, with poor results as the grafts, which were mostly harvested from non human primates, were all rejected within hours or days.

Since 1977, only 4 tentatives have been published. The last patient, transplanted by Starzl and coll. (1), had a longer survival thanks to the progresses in immunosuppressive therapy, and also because the liver is less strongly rejected than heart or kidney. However, the main reason for the relative scarcity of xenotransplantations and of experimental studies on the topic during the last decades was the increasing successes of allotransplantation. Nowadays, the increasing difficulties in finding organs of human origin triggers a renewed interest in xenotransplantation.

Xenotransplantation is invariably followed by a rejection. Experimentally, when the donor belongs to a species distant from the recipient, the rejection is extraordinarily fast and spectacular, occuring within minutes or hours. Such hyperacute rejection is observed in donor-recipient combinations that were termed "discordant" by Calne (2) in 1970. They are distinct from "concordant" combinations between closer species, that are followed by an acute rejection within 7 to 10 days.

The xenogeneic hyperacute rejection is clinically similar to that observed when an allotransplantation is unfortunately performed in a hyperimmunized recipient; xenogeneic acute rejection is clinically and immunologically similar to the acute rejection of allografts.

71

J. L. Touraine et al. (eds.), Rejection and Tolerance, 71–78.
© 1994 *Kluwer Academic Publishers.*

The mechanism of xenograft hyperacute rejection is complex. It involves the activation of the graft endothelial cells by antibodies and complement present in the recipient's serum. Activated endothelial cells produce various soluble mediators that participate in the formation of fibrin, in platelet agregation and in vasoconstriction. All these phenomena lead to hemorrhagic necrosis of the graft.

The recipient's complement plays a pivotal role that has been demonstrated by several experiments years ago: in 1967, Gewurz and the group of Good (3) showed that the transplantation of rabbit, sheep, pig or calf kidneys into dogs was followed by the decrease in complement components in the effluent blood of the graft. Schilling and coll (4) showed that isolated rat kidneys perfused with normal dog serum displayed lesions of hyperacute rejection within minutes, whereas in kidneys perfused with decomplemented sera or with sera depleted from immunoglobulins, the lesions were delayed. Similarly, isolated rabbit or guinea pig hearts perfused with decomplemented hman serum survive for a longer period of time than when perfused with normal human serum.

The isssue which is presently addressed by several groups of searchers, is that of the mechanism of complement activation during xenograft hyperacute rejection. In the guinea pig to rat combination, Miyagawa and coll (5) and Termignon and coll (6) showed that the alternative pahway of complement is engaged. The activation of the alternative pathway of the recipient's complement can occur through the direct contact between complement components and endothelial cell membranes. Indeed, the membranes may be altered, for example, by the release of heparan sulfate described by Platt and coll (7), during the process of cellular activation.

Preformed antibodies:

Preformed or natural anti-donor antibodies present in the recipient's serum can activate the direct pathway of complement once they have bound to the endothelial cells of the graft. Many groups (8, 9, 10, 11, 12, 13) favor this explanation and our present opinion is that, at least in the guinea pig to rat combination, and chiefly in the pig to human combination which is more interesting in terms of clinical applications, both direct and alternative pathways of complement are involved. Indeed, in an in vitro model of hyperacute rejection using pig endothelial cells in culture and human serum as source of natural antibodies and complement, we have shown that both C1q-deficient and factor

B-deficient sera lysed significantly fewer pig endothelial cells than normal sera (neither syngeneic pig sera nor decomplemented human sera were cytotoxic) (14).

Therefore, complement activation during hyperacute rejection involves both the alternative pathway and the direct pathway which is triggered by natural antibodies combined to xenoantigens borne by endothelial cells.

The antigens recognized by natural antibodies are not precisely known in most combinations. Platt and coll showed that human sera recognize 115-135 kD molecules on pig cells (15). We found that rat natural antibodies bound to 95-110 Kd antigens on membranes of guinea pig endothelial cells (16). The epitopes specifically recognized by the xenogeneic antibodies are oligosaccharides and are currently under investigation in many laboratories.

We observed that the cytotoxic power of rat serum towards guinea pig cells was correlated with the titer of rat anti-guinea pig antibodies (9). Plasma exchanges performed in rats prior to transplantation of a guinea pig heart, induced a decrease in the natural antibody titers and a significant prolongation of the graft survival: several hours versus15 min in the control group.

In order to assess the role of these natural antibodies more precisely, isolated guinea pig hearts were perfused by decomplemented rat serum or by fragments of immunoglobulins. Immunofluorescence studies showed the deposition of rat immunoglobulins on the coronary endothelium of guinea pig hearts. Fab' of rat natural IgM also bound to endothelial cells. We took opportunity of the inability of these Fab' fragments to activate complement, to mask the xenoantigens of the guinea pig hearts with these fragments prior to the transplantation into a rat. When guinea pig hearts had been perfused with a buffer solution or with IgG fragments, they were rejected in 15 min as usual: when they had been perfused with IgM Fab', the antigens were protected for some time and the rejection was significantly delayed up to 28 min (13). Of course, the graft was rejected as soon as the IgM fragments had been eluted from the graft endothelium.This experiment was not designed as a tentative treatment, but as a study of the role of natural antibodies in hyperacute rejection.

The study of acute rejection of xenografts requires that no hyperacute rejection occurs. This is achieved either by performing grafts that do not necessitate an immediate vascular reconnexion, such as skin grafts, or using concordant donor-recipient combinations such as, for example, hamster to rat.

While in vivo experiments showed similarities between acute xenogeneic and allogeneic rejections, xenogeneic MLRs are generally characterized by a weaker proliferation than allogeneic MLRs. This phenomenon is probably not due, as it was initially thought, to an inappropriate TCR repertory in recipients' respondig cells. At least two other findings can explain the weakness of in vitro xenogeneic proliferation: Bach and coll showed that the recipients' lymphoid cells may respond weakly to the cytokines produced by the cells from a distant species. In addition, when the donor and the recipient belong to widely disparate species, the ligands present on antigen-presenting cells of the donor may not be complementary of adhesion molecules on recipient's lymphoid cells.

The weakness of xenogeneic MLRs raises the hope that the xenogeneic acute rejection may be easy to prevent. However, this is not necessarily true, since no correlation between the rate of in vitro xenogeneic proliferation and the intensity of acute rejection has been established yet.

The choice of a donor: If such correlations existed, they could guide the choice of the potential donors. At first it was thought that using organs from primates such as monkeys would help solve the technical, physiological and immunological problems. Indeed, because of phylogenetic proximity, organs from primates were supposed to be appropriate substitutes in humans. In addition, the immunological rejection of primate organs is clinically and immunologically similar to the acute rejection of allografts. However, given the numerous technical, economical and ethical issues, the scientific community has begun to study the possibility of using animals more distant from human as organ donors:

- pigs, which are considered as the favorite potential organ donors, are less expensive than monkeys.

- the risk of transmission of viral diseases is not well known but is probably weaker than with non human primates, namely in terms of retroviruses.

- the use of pigs should raise fewer protests since this animal is already widely used as food in many countries; in addition, preliminary discussions with religious authorities ruling communities who do not consume pork meat, indicate that the transplantation of pig organs would not be forbidden if allowing to save human life.

- the physiology of pig kidney and liver is close to that of human.

The treatment of xenogeneic rejection: If non primates are chosen as donors, we will have to handle hyperacute rejection first, and if the patient overcomes this step, we will have to treat the acute rejection. Many experimental protocols have been designed to prevent or inhibit hyperacute rejection. Most of them are based on:

- recipient's depletion from natural antibodies by plasma exchanges or extracorporeal absorption on xenogeneic organs , or depletion of natural antibody producing CD5+ B cells using monoclonal antibodies (9, 17),

- inhibition of complement activation with infratoxic dosages of cobra venom factot (18, 19),

- inhibition of various soluble mediators produced by endothelial cells.

None of these treatments have been definitely convincing. It may be that some of them should be associated. However, two new methods could open new alleys in the prevention of hyperacute rejection:

- the use of transgenic donors,

- the accomodation of the graft prior to transplantation.

Transgenic animals: Human cells bear glycoproteins on their membranes such as CD35 (CR1), CD46 (Membrane Cofactor Protein), CD55 (Decay Accelerating Factor), CD59 (Protectin), and Homologous Restriction Factor, that are specific inhibitors of autologous complement and not of xenogeneic complement. It has already been shown than CHO cells transfected with human DAF or MCP genes (20) and murine cells transfected with human CD59 genes (21) are more resistant to lysis by human complement than non transfected cells. In vivo perfusion of soluble CR1 prolongs xenograft survival (22). Mice transgenic for DAF and MCP genes have been produced(23), and a sow bearing human DAF genes now lives in Cambridge (24).

Therefore, the idea would be to use as organ donors transgenic animals expressing one or several of these proteins which would inhibit human complement and probably hyperacute rejection.

Accomodation of the graft: A second new method would consist of accomodating the graft ex vivo prior to the transplantation. It has been shown that depletion of natural antibodies prior to transplantation and maintenance of low antibody levels, leads to a state in which the graft survives even after the anti-donor antibodies have returned to their initial level . Alexandre and coll (25) allowed porcine kidneys to survive in baboons after reappearance of natural xenoantibodies that had ben initially depleted. This situation, "...where temporary removal of an offending antibody before and for some time period after transplantation, allows survival when the antibody returns, in the presence of normal levels of complement..." has been named "accomodation" by Bach (26).

The accomodation phenomenon is presently studied in vitro by Zhao and coll (27), who showed that after 3 days' incubation with decomplemented normal human serum, pig endothelial cells are more resistant to human complement lysis (34%) than control cells preincubated with syngeneic serum (65%). The percentage of lysis by C1q-deficient serum is not significantly different whether the cells have been "accomodated" or not; in contrast, factor B-deficient serum is almost not cytotoxic to "accomodated" pig cells (2%) versus control cells (46%).

This observation suggests that the contact with xenogeneic antibodies before the transplantaton may inhibit the direct pathway of complement. Further experiments suggest that the recipients IgG and neither IgM nor IgA are responsible for this accomodation , and that an ex vivo perfusion of the graft with polyclonal IgG prior to the transplantation might effectively delay its hyperacute rejection.

If the dream of overcoming hyperacute rejection could be fulfilled, doctors would be left with the treatment of acute rejection which would perhaps require fewer imaginative efforts: progresses in immunosuppressive therapy, total lymphoid irradiation or even intrathymic graft of xenogeneic cells could be attempted as it already was in allogeneic situations.

REFERENCES

1- Starzl TE, Fung J, Tzakis A, Todo S, Demetris AJ, Marino IR, Dyle H, Zeevi A, Warty V, Michaels M, Kusne S, Ruddert WA, Trucco M. Baboon to human liver transplantation. The Lancet 1993; 341: 65-71.

2- Calne R. Organ transplantation between widely disparate species. Translant Proc 1970; 2: 550-553.

3- 11- Gewurz H, Clark DS, Cooper MD, Varco RL, and Good RA . Effect of cobra venom-induced inhibition of complement activity on allograft and xenograft rejection reactions. Transplantation1967 ; 5: 1296-1303.

4- Schilling A, Land W, Pratschke E, Pielsticker K, Brendel W. Dominant role of complement in the hyperacute xenograft rejection. Surg Gynecol Obstet 1976; 142: 29-35.

5- Miyagawa S. Hirose H. Shirakura R. Naka Y, Nakata S. Kawashima Y, Seya T. Matsumoto M. Uenaka A, and Kitamura H : The mechanism of discordant xenograft rejetion. Transplantation 1988; 46: 825-830.

6-Termignon JL, Calmus Y, Chéreau Ch, Kahan A, Houssin D, Weill BJ: In vitro analysis of complement activation in xenogeneic hyperacute rejection. Transplant Proc 1990; 22: 1060 - 1061.

7- Platt JL, Vercelotti GM, Lindman B, Oegema TR Jr, Bach FH, Dalmasso AP. Release of heparan sulfate from endothelial cells: implications for pathogenesis of hyperacute rejection. J Exp Med 1990; 171: 1363-1366.

8- Hammer C, Land W, rendel W. Experimental xenotransplantation in widely divergent species: mechanisms of the xenogeneic hyperacute rejection, their modification under the influence of active and passive enhancement. Res Exp Med, 1973; 14: 796-802.

9- Van de Stadt J, Meriggi F, Vendeville B, Weill B, Crougneau S, Filipponi F, Michel A, Houssin D. Prolongation of heart xenograft survival in the rat: effectiveness of cyclosporine in preventing early xenoantibody rebound after membrane plasmapheresis. Transplant Proc 1989; 21: 543-545.

10- Hammer C. Preformed natural antibodies and possibilities of modulation of hyperacute xenogeneic rejection. Transplant Proc 1989; 21: 522-524.

11- Platt JL, Fischel RJ, Matas AJ, Reif SA, Bolman R, Bach FH: Immunopathology of hyperacute xenograft rejection in a swine to primate model. Transplantation 1991; 52: 214-220.

12- Dalmasso A P, Vercellotti G M, Fischel R J, Bolman R M, Bach F H, and Platt JL. Mechanism of complement activation in the hyperacute rejection of porcine organs transplanted into primate recipients. Am J Pathol 1992; 140: 1157-1166.

13- Gambiez L, Salamé E, Chéreau C, Calmus Y, Ayani E, Houssin D. Weill BJ. Role of natural IgM in the hyperacute rejection of discordant heart xenografts. Transplantation 1992; 54: 577 - 583.

14- Zhao Z, Termignon JL, Cardoso J, Chéreau C, Gautreau C, Calmus Y, Houssin D, Weill B. Hyperacute xenograft rejection in the swine to human donor - recipient combination: in vitro analysis of complement activation. Submitted for publication .

15- Platt JL, Lindman BJ, Chen H, Spitalnik SL, Bach FH. : Endothelial cell antigens recognized by xenoreactive human natural antibodies. Transplantation 1990; 50 : 817-822.

16- Calmus Y, Ayani E, Cardoso J, Chéreau C, Kahan A, Houssin D, and Weill B. The target antigens of hyperacute xenogeneic rejection in the rat/guinea pig and guinea pig/rat discordant combinations. Transplantation, in press.

17- Cooper DKC, Human PA, Lexer G. Effects of cyclosporine and antibody absorption on pig cardiac xenograft survival in the baboon. J Heart Transplant 1988; 7: 238-246.

18- Kemp E, Steinbrüchel D, Starklint H, Larsen S, Henriksen I, and Dieperink H. Renal graft rejection: prolonging effect of captopril, ACE-inhibitors, prostacyclin and cobra venom factor. Transplant Proc 1987; 19: 4471-4474.

19- Tavakoli R, Michel A, Cardoso J, Ayani E, Maillet F, Fontaliran F, Crougneau S, Weill B, Houssin D. Prolonged survival of guinea pig to rat heart xenografts using repeated low doses of cobra venom factor. Transplant Proc 1993; 25: 407 - 409.

20- White D, Oglesby TJ, Tedja I, Liszewski K, Wallwork J, Van Den Bogaerde J, Atkinson JP. Protection of mammalian cells from human complement-mediated lysis by transfection of human membrane cofactor protein (MCP) or decay-accelerating factor (DAF). Ist International Congress on Xenotransplantation; 1991 August 25-28; Minneapoli. Abstr. 1B.1 p. 7.

21- Akami T, Arakawa K, Okamoto M, Sawada R, Naruto M, Oka T. The role of human CD59 antigen in discordant xenotransplantation between human and non primates. Transplant Proc 1993; 25: 394-395.

22- Pruitt SK, Baldwin W., Marsh HC, Lin SS, Yeh CG, Bollinger RR.The effect complement receptor type 1 on hyperacute xenograft rejection. Transplantation 1991; 52: 868-73.

23- Cary N, Moody J, Yannoutsos N, Wallwork J, White D. Tissue expression of human decay-accelerating factor, a regulator of complement activation expressed in mice: a potential approach to inhibition of hyperacute xenograft rejection. Transplant Proc, 1993; 25: 400-401.

24- White D : Down-regulation of hyperacute xenograft rejection by human RCA membrane-bound molecules. Conférence sur la xénotransplantation; 1993 March 3-5; Institut des Sciences du vivant Annecy.

25- Alexandre G, Gianello P, Latinne D.In: Hardy MA editor. Xenograft 25. Elsevier Science publishers, 1989: 259-266.

26- Bach FH. Transplant Proc 1992; 24:

27- Zhao Z, Chéreau C, Calmus Y, Houssin D, Weill B. In vitro accomodation of swine endothelial cells to human serum. Submitted for publication.

RISK FACTORS FOR REJECTION AND PREDICTIVE FACTORS FOR CHRONIC REJECTION IN
KIDNEY TRANSPLANTATION

Patrice DETEIX, Christine CARRIAS, Eliane ALBUISSON

To know the risk of rejection is one of the main goal for each physician in charge of

transplanted patients. Such a knowledge should allow us to adapt the immunosuppressive

therapy to the level of risk and to avoid to add several high risk factors for the same

allogenic kidney recipient. In the litterature two methods are used : to look for risk

factors in homogeneous but small one-center studies or in heterogeneous multi-center

studies with a large contingent of patients. Risk factors for rejection in kidney

transplantation can be classified in four groups : risk factors peculiar to the donor, to the

recipient, to the couple donor-recipient and to the post-transplant period. Risk factors

related to the donor are age, sex and living or cadaver status. Risk factors related to the

recipient are age, sex, race, primary disease, HLA antigens, blood transfusions prior to

transplantation and immunization. Risk factors related to the couple donor-recipient are

ABO and HLA compatibilities, cold ischemia and delayed graft function, crossmatch

procedures. Risk factors related to the evolution of the graft are the short term

evolution, infections with cytomegalovirus (CMV), immunosuppression and quality of

care.

Material and methods :

For this study we analysed the litterature and our one-center results ; 100 kidney

transplantations were performed between july 1987 and may 1992 using quadruple

immunosuppression with anti-thymocytes globulins (Institut Mérieux) during 10 days.

The shortest follow-up was 9 months. Seven patients were transplanted for the second

J. L. Touraine et al. (eds.), Rejection and Tolerance, 79–93.
© 1994 *Kluwer Academic Publishers.*

time. Ten patients came back to dialysis after rejection, 1 after recurrence of glomerulonephritis and 1 after transplantectomy with Kaposi in the graft. Two patients died after antirejection therapy, 2 died with sepsis and multiple organ failure (without rejection), 1 patient died of an acute lung cytomegalovirus infection. Five years actuarial survival is 94% for the patient and 82% for the graft (figure 1). The first rejection was not documented by biopsy, chronic rejection was documented on biopsy and clinical evolution. CMV infection was documented by positive viremia and/or positive viruria (rapid detection or viral cultures) and/or seroconversion and/or significant rise of the anti-CMV antibodies titers or the detection of specific anti-CMV IgM (ELISA). Viral monitoring was performed weekly from day 0 to day 21 then if clinical symptoms occured. Analysis of risk factors for acute rejection was performed with Kaplan-Meier survival curves compared with log-rank test, the end-point was the first rejection. We also performed comparison of qualitative and quantitative variables using either chi-square test or Mann-Whitney U test, the outcome variables were acute rejection and chronic rejection.

Results :

Fivty seven patients (57%) had acute rejection. We found (univariate analysis) significant statistical link between acute rejection and recipient age (less rejections in patients older than 60 years, chi-square = 3.87, p = 0.048), acute rejection and CMV infection (more rejections in patients with CMV infections, chi-square = 14.75, p < 0.0001), and between chronic rejection and acute rejection (more chronic rejection in patients with acute rejection, chi-square = 9.76, p = 0.0004), chronic rejection and CMV infection (more chronic rejection among patients with CMV infection, chi-square = 11.58, p < 0.0001). Patients with CMV infection experienced more rejections, 2 years

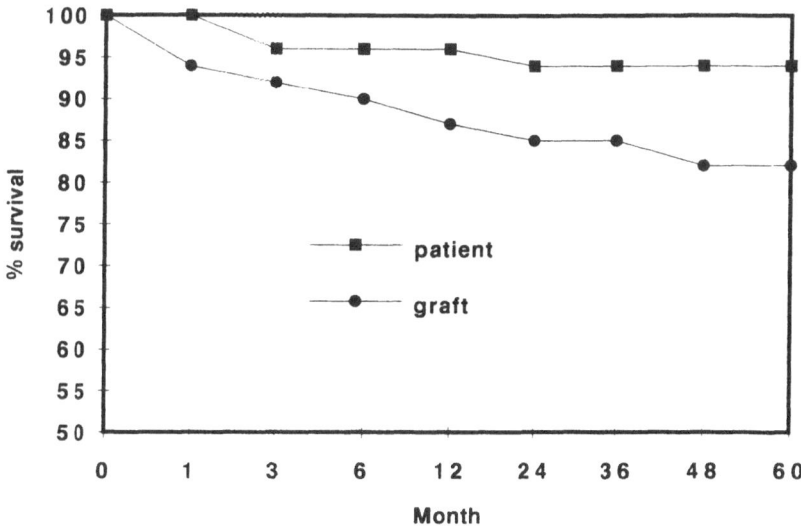

Figure 1. Actuarial patient and graft survival, one-center study.

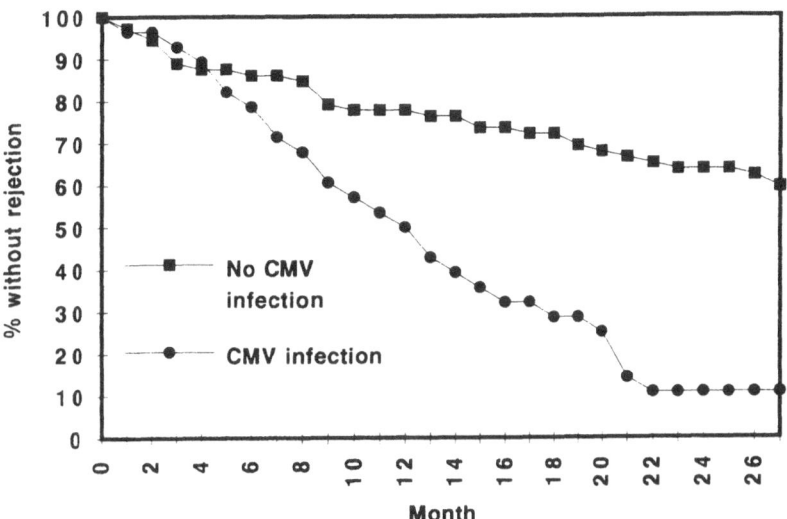

Figure 2. Recipients without rejection (Kaplan-Meier estimate) according to the absence or the presence of CMV infection. (log-rank : p < 0,0001)

after the transplantion 60% of the patients without CMV infection had no rejection while only 10% of the patients with CMV infection had no rejection (figure 2). Creatinine levels at 3 and 6 months were also statistically linked to acute rejection (Mann-Whitney U test, p < 0.0001).

Discussion :

In most of the published studies the outcome variable is the graft loss or the patient death. To find risk factors for rejection the outcome variable must be either rejection or graft loss by rejection or death of the patient directly related to rejection. Matas (1) has shown the importance to consider death with function in analyzing kidney transplant outcomes particularly when half-lives after the first year are compared. Difficulties appear also with the definition of the rejection, was a biopsy performed or was the diagnosis made on clinical grounds? Very few studies have chronic rejection as an outcome variable. When an event A is a risk factor for an outcome variable X, B can be a risk factor for A and X, B enhances the statistical link between A and X, the risk factor B is called confounding factor for A and X ; statistical tools as cross-stratification and multivariable analysis are used to avoid the action of confounding factors. Among multivariable methods proportional hazards regression (Cox) is widely used. We must carefully analyse the published results, Concato [2] in a recent review found 68% of violations of methodologic guidelines in a random sample of publications in the Lancet and the New England Journal of Medicine.

Donor risk factor for rejection

One year graft survival is lower when the donor is younger than 10 years [3,4], this appears even after exclusion of technical failure and whatever was the recipient age [5].

About old donors the results seem to be not so good [3,4,6] but Creagh [7] did not notice any difference in graft survival for donors older than 50 years. In the UNOS 1991 registry 1 year graft survival is lower with female donors who are older than male donor, the cause of brain death is more often traumatic for males and vascular for the women [6]. Cadaver versus living donor : one year graft survival is higher when the donor is a living related donor with 0 mismatch or 1 haplotype (cadaver donor : 79%, 0 mismatch living related donor : 94%, 1 haplotype : 90%) in the UNOS 1991 registry [6] and the difference still exists after one year with half-lives respectively at 7, 27 and 12 years. Sesso [8] found with the Cox model much less graft failure with identical and haplo-identical related living donor.

Recipient risk factor for rejection

Rate of first rejection and immunologic graft loss are higher with young recipients [4,9] quadruple immunosuppression reduces the risk of rejection in younger patients for Ettenger [10]. Howard [11] found no difference in graft survival between recipients younger or older than 50 years. No significant differences in graft outcome are associated with the recipient sex [9]. Concerning the race of the recipient Koyama [12] published in the UNOS registry lower 1 year graft survival and lower half-life after the first year in black people, more mismatches could be one of the explanations for those bad results. Lim and Cecka in 1992 published better results with patients whose primary disease was an IgA glomerulonephritis [13,14]. Sanfilippo in 1984 showed a beneficial effect of bilateral native nephrectomy with less graft lost from rejection and increase in overall graft survival [15]. Hendricks and Soulillou claimed in 1983 that recipients with the class II antigen DR6 had a lower graft survival than recipients without the DR6 antigen

[16,17]. The 1 year graft survival of non transfused patients in United States improved and surpassed the 1 year graft survival of transfused patients in 1989 [18]. Opelz (Collaborative Transplant Registry) found the same phenomenon, with or without cyclosporin the 3 years graft survival is now nearly the same with or without transfusions [19]. Nevertheless Baatard [20] in a recent one-center study found still a transfusion effect if the recipient received 3 or 4 blood transfusions before the transplantation. Lagaaij [21,22] reported in 1989 and later the beneficial effect of a single pre-transplantation transfusion with 1 HLA-DR antigen matched, we need confirmation by others groups. More and more patients are not transfused before the transplantation, the ratio of transfused to non transfused recipients is now near from one [18]. Pouteil-Noble [23] did not found any beneficial effect of platelets transfusions on 4 years graft survival. Sensitization against HLA antigens seems to be a deleterious risk factor for graft survival. Zhou [24] reported with the UCLA registry a diminution of 7% of graft survival in sensitized recipients, the HLA matching effect overcame the effect of sensitization. In the same study it appeared that the loss of transplants occured in the first three months, the half-life after three month was nearly the same whatever was the sensitization of the recipients.

Couple donor-recipient, risk factor for rejection

ABO compatible missmatches seem to have a light detrimental effect on 5 years graft survival [25]. HLA was the overriding factor that determined graft survival, matching has the highest and most significant relative risk of all the covariates in the study of UNOS 1991 registry by Cicciarelli ; 3 years graft survival was 84% with 0 mismatch and 68% with 6 mismatches [26]. Vereestraeten attracted attention on beneficial (donor

DR5+ recipient DR5- or donor DR7+ recipient DR7-) or detrimental (donor DR6-recipient DR6+ or donor DR7- recipient DR7+) HLA disparities, with a 20% more 2 years graft survival in recipients with beneficial disparities [27]. Opelz and the Collaborative Transplant Study have shown the importance of HLA antigen splits [28] and the great improvement of HLA matching effect when typing is made with molecular biology [29]. Cold ischemia and acute renal failure could be risk factors for rejection ; Preuschof reported much more vascular rejection on kidneys from older donors with a delayed graft function [30]. Crossmatch done before transplantation is usually a lymphocytotoxicity crossmatch (National Institute for Health assay) ; Birtch [31] has shown the relevance of a 51chromium release assay, Takahashi [32] has shown the significance of an antiglobulin crossmatch test to predict occurence of severe accelerated rejections in patients who received donor specific transfusions. Kerman [33] has compared the NIH assay with the anti human globulin test and with a flow cytometry crossmatch, the two last methods allowed to get better results for patients with a negative crossmatch ; the 1 year graft survival was repectively 66%, 77% and 83% for patients having a negative crossmatch with NIH assay, anti-Ig test and flow cytomotry test. Karuppan and Muller [34,35] laid stress on the importance of non-complement fixing antibodies (anti-HLA) in patients with acute rejection, detrimental effect of weakly positive B-cell cytotoxicity crossmatches (with T-cell cytotoxicity negative crossmatches) has been demonstrated, the patients with rejection had a T cell reactivity with the flow cytometer. Ting in a review [36] considered a T cell cytotoxicity crossmatch with IgG against class I HLA antigens in the current serum as the single definite contra-indication to transplantation. Guerin [37] has shown a favourable graft outcome in patients transplanted with a positive B-cell crossmatch on current serum.

Auto (non-HLA) antibodies are not detrimental [36].

Post transplantation risk factors for rejection.

CMV infection could have a detrimental effect on immunologic graft survival. Von Willebrand [38] demonstrated association between CMV infection, rejection and upregulation of HLA class II antigens in the graft. Fujinami [39] found a sequence homology and an immunologic cross reactivity between the early-2-protein of CMV and the beta chain of HLA class II antigens. In clinical studies Niaudet [40] claimed that CMV infection had no detrimental effect on graft survival, Lewis [41] found more acute rejections and a 1 year graft survival decreasing with CMV infections, Dittmer [42] found more vascular rejections associated with CMV infections. Pouteil-Noble [43] found a strong association between CMV infection and rejection and also between B-DR or DR HLA incompatibilities and CMV infection. Blancho [44] published an higher incidence of CMV infection in DR7 matched recipients. Therapy of CMV infections with interferon [45] can induce irreversible rejection. Early evolution could be a risk factor : Gulanikar [46] reported all the patients free of rejection at 3 months as free of rejection one year after the transplantation. Nicol [47] compared 48 patients with immunologic graft failure between 12 and 36 months after transplantation to 300 patients with graft survival at 3 years , among the group with graft failure 39% were free of rejection at 3 months and 27% had 2 or more rejections at 3 month against respectively 62% and 13% in the group with graft survival at 3 years. The appearance of survival curves in all the studies shows very well the higher rate of graft loss during the first three months, even now with very few technical failures, the evolution during the first three months seems to be a risk factor for more late rejections and chronic rejection. Obviously the kind of immunosuppression is a risk factor for rejection, everybody among physicians is looking for the best protocol with no rejections and no infectious complications. It is impossible to resume all the trials performed until now, most of the centers use cyclosporin, steroids and azathioprin. Norman [48] found less rejections, but identical 2 and 5 years graft survival when he compared patients receiving OKT3 and patients without the monoclonal antibody. Matas [49] has shown the beneficial effect of antilymphocyte globulin on the occurence of rejection in recipients with delayed graft function. Hanas [50] studied a new aspect of cyclosporin efficacy, a low cyclosporin concentration in the kidney tissue itelf could be a risk factor for rejection. The center effect which has disappeared in France [51] is still in United States (UNOS) a risk factor for rejection [52]. Graft survival following rejection is 10 to 30% lower in average and low centers. Risk factors for chronic rejection have been studied by Almond (53) in a recent one-center study. Acute rejection, cyclosporine dosage < 5mg/kg/day at one year and infection were the major risk factors found for the development of chronic rejection.

Busson [51] published a comparison of 9 studies on risk factors in kidney transplantation, HLA matching, sensitization and retransplantation, recipient age were found as risk factors in the majority of the studies. Major risk factors for rejection are a positive T cell crossmatch on the current serum and an ABO incompatibility without any preparation of the recipient. All others risk factors are relative. Shortage of organs brings us to take a few risks, it is not possible to have always a perfect match, no CMV infection and a recipient without HLA antibodies. Quality of care (monitoring) and immunosuppression have to overcome the effect of risk factors for rejection.

References :

1. Matas AJ, Gillingham KJ, Sutherland DER. Half-life and risk factors for kidney transplant outcome - importance of death with function. Transplantation 1993;55:757-761.

2. Concato J, Feinstein AR, Holford TR. The risk of determining risk with multivariable models. Ann Intern Med 1993;118:201-210.

3. Cecka JM, Terasaki PI. Matching kidneys for size in renal transplantation. Clin Transplantation 1990;4:82-86.

4. Pirsch JD, d'Alessandro AM, Sollinger HW et al. The effect of donor age, recipient age, and HLA match on immunologic graft survival in cadaver renal transplant recipients. Transplantation 1992;53:55-59.

5. De Jong MCJW, Hoitsma AJ, Koene RAP. Influence of donor age on graft rejection in paediatric kidney transplantation. Nephrol Dial Transplant 1990;5:308-309.

6. Cecka JM, Terasaki PI. The UNOS scientific renal transplant registry - 1991. In: Terasaki PI, Cecka JM, editors. Clinical Transplants 1991. Los Angeles: UCLA Tissue Typing Laboratory, 1992:1-11.

7. Creagh TA, McLean PA, Donovan MG, Walshe JJ, Murphy DM. Older donors and kidney transplantation. Transpl Int 1993;6:39-41.

8. Sesso R, Klag MJ, Ancao MS et al. Kidney transplantation from living unrelated donors. Ann Intern Med 1992;117:983-989.

9. Yuge J, Cecka JM. Sex and age effects in renal transplantation. In: Terasaki PI, Cecka JM, editors. Clinical Transplants 1991. Los Angeles: UCLA Tissue Typing Laboratory, 1992: 257-267.

10. Ettenger RB, Rosenthal JT, Marik J et al. Successful cadaveric renal transplantation in infants and young children. Transplant Proc 1989;21:1707-1708.

11. Howard RJ, Pfaff WW, Scornik JC, Salomon DR, Peterson JC, Brunson ME. Kidney transplantation in older patients. Clin Transplantation 1990;4:181-186.

12. Koyama H, Cecka JM. Race effects. In: Terasaki PI, Cecka JM, editors. Clinical Transplants 1991. Los Angeles: UCLA Tissue Typing Laboratory, 1992: 269-280.

13. Lim EC, Chia D, Terasaki P. Studies of sera from IgA nephropathy patients to explain high kidney graft survival. Hum Immunol 1991;32:81.

14. Lim EC, Terasaki PI. Outcome of renal transplantation in different primary diseases. In: Terasaki PI, Cecka JM, editors. Clinical Transplants 1991. Los Angeles: UCLA Tissue Typing Laboratory, 1992: 293-303.

15. Sanfilippo F, Vaughn WK, Spees EK. The association of pretransplant native nephrectomy with decreased renal allograft rejection. Transplantation 1984;37:256-260.

16. Hendriks G, Schreuder G, Claas F. HLA-DRw6 and renal allograft rejection. Br Med J 1983;286:85-87.

17. Soulillou JP, Bignon J. Poor kidney-graft survival in recipients with HLA-DRw6. N Engl J Med 1983;308:969-970.

18. Ahmed Z, Terasaki PI. Effect of transfusions. In: Terasaki PI, Cecka JM, editors. Clinical Transplants 1991. Los Angeles: UCLA Tissue Typing Laboratory, 1992: 305-312.

19. Opelz G. Disappearance of the transfusion effect in renal transplantation. In: Transplantation and clinical immunology, JL Touraine et all, editors, XXIV, Amsterdam, Excerpta Medica, 1992: 31-34.

20. Baatard R, Dantal J, Hourmant M et al. Effect of the number of pregraft blood transfusions in kidney graft recipients treated with bioreagents and cyclosporin A. Transplant Int 1991;4:235-238.

21. Lagaaij EL, Hennemann PH, Ruigrok M et al. Effect of one-HLA-DR-antigen-matched and completely HLA-DR-missatched blood transfusions on survival of heart and kidney allografts. N Engl J Med 1989;321:701-705.

22. Lagaaij EL, Persijn GG, Van Rood JJ, Claas FHJ. Blood transfusions: selection of HLA-DR matched blood donors. In: Transplantation and clinical immunology, JL Touraine et all, editors, XXIV, Amsterdam, Excerpta Medica, 1992: 9-15.

23. Pouteil-Noble C, Betuel H, Raffaele P, Robert F, Dubernard JM, Touraine JL. The value of platelet transfusions as preparation for kidney transplantation. Transplantation 1991;51:777-781.

24. Zhou YC, Cecka JM. Sensitization in renal transplantation. In: Terasaki PI, Cecka JM, editors. Clinical Transplants 1991. Los Angeles: UCLA Tissue Typing Laboratory, 1992: 313-323.

25. Stock P, Sutherland DER, Fryd DS et al. Detrimental effect of ABO-Compatible mismatching decreases 5-years actuarial graft survival after renal transplantation. Transplant Proc 1987;19:4522-4524.

26. Cicciarelli J, Cho Y. HLA matching: univariate and multivariate analyses of UNOS registry data. In: Terasaki PI, Cecka JM, editors. Clinical Transplants 1991. Los Angeles: UCLA Tissue Typing Laboratory, 1992: 325-333.

27. Vereerstraeten P, Andrien M, Dupont E, De Pauw L, Kinnaert P, Toussaint C. Individualization of high-and low-risk HLA-DR incompatibilities in renal transplantation. Clin Transplantation 1989;3:54-59.

28. Opelz G. Importance of HLA antigen splits for kidney transplant matching. Lancet 1988;2:61-64.

29. Opelz G, Mytilineos J, Scherer S et al. Survival of DNA HLA-DR typed and matched cadaver kidney transplants. Lancet 1991;338:461

30. Preuschof L, Lobo C, Offermann G. Role of cold ischemia time and vascular rejection in renal grafts from elderly donors. Transplant Proc 1991;23:1300-1301.

31. Birtch AG, McConnachie P, Lewis WI. Sensitization following donor-specific transfusions detected by Cr release assays - Cya modulation of early rejection effects. Transplant Proc 1987;XIX:805-807.

32. Takahashi H, Okazaki H, Taguma Y et al. Useful antiglobulin cross-match test for DST-sensitized patients. Transplant Proc 1987;19:794-799.

33. Kerman RH, Van Buren CT, Lewis RM et al. Improved graft survival for flow cytometry and antihuman globulin crossmatch-negative retransplant recipients. Transplantation 1990;49:52-56.

34. Karuppan SS, Lindholm A, Möller E. Fewer acute rejection episodes and improved outcome in kidney-transplanted patients with selection criteria based on crossmatching. Transplantation 1992;53:666-673.

35. Karuppan SS, Ohlman S, Möller E. The occurence of cytotoxic and non-complement-fixing antibodies in the crossmatch serum of patients with early acute rejection episodes. Transplantation 1992;54:839-844.

36. Ting A. Positive crossmatches-when is it to transplant? Transplant Int 1989;2:2-7.

37. Guerin C, Pomier G, Laverne S, Fleuru H, Le Petit JC, Berthoux F. Renal transplantation with a current T negative but historical T and/or B positive cross match. Nephrol Dial Transplant 1991;6:280-285.

38. Von Willebrand E, Pettersson E, Ahonen J, Häyry P. CMV infection, class II antigen expression, and human kidney allograft rejection. Transplantation 1986;42:364-367.

39. Fujinami RS, Nelson JA, Walker L, Oldstone MB. Sequence homology and immunologic cross reactivity of human cytomegalovirus with HLA-DR B chain : a means for graft rejection and immunosuppression. J Virol 1988;62:100.

40. Niaudet P, Raguin G, Lefevre JJ et al. Serological status of cytomegalovirus and outcome of renal transplantation. Kidney Int 1983;23:S50-S53.

41. Lewis RM, Johnson PC, Golden D, Van Buren ChT, Kerman RH, Kahan BD. The adverse impact of cytomegalovirus infection on clinical outcome in cyclosporine-prednisone treated renal allograft recipients. Transplantation 1988;45:353-359.

42. Dittmer R, Harfmann P, Busch R, Stenger KO, Bätge B, Arndt R. CMV infection and vascular rejection in renal transplant patients. Transplant Proc 1989;21:3600-3601.

43. Pouteil-Noble C, Ecochard R, Landrivon G et al. Cytomegalovirus infection - an etiological factor for rejection? Transplantation 1993;55:851-857.

44. Blancho G, Josien R, Douillard D, Bignon JD, Cesbron A, Soulillou JP. The influence of HLA A-B-DR matching on cytomegalovirus disease after renal transplantation. Evidence that HLA-DR7-matched recipients are more susceptible to cytomegalovirus disease. Transplantation 1992;54:871-874.

45. Kovaric J, Mayer G, Pohanka E et al. Adverse effect of low-dose prophylactic human recombinant leukocyte interferon-alpha treatment in renal transplant recipients. Transplantation 1988;45:402-405.

46. Gulanikar AC, MacDonald AS, Sungurtekin U, Belitsky P. The incidence and impact of early rejection episodes on graft outcome in recipients of first cadaver kidney transplants. Transplantation 1992;53:323-328.

47. Nicol D, MacDonald AS, Lawen J, Belitsky P. Early prediction of renal allograft loss beyond one year. Transpl Int 1993;6:153-157.

48. Norman DJ, Shield CF, Barry J et al. Early use of OKT3 monoclonal antibody in renal transplantation to prevent rejection. Am J Kidney Dis 1988;11:107-110.

49. Matas AJ, Tellis VA, Quinn TA, Glicklich D, Soberman R, Veith FJ. Individualization of immediate posttransplant immunosuppression. Transplantation 1988;45:406.409.

50. Hanas E, Tufveson G, Lindgren PG, Sjöberg O, Tötterman TH. Concentrations of cyclosporine-A and its metabolites in transplanted human kidney tissue during rejection and stable graft function. Clin transplantation 1991;5:107-111.

51. Busson M, Prevost P, Bignon JD et al. Multifactorial analysis of the outcome of 6430 cadaver kidney grafts. Transplant Int 1992;5:162-164.

52. Ogura K, Cecka JM. Center effects in renal transplantation. In: Terasaki PI, Cecka JM, editors. Clinical Transplants 1991. Los Angeles: UCLA Tissue Typing Laboratory, 1992: 245-256.

53. Almond PS, Matas A, Gillingham K et al. Risk factors for chronic rejection in renal allograft recipients. Transplantation 1993;55:752-757.

CHARACTERIZATON OF GRAFT INFILTRATING LYMPHOCYTES INVOLVED IN CARDIAC TRANSPLANT REJECTION

René J. Duquesnoy, Ricardo Moliterno, Melissa Chen-Woan, Christina Kaufman, Tony R. Zerbe and Adriana Zeevi, Division of Transplant Pathology, University of Pittsburgh Medical Center, Pittsburgh, PA 15261

INTRODUCTION

In vitro culturing of graft infiltrating lymphocytes has been useful in studying cell-mediated mechanisms of transplant immunity [1]. These cultures are generated in the presence of Interleukin-2 (IL-2) which induces proliferation of activated T lymphocytes expressing IL-2 receptors. In heart transplant patients, lymphocyte growth from endomyocardial biopsies correlates with the rejection grade assessed by histology [2]. During the first month after transplantation, about one-third of histologically negative biopsies show lymphocyte growth and this is associated with a higher incidence and earlier onset of a subsequent rejection episode [3,4]. During the first three months after transplantation, lymphocyte growth is also associated with a higher incidence of graft coronary disease [5]. These findings have led to the implementation of the biopsy growth

J. L. Touraine et al. (eds.), Rejection and Tolerance, 95–101.

Table 1

Lymphocyte Growth from Endomyocardial Biopsies For
Adult and Pediatric Heart Transplant Patients on
FK506 and CsA Immunosuppression

		Adult Patients		Pediatric Patients	
Histology	Drug	N	Frequency of growth	N	Frequency of growth
No rejection	CsA	350	41%	89	37%
No rejection	FK506	424	35%	60	18%
			$p<0.001$		$p<0.01$
Rejection	CsA	180	62%	76	65%
Rejection	FK506	132	51%	29	26%
			$p<0.02$		$p<0.001$

assay to supplement biopsy histology in the monitoring of heart transplant patients for rejection.

Donor-specific alloreactivity of biopsy grown lymphocytes has been determined in proliferation and cytotoxicity assays and increased alloreactivity has been observed during rejection [1]. These studies have also led to the concept of a sequential infiltration of class I followed by class II-specific lymphocytes through the vascular endothelium [6]. Our earlier observations have been reported in the proceedings of the 1990 CITIC meeting [7]. This summary describes our recent experience with the biopsy growth assay to monitor adult and pediatric patients on FK506 immunosuppression, the propagation of lymphocytes from arterial tissues of long-term heart transplant patients with graft coronary disease and the demonstration of heat-shock protein reactive lymphocytes in endomyocardial biopsies during rejection.

Biopsy growth monitoring of adult and pediatric heart transplant patients on FK506 immunosuppression.

FK506 is an efficient immunosuppressive drug which has particularly benefited liver and intestinal transplants. In heart transplant patients, FK506 based immunosuppression is associated with less histological rejection than Cyclosporine (CsA) based treatment. The overall frequency of histological rejection positive endomyocardial biopsies (EMB) was 26% (of 556 EMB) vs. 38% (of 541 EMB) in adult patients ($p<0.001$) and, 35% (of 89 EMB) vs. 47% (of 165 EMB) in pediatric patients ($p<0.05$). Biopsy growth from histologically positive and negative EMB was significantly less in the FK506 than the CsA groups (Table 1) [8]. The FK506 influence were especially apparent for the pediatric heart transplant patients. These findings are consistent with the clinical experience on the efficacy of FK506 in pediatric heart transplants.

Biopsy growth appears to correlate with plasma levels of FK506. A preliminary study on 10 patients has shown that FK506 levels were 1.06 ± 0.11 ng/ml when there was EMB growth and 2.06 ± 0.74 ng/ml when there was no growth ($p<0.01$) [8]. A similar experience has been described for liver transplant patients on FK506 [9]. These findings are consistent with the notion that monitoring FK506 levels is important for an effective immunosuppressive management of transplant patients.

Propagation of lymphocytes from arterial tissues and post-transplant obstructive vasculopathy. ·

Our initial findings that biopsy growth during the first three months after transplantation increases the risk of graft coronary disease suggested that cell-mediated immune mechanisms play a role in the pathogenesis of this obstructive vasculopathy presumably due to chronic rejection [5]. Recent studies on cultured arterial tissues from 23 allograft recipients (6 hearts, 6 livers and 11 kidneys) undergoing retransplantation have shown a correlation between lymphocyte growth and histologically diagnosed obstructive vasculopathy (100% {N=11} vs. 42% {N=12}, p<0.03) [10]. T cell phenotyping showed relatively high frequencies of CD4-CD8-, TCRγδ cells in lymphocyte cultures propagated from arterial tissues with vasculopathy. A functional characterization of such cells may lead to a better understanding of the cellular mechanisms of chronic rejection leading to graft coronary disease of heart transplant patients.

Presence of heat shock protein reactive T lymphocytes in cellular infiltrates of human cardiac allografts.

Recent reports have indicated that heat shock proteins (hsp) can be recognized by T cells during various immunologically mediated inflammatory processes including autoimmune disease. Also called stress proteins, hsp play an important role in maintaining cell integrity. They function as molecular chaperones by mediating assembly, folding and translocation of intracellular polypeptides and they are involved in protein degradation and interact with various receptors. Injurious stimuli to cells induce an increased production of hsp which could lead to their cell surface expression and subsequent recognition by the immune system. We have postulated that allograft infiltrating cells may recognize heat shock proteins, especially during rejection. This hypothesis was tested by incubating heart transplant biopsies with soluble Mycobacterium tuberculosis extracts (MTE), a source of hsp recognized by human T cells. Studies on 159 biopsies from 89 heart transplant patients have demonstrated that MTE can induce lymphocyte propagation from heart transplant biopsies. MTE-induced lymphocyte growth is associated with rejection (MTE alone: 56% vs. 29%; MTE+IL2: 88% vs. 37%). Two phenotype patterns seemed dominant for biopsy cells propagated with MTE. One consisted of a predominance of TCRαβCD4 cells and the other showed increased numbers of TCRγδ cells. Subsequent studies with recombinant hsp preparation has shown that hsp 65 and hsp 70 stimulate lymphocyte growth especially during rejection. Moreover, ongoing studies with a rat cardiac allograft model have indicated hsp reactive T cells during rejection. These findings provide first evidence for hsp reactive lymphocytes in cellular infiltrates during transplant rejection. We believe that the recruitment of hsp reactive T cells represents a second wave of graft infiltrating lymphocytes.

REFERENCES

1. Duquesnoy RJ, Trager JDK and Zeevi A. Propagation and characterization of lymphocytes from transplant biopsies. Critical Reviews in Immunology 1991;10:455-580.

2. Zeevi A, Fung J, Zerbe T, et al. Allospecificity of activated T cells grown from endomyocardial biopsies from heart transplant patients. Transplantation 1986;41:620, .

3.   Weber T, Kaufman C, Zeevi A, et al. Lymphocyte growth from cardiac allograft biopsy specimens with no or minimal cellular infiltrates: Association with subsequent rejection episode. J Heart Transplant 1989;8:233-40.

4.   Weber T, Zerbe T, Kaufman C, et al. Propagation of alloreactive lymphocytes from histologically negative endomyocardial biopsies from heart transplant patients: Association with subsequent histological evidence of rejection. Transplantation 1989;48:430-435.

5.   Kaufman C, Zeevi A, Kormos R, et al. Propagation of infiltrating lymphocytes and graft coronary disease in cardiac transplant recipients. Human Immunol 1990;28:228-36.

6.   Fung JJ, Zeevi A, Markus B, et al. Dynamics of allospecific T lymphocyte infiltration in vascularized human allografts. Immunological Research 1986;5:149.

7.   Duquesnoy RJ and Zeevi A: Clinical relevance of alloreactive T lymphocyte propagation from biopsies to allograft status. In: Transplantation and Clinical Immunology, Elsevier Science Publishers, pp. 3-11, 1991.

8.   Woan MC, Zerbe TR, Zeevi A, et al. Diminished lymphocyte growth from endomyocardial biopsies from cardiac transplant patients on FK506 immunosuppression. Transplantation Proc 1991;23:2941-42.

9.	Zeevi A, Eiras G, Kaufman C, et al. Correlation between bioassayed plasma levels of FK506 and lymphocyte growth from liver transplant biopsies with histological evidence of rejection. Transplant Proc 1991;23:1406-1408.

10.	Duquesnoy RJ, Kaufman CL, Zerbe TR, et al. Presence of CD4, CD8 double negative and TCRγδ positive T cells in lymphocyte cultures propagated from coronary arteries from heart transplant patients with graft coronary disease. J Heart & Lung Tx 1992;11:S83-86.

DISTINCT T CELLS MEDIATING ACUTE AND CHRONIC REJECTION

J. RICHARD BATCHELOR & M.Y. BRAUN

DEPARTMENT OF IMMUNOLOGY
ROYAL POSTGRADUATE MEDICAL SCHOOL
HAMMERSMITH HOSPITAL
DU CANE ROAD
LONDON W12 ONN

TEL: 081-74-3225

FAX: 081-740-3034

INTRODUCTION

The functions of T lymphocyte sub-populations in allograft rejection have been extensively studied in animal models of kidney transplantation, but in most instances, their roles have not been analysed in immunosuppressed animals. One of the interesting features of successful clinical renal transplants in immunosuppressed human patients is that rejection becomes less frequent and less acutely destructive with passage of time. Because of this, immunosuppression can be safely tapered to levels that still prevent rejection, but also avoid most, though not all, the toxic side effects of drug therapy. The explanation of this changing pattern of rejection remains unknown in cellular and molecular terms.

J. L. Touraine et al. (eds.), Rejection and Tolerance, 103–110.
© 1994 *Kluwer Academic Publishers.*

Over 10 years ago, Robert Lechler and I demonstrated in a rat renal allograft experimental system that if an MHC incompatible kidney was depleted of its indigenous population of passenger leucocytes, the immunogenicity of the incompatible graft was strikingly reduced [1]. In brief, the experimental model was to transplant an $(AS \times AUG)F_1$ kidney into an AS strain recipient, protect the graft from rejection by a regimen of immunological enhancement or a 10 day course of cyclosporin A, and leave the graft in place for 1-3 months. After this time, when the original passenger leucocytes present in the graft had been replaced by AS strain cells, the kidney was then retransplanted into another, non-immunosuppressed AS recipient. In this donor/recipient combination, the retransplanted graft is accepted indefinitely without undergoing clinical rejection [2,3].

However in other donor/recipient combinations, eg. AUG kidney into an AS, the retransplanted graft may suffer rejection, but in an attenuated form [4].

To account for this variation, we put forward the hypothesis that there are two pathways by which T cells can be sensitised to MHC incompatible tissues. The first or direct pathway involves a direct activation of the recipient's CD4+ T cells by the allogeneic dendritic cells within the graft. The second, or indirect pathway is identical to that followed by non-viable, "nominal" antigens ie. macromolecules are internalised by the recipient's antigen presenting cells, processed into peptides, bound by the recipient's MHC class II molecules, and presented at the cell surface of the presenting cell as a self-MHC restricted allogeneic peptide.

The hypothesis predicted some clear differences between the two pathways. Firstly, it seems highly probable that the direct pathway T cells dominate primary allograft rejection taking place in previously un-sensitised recipients. The reason for this is the very high frequency of cells able to respond by this pathway. It is known that in the MLC, the in vitro equivalent of the recognition stage of the allograft response, up to 10% of lymphocytes in the responder population are activated. Furthermore, if the sensitising population is depleted of allogeneic dendritic cells, the responding cells fail to incorporate labelled thymidine [5,6] suggesting that all the responding cells of the MLC are triggered by the direct pathway, which is not self-MHC restricted.

The indirect pathway contrasts with the direct in that in non-sensitised hosts, the frequencies of precursors responding to self-MHC bound peptides derived from nominal antigens is at least 2 or 3 log orders lower. Thus it is not to be expected that T cells sensitised by this pathway would play a large role in primary graft rejection. However, once T cell clones of the indirect pathway have been expanded after sensitisation, there is no reason why they should not be important effector cells. They are of course subject to immune response gene effects, and this may be one reason for the variation seen in different donor/recipient combinations. The other important distinction between the two pathways is that the T cells have quite different specificity.

When the above hypothesis was suggested, no clear examples of self-MHC restricted T cells specific for peptides derived from allogeneic MHC molecules were known. There are now numerous examples of them in mouse, rat, and human systems [7-9]. Their role in allograft rejection still remains to be fully defined.

In this paper, I will summarise recent studies on the functions of T cells sensitised by the direct pathway [10,11]

An AS (RT1^l) anti AUG (RT1^c) T cell line was raised in vitro. Its properties conformed to those of direct pathway T cells. It was specific for AUG class II MHC, was not self MHC restricted, gave minimal proliferative responses to third party stimulators, and was composed predominantly of CD4+ T cells. A T cell clone, L12.4, was derived from the line by limiting dilution, and was also shown to have the above properties. The T cell line showed a very weak cytolytic activity against ^{51}Cr labelled AUG T blasts, but L12.4 was non-cytotoxic. Both the T cell line and L12.4 secreted IL-2 in response to stimulation with AUG strain cells.

The effector function of these cells in kidney allograft rejection was then examined, using as target grafts kidneys harvested from normal AUG rats, and AUG kidneys that had been "parked" for >50 days in AS recipients, thus depleting them of AUG strain passenger cells. All recipients were male AS rats that had been irradiated (5Gy) one day before transplantation. At completion of the transplant, the rats were injected intravenously with T cells of the AS anti-AUG line, L12.4, T cells harvested from normal AS rats, or no cells.

The results were as follows. The irradiated AS recipients not given any T cells accepted kidneys from normal AUG donors for more than 50 days. There was a weak early rejection in 5 of 8 recipients but this resolved. Only 1 of the 8 rats developed chronic rejection, and died on day 42. The rats that were transplanted with kidneys from normal AUG donors, and which received 55-83 million normal AS T cells suffered acute rejection in 3 of 5 animals, but there were 2 animals that survived with normal blood ureas for the duration of the experiment (50 days). The group of rats transplanted with normal AUG kidneys and given 10 million of the AS anti AUG T cell line, or the same number of L12.4 cells rejected all the kidneys acutely. Subsequently, a dose response study has shown that even 1 million of the AS anti AUG T cell is sufficient to cause acute graft rejection of normal AUG kidneys.

In contrast to the above results, we found that AUG kidneys depleted of passenger leucocytes were not rejected even if as many as 10 million cells of the AS anti AUG T cell line or a similar number of L12.4 cells were given.

We interpret these results as showing that T cell sensitised by the direct pathway are potent initiators of acute allograft rejection, provided that the target kidneys still contain passenger dendritic cells of donor genotype. Once these have been replaced by recipient-derived cells, T cells of the direct pathway are no longer capable of causing graft rejection. The further implication arising from these experiments is that in those combinations in which rejection of passenger cell depleted kidneys does occur, the late and attenuated form of rejection is mediated by another population of T cells. We have speculated that this second population of T cells may be those sensitised by the indirect pathway.

Returning to the fate of T cells sensitised by the direct pathway, one possible interpretation of our results might be that the target kidney allograft did not express AUG MHC class II molecules, ie. the ligand of the T cell line and L12.4 Immunohistological studies demonstrated the expression of AUG class II, mainly on tubular epithelial cells. If these tubular cells were grown in vitro, in the presence of supernatants harvested from cultures of the AS anti AUG T cell line, abundant expression of AUG class II was demonstrated by cell fluorimetry.

The next question asked was whether class II expressing AUG tubular epithelial cells stimulated a proliferative response by the AS anti AUG T cell line, or L12.4. Interestingly, no proliferation occured, and further investigation showed that these T cells, if co-cultured with AUG renal tubular cells overnight, and then stimulated with AUG antigen presenting cells, failed to undergo a proliferative response. Specificity controls of the same T cells co-cultured overnight with AS strain renal tubular cells and then stimulated with AUG antigen presenting cells, proliferated normall. We therefore conclude that the direct pathway sensitised T cells have been induced to enter an anergic state by the AUG tubular epithelial cells.

In conclusion, the sum of this evidence suggests that T cells sensitised by the direct pathway are the dominant effectors in acute kidney allograft rejection in previously non-sensitised recipients. When the indigenous passenger leucocytes of the graft are replaced by recipient derived cells, the T cells of the direct pathway interact with class II molecules expressed on tubular epithelial cells, and perhaps other cell types, which induce anergy.

ACKNOWLEDGEMENTS

I am grateful to the MRC of the UK for financial support for the work described.

REFERENCES

1. Lechler RI, Batchelor JR. Restoration of immunogenicity to passenger cell-depleted kidney allografts by the addtion of donor strain dendritic cells. J Exp Med 1982; 155:31-37.

2. Batchelor JR, Welsh KI, Maynard A, Burgos H. Failure of long surviving, passively enhanced kidney allografts to provoke T-dependent alloimmunity. I. Retransplantation of (ASxAUG)F1 kidneys into secondary AS recipients. J Exp Med 1979; 150: 455-464.

3. Chui Y-L, Batchelor JR. Mechanisms underlying continued survival of rat kidney allografts after s short period of chemical immunosuppression. Transplantation 1985; 40: 150-153.

4. Lechler RI, Batchelor JR. Immunogenicity of retransplanted rat kidney allografts: effect of inducing chimerism in the first recipient and quantitative studies on immunosuppression on the second recipient. J Exp Med 1982; 156: 1835-1839.

5. Mason DW, Pugh CW, Webb M. The rat mixed lymphocyte reaction. Immunology 1981; 44: 75-79.

6. Steinman RM, Cohn ZA. Identification of a novel cell type in peripheral lymphoid organs of mice. J Exp Med 1974; 139: 380-384.

7. Song ES, Linsk R, Olson CA, McMillan M, Goodenow RS.
    Allospecific cytotoxic T lymphocytes recognize an H-2 peptide
    in the context of a murine major histocompatibility complex
    class I molecule. Proc Natl Acad Sci USA 1988; 85: 1927-1931.

8. Fangmann J, Dalchau R, Fabre JW. Allorecognition of isolated,
    denatured chains of class I and class II major histocompatibility
    complex molecules. Eur J Immunol 1992; 22: 669-677.

9. Chen BP, Madrigal A, Parham P. Cytotoxic T cell recognition of an
    endogenous class I HLA peptide presented by a class II HLA
    molecule. J Exp Med 1990; 172: 779-788.

10. Braun MY, McCormack A, Webb G, Batchelor JR. Mediation of acute
    but not chronic rejection of MHC-incompatible rat kidney grafts by
    alloreactive CD4 T cells activated by the direct pathway of
    sensitisation. Transplantation 1993; 55: 177-182.

11. Braun MY, McCormack A, Webb G, Batchelor JR. Evidence for clonal
    anergy as a mechanism responsible for the maintenance of
    transplantation tolerance. Eur J Immunol 1993 (In press).

ROLE OF ANTI-HLA IMMUNE RESPONSES IN ORGAN TRANSPLANT REJECTION

Zhuoru Liu, Elaine Reed, Paul Harris and Nicole Suciu-Foca

College of Physicians and Surgeons of Columbia University

Department of Pathology

630 West 168th Street

New York, New York 10032

Telephone: 212-305-6941

Fax: 212-305-3429

Introduction

The immune response to alloantigens can be either cell-mediated or humoral. Both types of immune reactions contribute to organ allograft rejection. T cell responses to alloantigens are vigorous with as many as 2 percent of host's T cells reacting against a single allogeneic MHC molecule.

An important question in transplantation is the molecular structure of the determinants on allogeneic MHC molecules which elicit T cell activation. Foreign MHC molecules differ from self molecules by polymorphisms in amino acid sequence at the top, sides and floor of the peptide binding groove. Evidence has been accumulated that one population of host T cells recognizes the peptide bound into the groove of the allogeneic MHC molecule, while another population recognizes peptides derived from the processing and presentation of the allogeneic MHC molecule by host APCs. These two distinct populations are the mediators of direct and indirect allorecognition, respectively. The direct recognition pathway is the primary mechanism accounting for acute rejection, while the indirect recognition pathway is

111

J. L. Touraine et al. (eds.), Rejection and Tolerance, 111–124.
© 1994 Kluwer Academic Publishers.

responsible for the development of humoral immunity to HLA and chronic rejection [1-5]. In the following we will discuss the molecular basis of allogeneic recognition, the cellular and humoral basis of rejection and anti-idiotypic mechanisms contributing to the down-regulation of the immune response.

Cellular Basis of Allogeneic Recognition.

A.   The Direct Recognition Pathway. Acute rejection episodes are mainly attributable to the recognition of donor HLA antigens by CD4 and CD8 cells which acquire effector function, killing allogeneic target cells from the transplanted tissue. This in vivo reaction is mirrored in vitro by the mixed lymphocyte culture reaction. MLC reaction (MLR) occurs only when the responding and the stimulating cells differ by MHC-class II antigens, activating the proliferation of CD4 cells.   During MLR, cytolytic T lymphocytes, which lyse target cells, are generated. These cells carry the CD8 phenotype and will kill target cells only if they differ from the responder by an MHC-class I antigens. The response is specific in that killing of third party cells occurs only if these targets share a class I MHC allele with the original stimulator. Transfectants expressing the respective antigen can be efficiently killed and antibodies against the target antigen can block the CML response.

MLC-reactivity, however, does not require processing of the allogeneic target by host APCs. Purified T cells of responder origin are stimulated by donor B cells, monocytes or dendritic cells. In fact, what the responding T cells recognize is an endogenous or exogenous peptide presented by donor MHC molecules. There is a wide array of evidence supporting this view, yet we will document it with data from our own laboratory, showing that: 1) alloreactive T cell clones discriminate between MHC antigens which differ by residues situated in the floor of the peptide-binding groove and 2) alloreactive TCC show species and cell-type specificity. The first conclusion emerges from experiments in which we stimulated T cells from a responder carrying the DRβ1*0407 allele with PBMCs from his HLA-half identical sibling who differed by a haplotype carrying the DRβ1*0406 allele. These two variants of DR4 differ by one amino acid at position 37 (which is at the bottom of the antigen binding groove) and 86 (which is on the side of the groove).

Some of the resulting TCCs were stimulated by PBMCs carrying the DRβ1*0406 allele but not by other variants of DR4. However, from the pattern of reaction seen with other TCCs we can infer that at least 3 distinct peptide/MHC complexes were recognized. Thus, TCC 10.4 reacted exclusively to the peptide bound to DRβ1*0406. TCC 20.1 also recognized a peptide bound to DRβ1*0406; however, this peptide/MHC complex is different from that recognized by TCC 10.4, resembling the complex presented by the DRβ1*0402 and 0405 molecule which also stimulate TCC 20.1. TCC 20.3 recognizes yet a different complex presented only by DRβ1*0406 and 0405. Mouse L cells transfected with the DRβ1*0406 gene did not elicit stimulation of any of the TCCs indicating that their response was directed against a species specific peptide, produced by human, but not by mouse cells (Table 1).

There was cross-stimulation of one clone (TCC 20.3) by DR9 homozygous cells. Because of the wide amino-acid differences between DR9 and DR4 alleles, this response is best explained by molecular mimicry between the DR9+ peptide complex and the DR4+ peptide complex. These data, therefore, indicate that direct recognition is triggered by complexes formed by allogeneic MHC molecules with peptides bound to the groove. These complexes are stimulatory because of molecular mimicry.

B.   The Indirect Recognition Pathway. In this pathway, T cells recognize graft MHC alloantigens that have been processed and presented by host APCs [1-5]. Indirect recognition is restricted by the host MHC class II molecule, which has bound a peptide derived from the processing of an allogeneic MHC molecule and, therefore, corresponds to the classical pathway of conventional antigen recognition by CD4 T

TABLE 1 PATTERNS OF ALLOREACTIVITY EXHIBITED BY TCCs FROM A DRβ1*0407 RESPONDER PRIMED TO A DRβ1*0406 STIMULATOR

STIMULATOR'S DRβ1*	TCC 10.4	TCC 20.1	TCC 20.3
401	-	-	-
402	-	++++	-
403	-	-	-
404	-	-	-
405	-	++++	++++
406	++++	++++	++++
407	-	-	-
408	-	-	-
101, 301	-	-	-
1501, 301	-	-	-
1101, 701	-	-	-
801	-	-	-
901	-	-	++++
1301,1401	-	-	-
L Cell 406 Transfectant	-	-	-

cells. The involvement of alloantigen-specific CD4 T helper cells, as mediators of alloantibody generation, suggests that the indirect pathway plays an essential role in chronic rejection, e.g. in the steady, but continuous attrition (2-5%/year) of organ allografts late after transplantation [1-7].

The indirect recognition pathway can be demonstrated experimentally by immunizing T cells with synthetic peptides corresponding to hypervariable regions of an allogeneic MHC molecule, for example DR [1,2]. T cells recognizing a synthetic peptide corresponding to the dominant epitope of the allogeneic MHC molecule will be restimulated by allogeneic cells expressing the respective antigen [1]. Stimulation requires, however, the presence in the culture of responder's APCs since the allopeptide has to be processed and presented by a host MCH class II molecule, for recognition to occur [1-5]. Alternatively, stimulation can be induced by allogeneic cells expressing both the host restriction element and the allogeneic MHC molecule from which the peptide derived [1[. Table 2 summarizes results of previous studies from our laboratory, documenting these conclusions [1,4,5]. The fact that recognition of an (DR1) allopeptide is MHC-class II restricted and requires processing was documented in experiments in which we showed that: 1) TCC recognized the peptide only when presented by syngeneic APCs or by APCs sharing with the responder an HLA-DR (DR11) allele; 2) the response was inhibited by mAb specific for HLA-DR and for CD4, and 3) glutaraldehyde fixation of APCs prevented peptide processing and presentation [1-5]. Taken together these data indicate that allogeneic MHC molecules, which are processed by host APC, trigger T cell alloreactivity.

Contribution of Direct and Indirect Recognition Pathways to T Cells Alloreactivity.
Since both the direct and indirect pathway are involved in allorecognition the relative contribution of each pathway to alloreactivity requires an analysis of the size of the corresponding populations of T cells engaged in an MLC response.

To address this question we stimulated in MLC T cells from an HLA-DR11/DR12 responder with cells carrying the DR1 antigen. After priming, T cells were challenged in an LDA test with six partially overlapping synthetic peptides derived from the sequence of the DRβ1*0101 molecule (residues 1-20, 11-30, 21-42, 31-50, 43-62, 51-70 and 66-90) and with cells carrying the DR1 or the DQ 1 antigen. The frequency of

T cells responding to the DR1 molecule, as expressed on allogeneic DR1 positive cells and on L-cell transfectants, was 1/328 and 1/361 respectively. The frequency of DQ1-reactive T cells was 1/1,529. Of the six synthetic peptides, only one, which corresponds to residue 21-42 was stimulatory, hence, representing the dominant DR1 epitope which T cells recognize. The frequency of peptide-reactive T cells was 1:43,992 [5]. These data, therefore, demonstrate that cells engaged in indirect recognition of peptides derived from the processing of the DR1 molecule are 100 times less frequent that cells engaged in the direct recognition pathway. The response to the peptide occurred only in the presence of responder APCs or of APCs sharing with the responder the DR12 antigen. These results demonstrate formally that allopeptides derived from the processing and presentation of donor MHC molecules by host-derived APC trigger alloreactivity.

Biassed Usage of TCR Vβ genes in Indirect Allorecognition. Because indirect allorecognition involves a self-MHC-class II-restricted response against the dominant epitope of a given allogeneic MHC molecule, the TCR usage in this response may be biased by its MHC restrictive element. To explore this hypothesis we immunized in vitro T cells from three unrelated individuals, sharing the DRβ1*1101 allele, with peptide 21-42 which comprises the dominant epitope of the DR1 molecule. In all three responders reactivity to peptide 21-42 was restricted by the DR11 molecule. The resulting T cell lines (TCL) showed a limited usage of Vβ genes. All the TCLs shared the expression of Vβ13.2 [4]. Since indirect recognition of allopeptide may play an important role in antibody-mediated allograft rejection, knowledge of the TCR-repertoire involved in the response to a given alloepitope may permit the development of strategies aimed at the specific ablation of T helper cells.

TCR-Usage in Lymphocytic Infiltrates of the Graft. In an effort to establish whether the repertoire of alloreactive cells infiltrating the graft or circulating in the blood differs, we monitored 15 cardiac allograft recipients over 1-6 months following transplantation, as follows. Peripheral blood lymphocytes were obtained at the time of biopsy, e.g. weekly over the first 2 months and monthly thereafter. PBMCs were primed in 7-day MLC with irradiated stimulating cells (splenocytes) from the donor and expanded for an additional week in medium supplemented with rIL2. After 2 weeks, when no donor cells were left in the cultures, primed recipient T cells were subjected to quantitative PCR-analysis of TCR-Vβ gene usage, as described [1,3-5]. Heart biopsies obtained concomitant with the peripheral blood were placed in cultures in complete tissue culture medium with rIL2. Lymphocyte growth was scored at 24 and 48 hours. After 48 hours, cultures were split: one part was used for quantitative PCR of TCR-Vβ gene expression and another was expanded further for functional testings.

Comparison of TCR expression in PBMC and in cells infiltrating the graft showed that the latter comprised only a fraction of the families found in the peripheral circulation. As illustrated in Table 3 the size of TCR families expanding in the graft (as expressed by percent of total cpm), was equal or greater than that encountered when recipient PBMC were primed to the donor in MLC. Testing of biopsy culture for anti-donor reactivity showed that T cells infiltrating the graft proliferated in response to donor stimulating cells. This oligoclonal T cell proliferation was characteristic of grade 1-3 rejection.

In some secondary rejection episodes we found that the TCR prevailing during the primary rejection, such as Vβ6, Vβ7 and Vβ 13.2 had expanded again (Table 3). This may indicate that the rejection was second-set in nature, e.g. that it represented a memory response directed against a previously recognized epitope. Supporting this view were pathology data, indicating that the secondary rejection was more severe, accompanied by vasculitis and by Ig, complement and fibrin deposition on the walls of the vessels. In most of these cases, anti-donor HLA antibodies were also found in patient's serum, depleted of soluble HLA antigens. The recurrence of the same TCR in a biopsy is, therefore, indicative of a more violent form of rejection.

TABLE 2   REACTIVITY (cpm 10^3) OF ALLOPEPTIDE SPECIFIC TCCs FROM A DR 11,12 RESPONDER TO DR1 PEPTIDE 21-42 AND TO ALLOGENEIC CELLS

	DR1 Peptide Yes No	DR11, 12 Not fixed	DR11, 12 Fixed	DR11,16	DR12, 8	DR1	DR1, 11
		DR Phenotype of PBMCs added to cultures					
TCC	+	53	1	49	0.1	0.1	38
	-	0.1		0.1	0.1	0.1	9
TCC+ syngeneic APC	-	0.6		0.3	0.1	29	35
TCC + Syngeneic APC + Anti-DR MAb	+	0.6		0.5	0.1	0.1	0.1

TABLE 3 TCR DISTRIBUTION IN THE PERIPHERY AND IN THE GRAFT (%)

TCR	No Rejection (Day 87)			Rejection (day 138)			Anti-donor MLC on Day
	Biopsy	Periphery	Ratio	Biopsy	Periphery	Ratio	61, 68, 87, 138
Vβ1	9	13	0.69	11	17	0.64	3,14,11,15
Vβ2	3	15	0.2	20	16	1.25	3,4,3,8
Vβ3	5	11	0.45	0	19	0	2,10,6,6
Vβ4	0	3	0	0	1	0	0,1,1,1
Vβ5.1	0	2	0	0	1	0	2,2,1,1
Vβ5.2	0	0	0	6	1	6	9,6,4,9
Vβ6	24	9	2.66	34	12	2.83	21,18,24,34
Vβ7	35	9	3.88	19	10	1.9	10,7,9,8
Vβ8	0	3	0	0	3	0	4,5,3,2
Vβ9	0	1	0	0	0	0	1,0,0,0
Vβ10	0	0	0	0	0	0	0,0,0,0
Vβ11	0	1	0	0	0	0	2,3,1,1
Vβ12	8	1	8	0	0	0	0,1,2,1
Vβ13	2	3	0.66	0	1	0	2,6,4,3
Vβ13.2	8	6	1.3	11	6	1.83	3,3,2,1
Vβ14	0	1	0	0	1	0	3,3,2,1
Vβ15	2	2	1	0	3	0	17,5,7,10
Vβ16	0	0	0	0	1	0	1,1,1,1
Vβ17	0	0	0	0	0	0	2,2,0,1
Vβ18	0	0	0	0	0	0	2,2,1,1
Vβ19	2	12	0.16	0	3	0	2,1,3,2
Vβ20	3	5	0.6	0	3	0	19,1,3,3

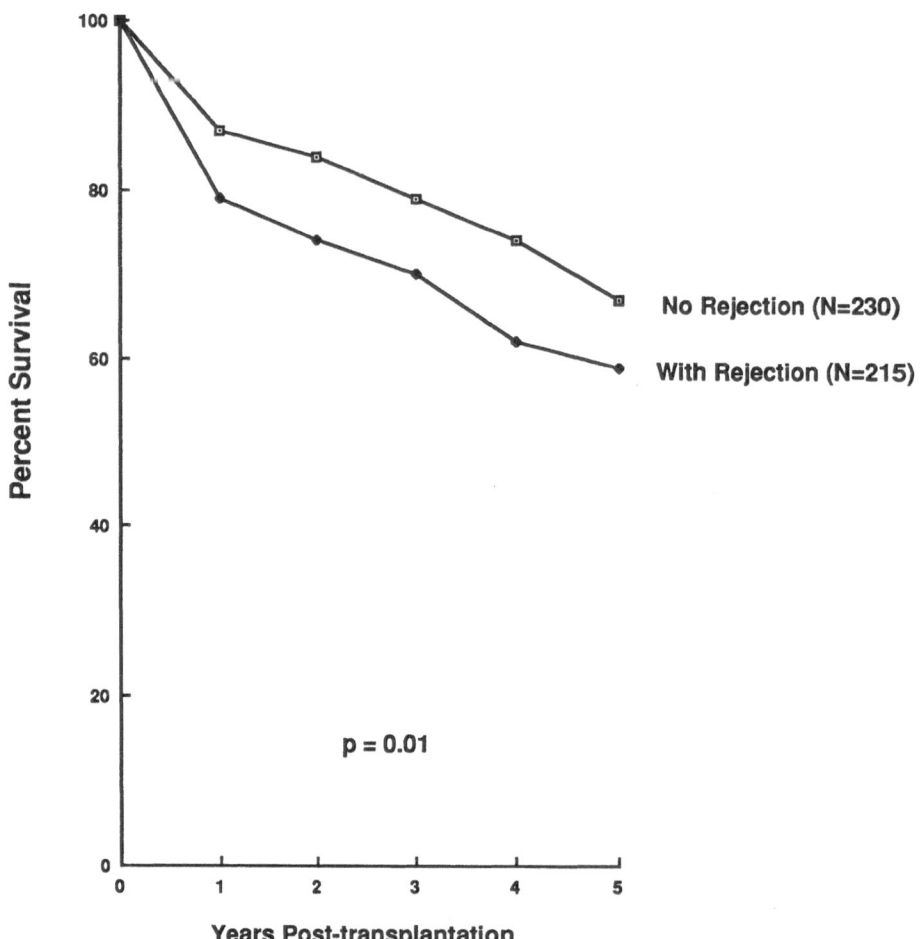

**Fig. 1   Actuarial Survival of Heart Allografts in Recipients
With and Without Acute Rejection Episodes
During the First 30 Weeks Post-transplantation**

Fig. 2   Actuarial Survival of Heart Allografts in Recipients with and without Presensitization

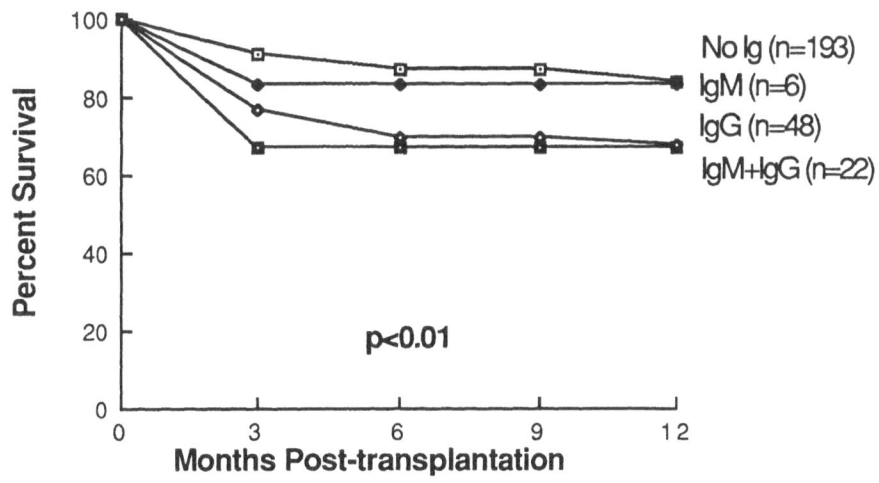

Table 4   Association Between Early (<3 Months) Acute Rejection and Anti-HLA Antibodies

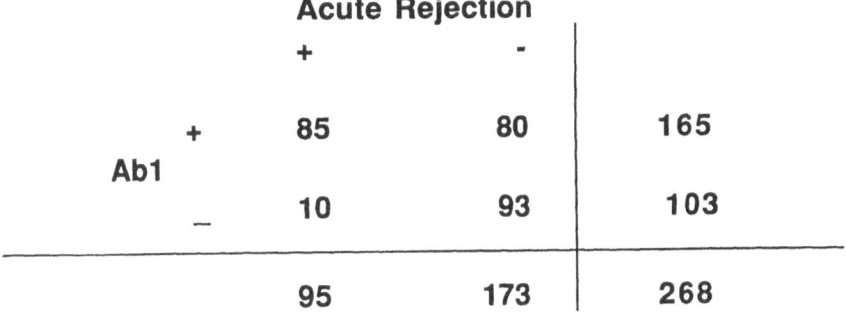

		Acute Rejection		
		+	-	
Ab1	+	85	80	165
	−	10	93	103
		95	173	268

p<0.0001

In other sequential biopsies there was no preferential expansion of a particular TCR, seemingly indicating that the antigenic focus of T cell reactivity has changed over time.

Clonal expansion, as measured by quantitative PCR of TCR Vβ genes, was also mirrored in a rise in the titer of anti-TCR antibodies. We quantitated anti-TCR antibodies by ELISA using as antigen synthetic peptides derived from the CDR2 region of Vβ8 and Vβ2 (Marchalonis et al, in preparation). In most instances, the titer of the antibodies increased in the proximity of rejection, suggesting that the TCR per se may represent the target of network regulation.

Relationship Between Acute and Chronic Rejection. Chronic rejection may represent the end-result of multiple rejection episodes and/or it may constitute a distinct pathologic entity. To determine the impact of acute rejection on long-term outcome we calculated the actuarial heart allograft survival at five years in patients with or without an acute rejection episode during the first year. Survival was significantly lower ($p < 0.01$) in patients who had at least one rejection during the first year post-transplantation (Fig. 1).

Next, we explored the relationship between the occurence of a rejection episode and the development of circulating anti-HLA antibodies following transplantation. There was a positive association between anti-HLA antibodies and acute rejection, indicating that these two events are inter-related (Table 4). The actuarial heart allograft survival of patients developing anti-HLA antibodies of IgG class was significantly lower than that observed in patients without antibodies or with antibodies of IgM class (Fig. 2).

T helper cells mediating the differentiation and affinity maturation of anti-HLA Ig, therefore, contribute to antibody-mediated humoral rejection.

There was heterogeneity, however, within the antibody producing group, in that some patients tolerated the graft for 5 years or more in spite of having shown anti-HLA antibodies. It is possible that such patients develop, anti-anti-HLA or anti-idiotypic antibodies. To explore this possibility we tested Ab1 negative sera from anti-HLA antibody producers, for Ab2 activity. In both cardiac and renal transplantation we found that the development of Ab2 correlates with better survival rates at 5 years [6,7,8].

Summary and Conclusions

Allograft rejection is a complex phenomenon in which both the cellular and the humoral arm of the immune response are involved. Our studies indicate that the earliest event occuring following transplantation resides in T cell recognition of allogeneic molecules via the direct pathway. This event is due primarily to molecular mimicry between complexes of self MHC plus peptide to which the host's immune response has been previously exposed and allogeneic MHC molecule(s). Direct recognition eventually results in acute rejection episodes, damaging the graft. During acute rejection there is a relatively oligoclonal proliferation of T cells which may be positively or negatively regulated by anti-TCR antibodies.

HLA antigens shed from the injured cells during acute rejection are processed and presented by host APCs to syngeneic T cells. Such T cells participate in the self-MHC-restricted pathway of indirect recognition which generates the help required for DTH and antibody-mediated rejection

Anti-HLA antibodies accompany severe (probably "memory"-type) acute rejection episodes and are likely to be the primary mediators of chronic rejection. We believe that suppression of anti-HLA antibodies by anti-idiotypic antibodies to HLA is an important feed-back mechanism which ultimately determines the long-term outcome of organ allografts.

Acknowledgements

This work was supported in part by the American Cancer Society Grant # IM-694 and the National Institutes of Health Grant RO1-A125210-06.

References

1. Liu Z, Braunstein N, Suciu-Foca N. T cell recognition of allo-peptides in context of syngeneic MHC. J Immunol 148: 35-40, 1992.

2. Harris P, Liu Z, Suciu-Foca N. MHC class II binding of peptides derived from HL DR1. J Immunology 148:2169-2174, 1992.

3. Liu Z, Sun YK, Xi YP, Harris P, Suciu-Foca N. T Cell Recognition of self-human histocompatibility leucocyte antigens (HLA) -DR peptides in context of syngeneic HLA-DR molecules. J Exp Med 175: 1663-1668, 1992.

4. Liu Z, Sun YK, Xi YP, et al. Limited usage of TCR Vβ genes by allopeptide spec T cells. J Immunol 150:3180-3186, 1993.

5. Liu Z, Sun YK, Xi YP, et al. Contribution of direct and indirect recognition pathw₂ T cell alloreactivity. In press, J Exp Med 1993

6. Suciu-Foca N, Reed E, D'Agati VD, et al. Soluble HLA-antigens, anti-HLA antibodies and anti-Idiotypic antibodies in the circulation of renal transplant recipien Transplantation 51:593-601, 1991.

7. Suciu-Foca N, Reed E, Marboe C, et al. Role of anti-HLA antibodies in heart transplantation. Transplantation 51: 716-724, 1991.

8. Reed E, Ho E, Cohen DJ, et al. Anti-idiotypic antibodies specific for HLA in heart and kidney allograft recipients. In press, J Immunol Res 1993.

TOLEROGENICITY OF THYMIC EPITHELIAL CELLS: STUDIES WITH ALLOGENEIC AND XENOGENEIC CHIMERAS

Jonathan Sprent, Hiroshi Kosaka*, and Charles D. Surh

Department of Immunology, IMM4A
The Scripps Research Institute
10666 North Torrey Pines Road
La Jolla, California 92037

*Present address:
Hiroshi Kosaka, M.D., Ph.D.
Tsukuba Life Science Center
3-1-1 Koyadai, Tsukuba
Ibaraki 305, JAPAN

INTRODUCTION

Self tolerance is under the strict control of T lymphocytes and is imposed during early T cell differentiation in the thymus [1-5]. Which particular cell types in the thymus induce self tolerance (negative selection) is controversial [5,6]. The prevailing view is that tolerance induction is largely a reflection of T cells encountering the contingent of bone-marrow-derived cells in the medulla [7-9]. These cells, especially dendritic cells [9], have a proven role in tolerance induction and are strategically positioned at the cortico-medullary junction. The role of thymic epithelial cells (TEC) in tolerance induction is less clear. In this paper we review our recent studies on the tolerogenicity of TEC in bone marrow (BM) and fetal liver (FL) chimeras. For allogeneic (mouse → mouse) chimeras, we present evidence that TEC are strongly tolerogenic for some T cells but only weakly tolerogenic for others. For

125

J. L. Touraine et al. (eds.), Rejection and Tolerance, 125–140.

xenogeneic (rat → mouse) chimeras, by contrast, TEC are almost nontolerogenic.

TEC and split tolerance.

Early studies on the effects of depleting BM-derived cells from fetal thymuses with deoxyguanosine (dguo) led to the conclusion that TEC are essentially nontolerogenic [7,8]. In particular, it was reported that T cells differentiating in allogeneic dguo-treated thymuses display no detectable tolerance in terms of CD8$^+$ cytotoxic T lymphocyte precursors (CTLp) [7]. This applied to responses measured in vitro. Under in vivo conditions, however, several investigators have found that intrathymic contact with MHC alloantigens expressed selectively on TEC, especially medullary TEC, is sufficient to induce quite strong tolerance in terms of skin graft rejection [10-12]. At the level of CD4$^+$ cells, tolerance is also apparent in vitro in mixed lymphocyte cultures [13]. Collectively, these data indicate that the tolerogenicity of TEC depends critically upon the assay used for measuring tolerance. To seek further information on this issue we have studied tolerance induction in bone marrow chimeras (BMC).

Tolerogenicity of TEC in bone marrow chimeras.

The rationale for studying tolerance in BMC is that pretreatment of the host mice with irradiation, especially supralethal irradiation, destroys virtually all host BM-derived cells. This means that, after BM reconstitution, the chimeras show complete repopulation with donor-derived cells. The donor stem cells repopulating the host thymus thus encounter host MHC antigens displayed selectively on TEC (and other non BM-derived cells). To ensure complete removal of host BM-derived cells, we prepare parent → F$_1$ BMC with two rounds of irradiation and (T-depleted) BM reconstitution, using a total dose of 2300 cGy [14-18]; anti-T cell antibodies are injected initially to remove residual radioresistant T cells. Within 1-2 months these chimeras show complete reconstitution with donor-derived cells; host BM-derived cells are undetectable throughout the body, including the thymus [14]. Host MHC expression is restricted to non BM-derived cells and is conspicuous on TEC, especially medullary TEC [18]. In extrathymic tissues, MHC expression is limited to low-level staining of various stromal cells (with the exception of follicular dendritic cells which show quite strong staining) [15,16].

Since host MHC expression in BMC is evident in both the intrathymic and extrathymic environments, studying tolerance imposed in the thymus necessitates examining thymocytes rather than peripheral T cells. We have concentrated on examining tolerance at the level of CD8$^+$ T cells [17]. To prepare mature "single-positive" (SP) CD4$^-$8$^+$ cells from thymus, we use a combination of antibody plus C treatment followed by positive panning. This treatment yields a pure population of mature (HSA$^-$) CD8$^+$ SP thymocytes. The results of comparing the function of SP CD8$^+$ cells prepared from the thymus of parent → F$_1$ BMC vs. normal parental strain mice can be summarized as follows (Table 1) [17].

In the case of primary mixed lymphocyte reactions (MLR) in vitro, CD8$^+$ SP thymocytes from the chimeras respond quite well to third-party spleen antigen-presenting cells (APC) but show almost complete unresponsiveness to host-type APC. By this parameter, the chimera CD8$^+$ cells show near-complete tolerance to host class I antigens. Different results apply when lymphokines are added to the cultures. Under these

Table 1.   T cell tolerance in supralethally-irradiated parent → F$_1$ BMC:
different levels of tolerance of CD8$^+$ cells in thymocytes vs.
LN

Assay for measuring tolerance	Extent of tolerance relative to T cells from normal parental strain mice	
	CD4$^-$8$^+$ LN	CD4$^-$8$^+$ thymocytes
MLR, no lymphokines	very strong	very strong
MLR, with lymphokines	strong	limited
CTL, bulk cultures	moderate	limited
CTL, limiting dilution	limited	very limited
GVHD on transfer	very strong	very strong

The data are summarized from ref. 17.

conditions, the chimera CD8$^+$ thymocytes display only partial tolerance to
host antigens: responses are lower than to third-party antigens but only
by a factor of 3-4 fold. The capacity of lymphokines to abrogate
tolerance is also apparent in CTL assays. Thus, when CTL are generated in
bulk cultures with high doses of lymphokines (EL-4 supernatant), CTL
responses to host-type target cells are only 2-3 fold less than to third-
party targets. Even less tolerance is evident when CTLp are quantitated

Table 2.   Different levels of tolerance in adult irradiated SCID mice
            reconstituted with allogeneic vs. xenogeneic FL cells

| Assay | Adult irradiated (250 cGy) SCID mice reconstituted with: | |
	Allogeneic (AKR/J or B6) FL cells	Xenogeneic (Lewis rat) FL cells
Incidence of spontaneous lethal GVHD	undetectable	90-100%
Lethal GVHD on adoptive transfer to adult irradiated SCID hosts	none	90-100%
Splenomegaly on transfer to neonatal SCID hosts	undetectable	marked
MLR of lymph node T cells to host APC in vitro	weak	strong
CTLp frequency to host antigens by limiting dilution analysis	low	low

A summary of unpublished data of C.D. Surh and J. Sprent

by limiting dilution analysis. In this assay — which involves exposure to
lymphokines plus antigen for 7 days — the reduction in CTLp specific for
host antigens is only about 20% relative to normal parental strain mice.

Collectively, these data on in vitro responses of CD8$^+$ thymocytes indicate that tolerance to host antigens is marked in the absence of exogenous lymphokines but quite limited when the cells are supplemented with lymphokines. The key question is whether tolerance is evident under in vivo conditions. To examine this question, we tested whether $CD8^+$ SP thymocytes from the chimeras are capable of inducing lethal graft-versus host disease (GVHD) after transfer to irradiated host-type F_1 recipients. The results are clear cut: the chimera $CD8^+$ cells produce a high incidence of lethal GVHD in third-party irradiated hosts but fail to kill host-type F_1 recipients, even in high doses. The complete tolerance seen in this GVHD assay is also observed when the chimera $CD8^+$ thymocytes are first "parked" for 2 weeks in a neutral environment (irradiated donor-strain mice). Thus, tolerance does not seem to be a reflection of persistent contact with host antigens in the chimera hosts [19]. It should be mentioned that, in all of the assay systems described above, complete tolerance is observed in double chimeras, i.e. in chimeras reconstituted with BM cells taken from both parental strains. Thus, the presence of host-type BM-derived cells (BM-derived cells of the opposite parental strain) leads to complete tolerance induction.

The above findings reinforce the view that TEC are strongly tolerogenic, but only in certain assays. To explain this split tolerance, some workers [20] argue that TEC are intrinsically just as tolerogenic as BM-derived cells but express only a limited range of self peptides: TEC produce strong tolerance to these peptides but cannot induce tolerance to other self peptides, e.g. to peptides present on BM-derived cells but not on TEC. Since there is no direct evidence that there are more than minimal differences in the range of self peptides on BM-derived cells vs TEC, we prefer the idea that the tolerogenicity of TEC is restricted to high-affinity T cells, low-affinity cells being spared [14,17,21]. Our rationale for this idea is as follows.

We view high-affinity T cells as cells able to respond well to antigen in the absence of added lymphokines [21,22]. These cells undergo strong signalling during interaction with APC and are induced to synthesize their own growth factors (plus the receptors for these factors). These helper-independent (HI) T cells function effectively under in vivo conditions and are largely responsible for such in vivo effector functions as skin graft rejection and GVHD. We view low affinity T cells as crippled cells. These cells receive suboptimal signals from APC during antigen recognition and are driven to synthesize only the receptors for growth factors (e.g. IL-2R) and not the growth factors (e.g. IL-2) themselves. The function of these crippled cells depends critically upon the availability of "help" (growth factors) released from neighboring cells. These helper-dependent (HD) cells function well under artificial conditions in vitro, e.g. in the presence of lymphokines in CTL assays [23], but probably make only a minor contribution to typical immune responses occurring in vivo.

In the case of tolerance induction, we argue that the high-affinity of HI T cells makes these cells hypersusceptible to tolerance induction during early differentiation in the thymus. Tolerizing (deleting) these cells does not require professional APC (BM-derived cells), and contact with TEC is sufficient to cause clonal deletion. The situation with HD cells is different. Because of their low affinity, these cells are more difficult to tolerize. Clonal deletion of these cells is under the strict control of professional APC: contact with antigen expressed only on TEC and not on BM-derived cells fails to delete low-affinity T cells and these cells are allowed to escape to the periphery.

Based on the above line of reasoning, our overall conclusion is that TEC are strongly tolerogenic for T cells, but only for high-affinity cells. Tolerance induction of low-affinity cells requires contact with antigen on professional APC.

Post-thymic tolerance in chimeras.

Since host class I expression in chimeras is apparent in both the intrathymic and extrathymic environments, the question arises whether the low-affinity T cells escaping tolerance induction in the thymus succumb to tolerance in the post-thymic environment. This does indeed appear to be the case (Table 1). Thus, for CTLp, the precursor frequency of host-specific T cells is much lower in spleen and lymph nodes than in the thymus [17]. The same finding applies to lymphokine-dependent proliferative responses [17].

These findings indicate that tolerance induction of CD8$^+$ cells in chimeras is a two-step process: some cells undergo tolerance induction (deletion) in the thymus but others are tolerized in the periphery. These data might be taken as support for the popular idea that post-thymic mechanisms of tolerance are required for normal self tolerance induction [24-26]. Our own view is that the post-thymic tolerance we observe in chimeras is highly artificial and reflects that the low-affinity T cells escaping deletion in the thymus are actually semi-tolerized [14,17]. These residual low-affinity cells can be rescued from tolerance by exposure to lymphokines in vitro (e.g. in CTL assays) and also by depriving the cells from contact with antigen, (e.g. by parking the cells in a neutral environment). When left in situ in the chimeras, however, exit of the cells into the post-thymic environment leads to exposure to host antigens in the relative absence of lymphokines. Semi-tolerance then proceeds to full tolerance and the cells die. Why is this situation artificial? The point to emphasize is that, in the normal (nonchimeric) thymus, antigen is expressed on BM-derived cells as well as on TEC. T cells escaping tolerance induction by TEC would thus be deleted by the adjacent BM-derived cells. For this reason, the split tolerance we see in chimeras is probably irrelevant to tolerance occurring in the normal thymus.

Tolerance in rat → mouse chimeras.

The above data refer to tolerance induction across allogeneic (H-2) barriers. Recently, we have been studying tolerance of xenogeneic rat T cells differentiating from stem cells in mice, specifically in SCID mice. These mice are devoid of mature T and B cells because of a failure to rearrange TCR and Ig genes [27]; the SCID thymus is atrophic, and thymopoiesis is limited to incomplete differentiation of $CD4^-8^-$ stem cells. Since the SCID defect is restricted to stem cells, full restoration of T and B cells can be induced by injecting the mice with stem cells [27]. Interestingly, this also applies to rat stem cells. Thus, providing the hosts are conditioned with light irradiation (250 cGy), injecting adult SCID mice with rat FL cells (4×10^7 day-15 Lewis FL i.v.) leads to complete repopulation with a full spectrum of rat-derived T and B cells [28]. The thymus enlarges to near-normal size and contains the usual ratio of thymocyte subsets; > 90% of the cells in the thymus are of rat origin, and the few residual mouse-derived cells are TCR⁻. Repopulation with rat-derived cells also applies to myeloid and erythroid cells as well as to BM-derived APC. To avoid confusion it should be mentioned that the paucity of host-derived hemopoietic cells in rat → SCID chimeras is largely a reflection of the heightened sensitivity of SCID cells to irradiation [27,29], a dose of 250 cGy being sufficient to destroy most host stem cells.

Rat → SCID chimeras prepared from Lewis rat FL cells appear quite healthy for the first 2 months post-reconstitution. Thereafter, the mice gradually deteriorate with weight loss and ruffled fur (C.D. Surh and J. Sprent, unpublished). Skin lesions suggestive of GVHD appear at about 3 months. These lesions progress and by 4-5 months the mice display a pattern of florid cutaneous GVHD with severe dermatitis and widespread loss of hair. This syndrome is eventually lethal and few mice survive beyond 6 months. Diarrhea is mild, and GVHD is largely confined to the skin.

Initially, we thought that the GVHD developing in rat → SCID chimeras might reflect minor contamination of the rat FL cells with mature T cells. We now think this is unlikely for two reasons (C.D. Surh and J. Sprent, unpublished). First, severe GVHD occurs with transfer of even very early (day 13) FL cells. Second, thymectomizing the SCID hosts before FL injection prevents GVHD. This latter finding indicates that the development of GVHD is thymus dependent and implies that GVHD reflects a failure to induce tolerance of newly-formed T cells. Our data on the lack of tolerance in rat → SCID chimeras can be summarized as follows (Table 2); these data have yet to be published.

In the case of GVHD, transferring either peripheral T cells or thymocytes from rat → SCID chimeras into secondary SCID hosts leads to rapid induction of GVHD and death. This is especially pronounced when the chimera T cells are transferred to neonatal SCID hosts. In this situation the recipients develop marked splenomegaly and die within a few weeks. Similar lack of tolerance applies to primary MLR in vitro (carried out in the absence of lymphokines using unseparated lymph node T cells as responders). Interestingly, the chimera T cells show quite strong tolerance in terms of CTL assays. This finding implies that the lack of tolerance in the chimeras applies only to CD4$^+$ cells and not to CD8$^+$ cells.

In interpreting these data, it should be emphasized that reconstituting SCID hosts with H-2-different mouse FL cells, e.g. AKR/J or B6 FL, fails to cause GVHD (Table 1). Moreover, the donor T cells recovered from these allogeneic chimeras show quite strong tolerance to the host in functional studies. Lack of tolerance induction thus seems to be unique to rat stem cells.

Since rat → SCID chimeras prepared with 250 cGy show a profound lack of host-derived APC, the question arises whether supplementing the chimeras with host hemopoietic cells would promote tolerance induction. In support of this idea we find that, when rat → SCID chimeras are prepared with a mixture of rat and SCID FL cells, GVHD is much less evident. To prevent GVHD completely, however, it is necessary to supplement the SCID FL cells with normal B cells (taken from H-2 compatible BALB/c mice). These data apply to adult SCID mice conditioned with 250 cGy. What happens when rat FL cells are transferred to nonirradiated SCID mice? In this situation, the overwhelming numbers of host APC would be expected to be strongly tolerogenic for rat T cells. In practice, however, rat FL cells fail to differentiate in nonirradiated adult SCID mice, presumably because of rejection by host NK cells [30,31]. In neonatal SCID mice, by contrast, NK function is limited, and rat FL cells differentiate into mature T cells without conditioning the hosts with irradiation. The key finding with these neonatally injected SCID mice is that the rat T cells arising in these hosts show full tolerance and fail to cause GVHD; significantly, these rat → neonatal SCID chimeras show prominent survival of host hemopoietic cells. These data on neonatal SCID mice provide further evidence that tolerance induction in rat → SCID chimeras is largely under the control of BM-derived cells.

Concluding comments.

It is notable that restoration of adult irradiated SCID mice with H-2-different mouse FL cells leads to strong tolerance and no signs of GVHD. This finding is in agreement with the studies on parent → F_1 chimeras and provides further evidence that contact of early T cells with TEC (or other non BM-derived cells) is sufficient for tolerance induction. This does not seem to apply to rat T cells, however, because reconstituting adult irradiated SCID mice with rat FL cells fails to cause tolerance and the recipients eventually die from GVHD. Tolerance of rat T cells in SCID mice depends critically upon contact with large numbers of host APC. This occurs when rat FL cells differentiate in nonirradiated neonatal SCID hosts.

Why mouse TEC tolerize mouse T cells but fail to tolerize rat T cells is unclear. The possibility we are exploring is that rat T cells interact poorly with mouse TEC because of mismatching of their respective cell-surface adhesion molecules. The main problem with this idea is that positive selection of T cells in rat → SCID chimeras seems to be normal. Thus, one is forced to argue that mismatching of adhesion molecules on rat T cells and mouse TEC selectively impairs negative selection without affecting positive selection. Resolving this issue will presumably hinge on defining the range of adhesion molecules involved in positive and negative selection. At present, direct evidence on this crucial issue is rather sparse.

ACKNOWLEDGEMENTS. The typing skills of Ms. Barbara Marchand are gratefully acknowledged. This work was supported by grants CA38355, CA25803, and AI21487 from the United States Public Health Service. C.D. Surh is the recipient of a Leukemia Society of America Special Fellowship. Publication no. 8195-IMM from The Scripps Research Institute.

REFERENCES

1. Kappler JW, Roehm N, Marrack P. T cell tolerance by clonal elimination in the thymus. Cell 1987;49:273-280.

2. Kappler JW, Staerz U, White J, Marrack P. Self-tolerance eliminates T cells specific for Mls-modified products of the major histocompatibility complex. Nature (Lond). 1988;332:35-40.

3. MacDonald HR, Schneider R, Less RK, Howe RC, Acha-Orbea H, Festenstein H, Zinkernagel RM, Hengartner H. T-cell receptor $V\beta$ use predicts reactivity and tolerance to Mls[a]-encoded antigens. Nature 1988;332;40-45.

4.   von Boehmer H. Developmental biology of T cells in T cell receptor transgenic mice. Ann Rev Immunol 1990;8:531-556.

5.   Sprent J. T lymphocytes and the thymus. In: Paul WE, editor. Fundamental Immunology, Third Edition. New York: Raven Press, 1993, in press.

6.   Houssaint E, Flajnik M. The role of thymic epithelium in the acquisition of tolerance. Immunol Today 1990;11:357-360.

7.   von Boehmer H, Schubiger K. Thymocytes appear to ignore class I major histocompatibility complex antigens expressed on thymic epithelial cells. 1984;14:1048-1052.

8.   Jenkinson EJ, Jhittay P, Kingston R, et al. Studies on the role of the thymic environment in the induction of tolerance to MHC antigens. Transplant 1985;39:331-333.

9.   Matzinger, P, Guerder S. Does T-cell tolerance require a dedicated antigen-presenting cell? Nature 1989;338:74-76.

10.   Salaun J, Bandiera A, Khazaal I, et al. Thymic epithelium tolerizes for histocompatibility antigens. Science 1990;247:1471-1474.

11.   Houssaint E, Flajnik M. The role of thymic epithelium in the acquisition of tolerance. Immunol Today 1990;11:357-360.

12.   Hoffman MW, Allison J, Miller JFAP. Tolerance induction by thymic medullary epithelium. Proc Natl Acad Sci USA 1992;89:2526-2530.

13.   Webb S, Sprent J. Tolerogenicity of thymic epithelium. Eur J Immunol 1990;20:2525-2528.

14.   Gao E-K, Lo D, Sprent J. Strong T cell tolerance in parent $\rightarrow$ F_1 bone marrow chimeras prepared with supralethal irradiation. Evidence for clonal deletion and anergy. J Exp Med 1990;171:1101-1121.

15. Gao, E-K, Kosaka H, Surh CD et al. T cell contact with Ia antigens on nonhemopoietic cells in vivo can lead to immunity rather than tolerance. J Exp Med 1991;174:435-446.

16. Kosaka H, Surh CD, Sprent J. Stimulation of mature unprimed CD8[+] T cells by semiprofessional antigen-presenting cells in vivo. J Exp Med 1992;176:1291-1302.

17. Kosaka H, Sprent J. Tolerance of CD8[+] cells developing in parent → F_1 chimeras prepared with supralethal irradiation: step-wise induction of tolerance in the intrathymic and extrathymic environments. J Exp Med 1993;177:367-378.

18. Surh CD, Gao E-K, Kosaka H et al. Two subsets of epithelial cells in the thymic medulla. J Exp Med 1992;176:495-505.

19. Ramsdell F, Fowlkes BJ. Maintenance of in vivo tolerance by persistence of antigen. Science 1992;257:1130-1134.

20. Bonomo A, Matzinger P. Thymus epithelium induces tissue-specific tolerance. J Exp Med 1993;177:1153-1164.

21. Sprent J, Gao E-K, Webb SR. T-cell reactivity to MHC molecules: immunity versus tolerance. Science 1990;248:1357-1363.

22. Sprent J, Schaefer M. Antigen-presenting cells for CD8[+] T cells. Immunol Rev 1990;117:213-234.

23. Mizuochi T, Munitz TI, McCarthy SA, et al. Differential helper and effector responses of Lyt-2[+] T cells to H-2K[b] mutant (K[bm]) determinants and the appearance of thymic influence on anti-K[bm] CTL responsiveness. J Immunol 1986;137:2740-2747.

24. Mueller DL, Jenkins MK, Schwartz RH. Clonal expansion versus functional clonal inactivation: a costimulatory signaling pathway

140

determines the outcome of T cell antigen receptor occupancy. Ann Rev Immunol 1989;7:445-480.

25.   Kroemer G, Martinez-A C, eds. Clonal deletion and anergy: from models to reality. Res Immunol 1992;143:267-370.

26.   Miller JFAP, Morahan G. Peripheral T cell tolerance. Ann Rev Immunol. 1992;10:51-69.

27.   Bosma MJ, Carrol AM. The SCID mouse mutant: definition, characterization and potential uses. Ann Rev Immunol 1991;9:323-350.

28.   Surh CD, Sprent J. Long-term xenogeneic chimeras: Full differentiation of rat T and B cells in SCID mice. J Immunol 1991;147:2148-2154.

29.   Fulop GM, Phillips RA. The scid mutation in mice causes a general defect in DNA repair. Nature (Lond.). 1990;347:479-482.

30.   Dorshkind K, Pollack SB, Bosma NJ, Phillips RA. Natural killer (NK) cells are present in mice with severe combined immunodeficiency (scid). J Immunol 1985;134:3798-3801.

31.   Murphy WJ, Kumar V, Bennett M. Rejection of bone marrow allografts by mice with severe combined immune deficiency (SCID): evidence that natural killer cells can mediate the specificity of marrow graft rejection. J Exp Med 1987;165:1212-1271.

HLA Matching in Liver Transplant Immunity

René J. Duquesnoy, Division of Transplant Pathology, University of Pittsburgh Medical Center, Pittsburgh, PA 15261

INTRODUCTON

The role of HLA in transplantation has been generally viewed that HLA matching is good for transplant outcome. This is demonstrated with the higher survival rates of kidney and heart transplants from donors with increased HLA matching. However, this concept seems less applicable to liver transplantation and it has become apparent that the effect of HLA is considerably more complex.

The role of HLA in transplantation should be assessed analogous to the way we view the physical characteristics of H_2O. Cooling of H_2O results in ice and heating of H_2O produces steam. Each of these physical forms of H_2O has very unique features. However, mixing ice and steam will lead to only lukewarm water. To critically understand its role in transplantation, HLA cannot be studied like lukewarm water. The functional characteristics of HLA are complex and different properties of HLA need to be assessed separately. HLA serves not only as a system of transplantation antigens involved in rejection but it also plays a crucial role in antigen presentation leading to T cell-mediated responses relevant to transplant immunity. This summary deals with recent experience how HLA matching affects liver transplant outcome.

J. L. Touraine et al. (eds.), Rejection and Tolerance, 141–148.
© 1994 Kluwer Academic Publishers.

HLA matching and liver transplant survival.

It is well known that HLA matching prolongs kidney and heart transplant survival by reducing the incidence and severity of rejection. However, a study published by Markus et al [1] in 1988 revealed the surprising finding that HLA matching was associated with lower survival rates of liver transplants. These observations were made with cyclosporine-treated patients and of special interest was the negative effect of HLA-DR matching on liver transplant outcome. Similar results have recently been reported for FK506 treated patients in Pittsburgh [2] and liver transplant recipients in the Eurotransplant program [3].

Dualistic role of HLA in liver transplantation.

In the original report by Markus et al [1], the concept was proposed that HLA matching has a dualistic effect on liver transplantation. In one way, it may diminish transplant rejection but conversely, HLA matching could promote MHC-restricted immunologically-mediated injury associated with viral infection and autoimmunity. As been observed for other organ transplants, HLA is an important system of transplantation antigens involved in cellular rejection of liver transplants. This has been demonstrated not only with the isolation of HLA-specific alloreactive T lymphocytes from rejecting liver transplants [4], but also by associations between HLA-DR mismatching with a higher rate of graft failures due to rejection [1], and cholangitic/cholestatic rejection [5].

To better understand the role of HLA in transplantation, one must consider that besides rejection, other immune mechanisms will contribute to allograft failure. Such immune responses could be directed towards viral or other microbial antigens or are associated with autoimmune disease and many could operate through MHC-restricted mechanisms. Of clinical relevance are infections with hepatitis B virus, cytomegalovirus and Epstein Barr virus. Cytotoxic T cells specific for these viruses have been shown to function through HLA-restricted mechanisms. Such lymphocytes would be more efficient in causing injury if the infected target cells in the allograft expresses shared HLA antigens [6].

In many liver transplant recipients, the pathogenesis of the original disease has an immunologic basis. Several liver diseases show HLA associations suggesting that their etiology involves MHC-restricted immune mechanisms. With replacement of the diseased liver by a normal allograft it can be expected that immune cells responsible for the original disease will remain in the recipient. If such lymphocytes operate through HLA-restricted effector mechanisms they would be more efficient in causing injury to liver allografts that share HLA antigens with the recipient [6]. Relevant to this concept are findings by Houssin's group [7] showing that HLA class I matching is associated with recurrent viral hepatitis B after liver transplantation.

Effect of HLA-DR matching on CMV hepatitis and chronic liver transplant rejection.

Manez et al [8] have recently reported that HLA-DR sharing between donor and recipient is associated with higher incidence and earlier onset of CMV hepatitis of liver transplant patients. No associations were found for HLA-A and HLA-B antigen sharing. Class I restricted immune responses to CMV are mediated by CD8 positive T cells which are believed to play a major role in the development of protective immunity to CMV infection [9]. Conversely, class II MHC-restricted CMV-specific T cells have generally the CD4 phenotype and can be expected to produce lymphokines which mediate inflammatory processes leading to hepatic injury. During CMV hepatitis, there is *de novo* expression of HLA-DR molecules on hepatocyte membranes [10]. These HLA-DR molecules on infected hepatocytes could present CMV antigen to graft infiltrating CMV-specific lymphocytes. This process would be more efficient with antigenically compatible HLA-DR molecules and this would enhance the intragraft activation of CMV-specific T cells and subsequent cell-mediated inflammatory processes.

The studies by Manez et al [8] have also demonstrated a higher incidence and earlier onset of chronic rejection in liver transplant patients who experienced CMV hepatitis. O'Grady et al [11] reported an association between CMV infection and vanishing bile syndrome, a manifestation of chronic rejection, and that HLA-DR matching of the liver donor presented an additional risk. These investigators concluded that HLA-DR status was not a predisposing factor to CMV infection. The data by Manez et al [8] suggest instead that HLA-DR matching increases the risk for CMV hepatitis which then leads to a higher incidence of chronic rejection. In kidney transplants, CMV disease has been found in association with HLA antigen matching [12-14].

The development of vanishing bile duct syndrome is related to a persistent CMV infection of the liver allograft [15]. Although no data are available about infiltrating CMV-specific lymphocytes in liver allografts, evidence has been obtained for the persistence of primed CMV-specific T cells in bronchoalveolar lavages from lung transplant patients [16]. Relevant are findings that CMV infection is associated with a higher risk for chronic rejection of lung allografts [17]. Altogether, one might speculate that the persistence of intragraft CMV-specific cellular immunity may accelerate chronic rejection of liver allografts.

The studies by Manez et al [8] indicated that HLA-DR matching is associated with an earlier onset but not a higher frequency of chronic liver transplant rejection. Since the HLA-DR matching effect was also seen in patients without CMV hepatitis, one must conclude that additional HLA-DR restricted immune responses to other antigens including viruses and autoantigens must be involved. Donaldson et al [18] have suggested that HLA-DR restricted responses to HLA class I antigen mismatches may play a role in the development of chronic rejection.

SUMMARY

The findings summarized in this report are consistent with the concept of the dualistic role of HLA in liver transplantation. HLA is an important system of transplantation antigens involved in humoral and cellular immune rejection. Matching for HLA would reduce the rejection mediated injury of liver allografts. On the other hand, HLA plays an important role in the immune responses to other antigens including these involved in infection and autoimmune disease. Matching for HLA may promote such antigen-specific immune mechanisms of liver graft injury. Most intriguing is the relationship between HLA and chronic rejection, a significant complication for long-term liver transplant survivors. Although HLA-specific immunity seems an important factor for chronic rejection, other immunological mechanisms which may well be HLA restricted, must be considered. A better understanding of the different roles of HLA in various immunological processes within the allograft may lead to improved management strategies for transplant recipients.

REFERENCES

1. Markus BH, Duquesnoy RJ, Gordon RD, Fung JJ, Vanek M, Klintmalm G, Bryan C, Van Thiel DH and StarzL TE: Histocompatibility and liver transplantation: A dualistic effect of HLA: Transplantation 1988;46:372-377.

2.   Kobayashi M, Yagihashi A, Noguchi K, Terasawa N, Konno A, Hayashi S, Starzl TE and Iwaki Y: HLA-DR matching effect in orthotopic liver transplantation under FK506. Transplant Proc 1993;25:228-229.

3.   Thorogood J et al: Relationship between HLA compatibility and first liver allograft survival. Transplant Proc 1993; In press.

4.   Markus BH, Demetris AJ, Saidman S, Fung JJ, Zeevi A, Starzl TE and Duquesnoy RJ: Alloreactive T lymphocytes cultured from liver transplant biopsies: Associations of HLA specificity with clinicopathological findings. Clin Transplant 1988;2:70-75.

5.   Gubernatis G, Kemnitz J, Tusch G and Richlmayr R: HLA compatibility and different features of liver allograft rejection. Transplant Int 1988;1:155-160.

6.   Duquesnoy RJ, Saidman S, Markus BH, Demetris AJ and Zeevi A: Role of HLA in intragraft cellular immunity in human liver transplantion. Transplant Proc 1988;20(1):724-727.

7.   Calmus Y, Hannoun L, Dousset B, Wolff P, Miquet JP, Duffoel M, Gillet M, Cinqualbre J, Poupon R and Houssin D: HLA class I matching is responsible for the hepatic lesions in recurrent viral hepatitis B after liver transplantation. Transplant Proc 1990;22:2311-2313.

8.   Manez R, Whiter LT, Linden P, Kusne S, Martin M, Kramer D, Demetris AJ, Van Thiel DH, Starzl TE and Duquesnoy RJ: Influence of HLA matching and

cytomegalovirus hepatitis and chronic rejection after liver transplantation. Transplantation 1993;55:1067-1071.

9. Quinnan GV, Burns WH, Kirmani N, et al: HLA-restricted cytotoxic T lymphocytes are an early immune response and important defense mechanism in cytomegalovirus infections. Revs. Infect. Dis. 1984;6:156-169.

10. Steinhoff G, Wonigeit K and Pichlmayr: Analysis of sequential changes in major histocompatibility complex expression in human liver grafts after transplantation. Transplantation 1988;45:394-401.

11. O'Grady JG, Sutherland S, Harvey F, Et al: Cytomegalovirus infection and donor/recipient HLA antigens: Interdependent co-factors in pathogeneis of vanishing bile duct syndrome after liver transplantation. The Lancet 1988;2:302.

12. May AG, Betts RJ, Freeman RB and Andrus Ch: An analysis of cytomegalovirus infection and HLA antigen matching on the outcome of renal transplantation. Ann Surg 1978;187:110.

13. Pouteil-Noble C, Betuel H, Raffaele P, et al: Influence de al compatibilité HLA sur l'infection a cytomégalovirus en transplantation rénale. La Presse Médicale 1991;27:20.

14. Blancho G, Josien R, Douillard D, Bignon JD, Cesbron A and Soulillou JP: Influence of HLA-A-B-DR matching on CMV disease after renal

transplantation: HLA-DR7 matched recipients are more susceptible to CMV disease. Transplantation 1992;54:871-875.

15.   Arnold JC, Portman BC, O'Grady JG, Naoumou NV, Alexander GJM and Williams R: Cytomegalovirus infection persists in the liver graft in the vanishing bile duct syndrome. Hepatology 1992;16:285-202.

16.   Zeevi A, Uknis ME, Spichty KH, Tector M, Keenan RJ, Rinaldo C, Yousem S, Duncan S, Paradis I, Dauber J, Griffith B and Duquesnoy RJ: Proliferation of cytomegalovirus primed lymphocytes in bronchoalveolar lavages from lung transplant patients. Transplantation 1992;54:635-639.

17.   Keenan RJ, Lega ME, Dummer JS, Paradis IL, Dauber JH, Rabinowich H, Yousem S, Hardesty RL, Griffith BP, Duquesnoy RJ and Zeevi A: Cytomegalovirus serologic status and postoperative infection correlates with risk of developing chronic rejection after pulmonary transplantation. Transplantation 1991;51;433.

18.   Donaldson PT, O'Grady J, Portmann B, Davis H, Alexander GJM, Neuberger J, Thick M, Calne RY and Williams R: Evidence for an immune response to HLA class I antigens in the vanishing bile duct syndrome after liver transplantation. The Lancet 1987;:945-948.

Transgenic pigs as potential donors for xenografts.

John Dunning,
Senior Registrar in Cardiac Surgery,
Papworth Hospital,
Cambridge.

David White,
Lecturer in Department of Surgery,
University of Cambridge.

John Wallwork,
Director of Transplantation,
Papworth Hospital,
Cambridge.

The field of organ transplantation has grown dramatically over the last 35 years, and one of the key advances that has led to this growth is the introduction of Cyclosporin A as an effective immunosuppressive agent (1). So successful has allotransplantation become with improvement in terms of survival (2), quality of life (3, 4) and cost benefit (5) that ever greater numbers of patients are being referred by physicians for consideration of transplantation. This has resulted in a relative shortage in the number of donor organs and in no area is this more marked than in the field of cardio-pulmonary transplantation. In the United Kingdom 454 patients received thoracic organ transplants in the year ending 31 December 1992 while the waiting list grew to 706 patients (6) and the number of patients passing through the assessment procedure is more than three times that number. 25 -

J. L. Touraine et al. (eds.), Rejection and Tolerance, 149–160.
© 1994 *Kluwer Academic Publishers.*

30% of patients waiting for heart or lung transplants die before suitable organs become available for them.

A similarly bleak picture is seen for kidney transplantation. The disparity in numbers between the waiting list and operations performed is shown in figure 1. It is estimated that between 2500 and 4000 kidneys are required annually to meet the demand (7), while a recent audit of intensive care units in England suggested an absolute maximum of 1700 potential donors (8). Even were all of these patients consented for donation and medically suitable there would still be a shortfall in the supply compared to the demand.

The true need may be even higher than estimated since waiting lists are kept artificially low in the knowledge that there is a limited donor resource. With the unprecedented success of transplantation the operations are sought not only to save life as was initially the case, but also to improve the quality of life. Hence the indications for transplantation are widening with a dwindling donor resource.

Public education has ensured that fewer potentially transplantable organs are lost through ignorance and prejudice, but even so the shortage becomes worse each year. Artificial organs such as renal dialysis machines provide partial answers, but progress in the development of totally implantable artificial organs has perhaps been disappointing particularly in view of the huge resource invested in this area. The artificial heart is probably the most successful of the artificial organs, but even though it is a relatively simple pump problems remain with the power supply, biocompatibility, thrombosis and infection. It is likely that this will be developed to a state of clinical

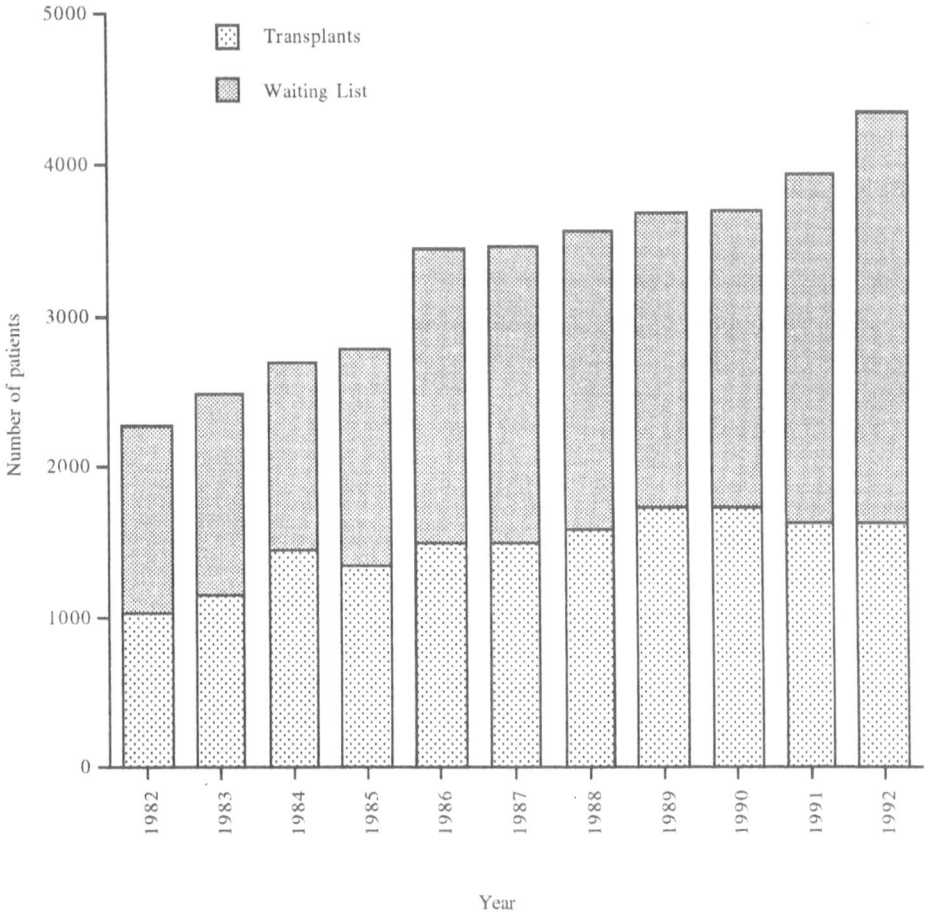

Figure 1: <u>Comparison of renal transplant waiting list and number of</u>
<u>transplants performed</u>

usefulness in the near future, but there is currently no prospect of a totally
artificial alternative to the more complex metabolic organs such as the lungs,
liver or kidney.

It is our belief that the field of xenotransplantation, that is the transplantation
of organs between species provides the best solution to the shortage of

transplantable organs. The use of animals already bred and slaughtered in large numbers for food poses fewer ethical problems than those posed using a closely related primate species for donor organs. In addition the use of an animal such as the pig which is bred easily in captivity with high parity ensures a ready supply of organs.

The phenomenon of hyperacute xenograft rejection (HXR) occurring within minutes of revascularisation of a transplanted organ has prevented the use of discordant animal organs to date. This phenomenon has several elements including the recognition of foreign tissue by preformed naturally occurring antibodies (PNAB) and the activation of the complement cascade by either alternative or classical pathways. Debate centres on the relative importance of these mechanisms in causation of the violent rejection seen in discordant species combinations. To some extent the use of non-human primate organs may overcome the problem since HXR is not seen in such combinations, but first set rejection still occurs. In addition it is unlikely that these animals can provide the organs in the quantity required or of an appropriate physical size and there may be deep-rooted moral objections to the use of animals which are so closely related to man.

A great deal has been written describing the discordant xenograft rejection process. Preformed naturally occurring anti-species IgM antibody binds to donor endothelium and activates complement via the classical pathway (9) although in some species combination it would appear that alternative pathway complement activation assumes greater importance. Although it is probable that antigenic determinants are glycoproteins this remains unproven at present. Tissue factor and plasminogen activator inhibitor are synthesised and heparan sulphate is lost (10). These processes promote the accumulation of fibrin and in addition platelet activating factor is released stimulating the adhesion of platelets (11). Neutrophil polymorphs are retained in the organ by their cell surface complement receptors and play an important role in the intravascular compartment in the generation of further inflammatory mediators and the disruption of the endothelial barriers to blood cells and proteins. The resultant platelet thrombi cause ischaemia and failure of the transplanted organ.

Discordant xenograft survival may be prolonged from minutes to hours in experimental models using techniques such as plasmapheresis or xenoabsorption to remove PNAB. Complement depletion with cobra venom factor (CVF) has a similar effect. Graft survival may also be prolonged by depletion of cellular fractions but none of these techniques have produced a xenograft which functions for more than a few hours and none can be envisaged in clinical use to provide long term maintenance of xenografted organs.

Although the role of PNAB is established another area which is becoming more clearly defined is the role of complement through both the classical and alternative pathways. It appears that the regulators of complement activation which are present on all cell surfaces are species specific and those in a xenografted organ fail to inhibit recipient complement activity. A novel approach to complement control would be to express appropriate recipient species RCA's on the xenograft cells. Indeed such an approach is already in use in nature in several micro-organisms. Schistoma Mansoni do not activate the human complement cascade after they have been in the human blood stream. The failure to activate complement is blocked by antibody against DAF (Decay Accelerating Factor - a complement control protein) suggesting that the parasites insert host DAF into their surfaces (12). Similarly the vaccinia virus is able to encode for secretory proteins which bind host C3 and C4 products to protect against attack by complement (13).

There is experimental evidence to suggest that the manipulation of RCA's will protect an organ against xenogeneic complement. The transfection of cell lines with gene constructs coding for human DAF and MCP (Membrane Cofactor Protein) have provided almost complete protection against human complement but not rabbit complement (14).

It is hoped that the introduction of cDNA constructs into the genome of an animal could produce transgenic animals which would express human DAF and MCP and thus protect transplanted donor organs from hyperacute complement mediated rejection. Mice transgenic for human DAF have already been produced although expression is variable (15, 16) and a transgenic breeding programme in pigs incorporating the DAF cDNA construct has been undertaken. Again expression is somewhat variable. To date 27 live transgenic pigs have been born from a total of 150 piglets. This holds promise for the future.

Clearly there is a long way to go before the RCA's are reliably expressed throughout all organ systems and on the vascular endothelium and there will need to be detailed experimental assessment before the clinical application of discordant xenografting. However this approach seems likely to produce a useful strategy for the establishment of clinical xenograft programmes (15, 17) and it may be as early as five years from now that the first successful transplants are performed using organs from transgenic animals.

If hyperacute rejection could be completely prevented it is not clear what would be the fate of the discordant xenograft, although studies of concordant grafts suggest that there would be many features in common with allograft rejection. Destruction by newly generated antibody and cellular rejection both occur although of course both these processes may be controlled by existing immunosuppressive techniques.

Assuming that HXR can be overcome an animal must be selected as a potential donor for man. The ideal animal must fulfil several criteria. It must be available in large numbers and able to breed easily in captivity. Clearly it must be of an adequate size to produce organs anatomically and physiologically similar to man. For preference it should already be bred as a food source since this is likely to be more readily acceptable to the public than taking an animal which is naturally wild and establishing new breeding colonies which may have highly organised social structures.

The pig has long been quoted as an animal which meets these requirements producing large litters, with rapid growth of offspring, needing relatively small areas for rearing and having low breeding and maintenance costs. In addition there is relatively easy availability of gnotobiotic animals which may be an important consideration when transplanting organs across species barriers. Clearly the transmission zoonoses with the organ is undesirable.

Table 1: The clinical application of xenotransplantation

Year	Organ	Donor	Cases	Survival
1964	Kidney	Chimpanzee	12	<9months
1964	Kidney	Monkey	1	10 days
1964	Kidney	Baboon	1	4.5 days
1964	Kidney	Baboon	6	<2 months
1964	Heart	Chimpanzee	1	2 hours
1968	Heart	Sheep	1	0
1968	Heart	Pig	1	4 minutes
1969	Heart	Chimpanzee	1	Short time
1969-73	Liver	Chimpanzee	3	<14 days
1977	Heart	Baboon	1	5 hours
1977	Heart	Chimpanzee	1	4 days
1984	Heart	Baboon	1	20 days
1992	Liver	Baboon	1	70 days
1992	Heart	Pig	1	<24 hours
1993	Liver	Baboon	1	30 days

Other diseases too may be transmitted in the transplant organ and neoplasia must also be considered. The best information comes from a large post-mortem series performed in the United States which reported an incidence of swine neoplasia of 0.004% of which the majority were malignant lymphomas and embryonal nephromas. However this data is far from perfect since the animals were all relatively immature having come to slaughter for food.

Congenital anomalies may also prove to be an important consideration but in the same series were reported as around 0.5% for congenital cardiac defects, and it seems unlikely that any of these considerations will ultimately prove a bar to the successful use of the pig as a cardiac xenograft donor. The question of whether or not the more complex synthetic organs such as the liver or pancreas will ever be usable remains open at this time.

Clinical experience of xenotransplantation has been limited to around 30 cases (Table 1) and with two notable exceptions in 1993 these attempts have been limited to concordant combinations. Although none of these grafts survived beyond nine months, and indeed most for a much shorter period a great deal of useful information has been revealed. It is clear that one species organs can function usefully in another species body although what the long term implications of for example a chronically different albumen level will prove to be remain a matter of speculation. It appears that the most likely organ to function usefully at present is the heart and comparative physiological studies of human and porcine hearts have shown similar haemodynamic function suggesting that they may work successfully in man.

Conclusion:

The success of allotransplantation has improved dramatically over the last 35 years. Much of this success has been due to improvements in immunosuppression. New drugs with novel modes of action may further improve graft and patient survival, but allotransplantation remains limited by donor organ supply and xenotransplantation is probably the only way to provide an adequate number of organs for all those in need. Currently available drugs have not been shown to confer any advantage in the prevention of hyperacute xenograft rejection dictating novel approaches based on examples from the natural world. Genetic modification of donor animals may prove the solution and transgenic breeding programmes are already established. Other obstacles both physiological and moral must be overcome before widespread acceptance of xenotransplantation but there is growing impetus in this direction. It is only a matter of years before clinical xenotransplantation programmes are established.

References:

1.   Calne R, Rolles K, White D, et al. Cyclosporin A initially as the only immunosuppressant in 34 recipients of cadaveric organs: 32 kidneys, 2 pancreases and 2 livers. Lancet 1979;(ii):1033-1036.

2.   Kaye M. The registry of the International Society for Heart and Lung Trnsplantation: Ninth official report-1992. J Heart Lung Trans 1992;11(4):599-606.

3.   Caine N, O'Brien V. Quality of life and psychological aspects of heart transplantation. In: Wallwork J, ed. Heart and Heart-Lung Transplantation. Philadelphia: W B Saunders Company, 1989: 389-422.

4.   Caine N, Sharples L, English T, Wallwork J. Prospective study comparing quality of life before and after heart transplantation. Trans Proc 1990;22(4):1437-1439.

5.   Buxton M, Acheson R, Caine N, Gibson S, O'Brien V. Costs and benefits of heart transplant programmes at Harefield and Papworth hospitals: Final report. In: London: HMSO, 1985.

6.   UKTS Users Bulletin: Winter 1992/93. In: Bristol, UKTSSA, 1993.

7.   Hoffenberg R. Working party on the supply of donor organsfor transplantation. In: London: HMSO, 1987.

8.   Gore S, Hinds C, Rutherford A. Organ donation from intensive care units in England. Brit Med J 1989;299:1193-1197.

9.   Fischel RJ, Kim W, Cahill D, Matas AJ. The cellular response to xenotransplantation. Curr Surg 1990;47(5):345-7.

10.   Platt J, Vercolotti G, Lindman B, Oegema T, Bach F, Dalmaso A. Release of heparan sulfate from endothelial cells. J Exp Med 1990;71:1363-1368.

11.   Reding R, Maldague P, Massion P, Lambotte L, Otte J. Differential effect of plasma exchange and platelet activating factor antagonist WEB 2170 on hyperacute vascular rejection of discordant xenografts in rodents: preliminary results. Min Chir 1991;46:167-168.

12.   Pearce EJ, Hall BF, Sher A. Host-specific invasion of the alternative complement pathway by schistosomes correlates with the presence of a phospholipase C-sensitive surface molecule resembling human decay accelerating factor. J Immunol 1990;144(7):2751-2756.

13. Kotwaj GJ, Moss B. Vaccinia virus encodes a secretory polypeptide structurally related to complement control proteins. Nature 1988;335:176-178.

14. Oglesby TJ, White D, Tedja I, et al. Protection of mammalian cells from complement-mediated lysis by transfection of human membrane cofactor protein and decay accelerating factor. Trans Ass Am Phys 1991;104:164-172.

15. White D, Oglesby TJ, Liszewski K, et al. Expression of human decay accelerating factor or membrane cofactor protein genes on mouse cells inhibits lysis by human complement. Trans Proc 1992;24(2):474-476.

16. White DJG. Transplantation of organs between species. Int Arch All Immunol 1992;98:1-5.

17. Platt JL, Bach FH. The barrier to xenotransplantation. Transplantation 1991;52(6):937-47.

PERCUTANEOUS ASPIRATION AND DRAINAGE OF FLUID COLLECTIONS AFTER PANCREATIC OR RENAL TRANSPLANTATION

C. Pangaud, D. Lyonnet - Service de Radiologie Pavillon P
Hôpital Edouard Herriot - LYON

Percutaneous Aspiration and Drainage of Abdominal Fluid Collections after Pancreatic Transplantation.

Whole or segmental PT is sometimes complicated by the development of intra-abdominal fluid collections. Detection of fluid after PT can be accomplished with US, CT, or RM. Indications for radiologic procedures of the abdomen and pelvis after transplantation are fever, abdominal pain, abdominal distension, suspected hemorrhage. Fluid can be localized in a peripancreatic location or it can present as free ascites of a variable amount. The sizes of the collections are variable and are sometimes difficult to precisely measure because of their irregular shape. MR imaging is the preferred imaging technique for estimating volume and shape of the fluid collection. T1 and T2 signal intensity sometimes allows to charaterize the fluid. But CT is the most common technique for symptomatic pancreas recipients, often more useful than US when an adynamic ileus is present, and the occurence of multiple fluid collections and interloop free peritoneal fluid makes CT more effective than US. CT scans are done after bowel opacification, with or whithout contrast medium injection.

The most common abnormality identified by US after PT is the presence of focal peripancreatic fluid in 50 to 60% of examinations. The large fluid collections most commonly represent sterile pseudocysts (exocrin pancreatic secretions) often in association with polymer injection of the pancreas duct in segmental PT, or abscesses. Technical failures are still a major obstacle to successful pancreas transplantation, of which thrombosis and infection are the two most frequent. There is a high incidence of intra-abdominal infection after pancreas transplantation (near 20%) with a high mortality rate in this group (20-30%). Infections occur with all techniques, but the incidence is highest with enteric drainage which carries a high risk of contamination at the site of the bladder anastomosis. The lowest incidence of infection is with duct injection. Other fluid collections include hematoma, lymphocele.

Percutaneous aspiration and drainage : techniques

Guided percutaneous aspiration of fluid collections is a safe and effective technique for obtaining samples of fluid. US or CT guided aspiration can be

J. L. Touraine et al. (eds.), Rejection and Tolerance, 161–163.

performed. An anterior or lateral approach is used. The needle course is planned in order to avoid the ponction of intestinal loops. Sizes of needles include 18 to 22 G. Under local anesthetic, the needle is placed into the collection, and fluid samples are aspirated. Percutaneous drainage can be accomplished with Seldinger technique : we use a sheathed needle to provide an access to the collection (18G), then a J guidewire is passed through the sheath, and a pigtail catheter (7 to 12 F) can be positioned deeper into the collection, sutured to the skin. The trocar technique allows rapid insertion of the catheter without the difficulties of a cumbersome catheter exchange when using Seldinger technique. Procedures are performed under CT guidance, sometimes with the adjunction of fluoroscopy. The final catheter position can be confirmed radiographically with contrast material. All patients undergo antibiotic treatment at the time of catheter placement.

Results

US or CT guided percutaneous abdominal aspiration of abdominal fluid collections is generally successful in all cases without complications. Bacteriological results may not completely reflect the character of the fluid because all patients are treated for abdominal sepsis with broad-spectrum antibiotics at the time of catheter drainage. Percutaneous catheter drainage is not very successful in treating large and/or intraperitoneal infected abdominal fluid collections after pancreatic transplantation with the graft in-situ. Continued immunosuppression and necrotic activity of the pancreatic enzymes compromise the therapeutic effect of adequate catheter drainage : percutaneous aspiration or drainage of these abscesses often is followed by surgical exploration with the graft removal, concomittent debridement of necrotic tissue and use of large-bore catheters for drainage. Nonetheless, PCD has been shown to be useful as an adjunct to surgical drainage and more recently to preclude surgical drainage in some of these immunocompromised patients, factors of decision including a precise anatomic definition (fluid collection and transplant), a safe percutaneous access route using large-bore catheter, an attentive post-procedural management. In our serie, PCD as exclusive treatment of multiple infected collections was successful in one patient with a segmental graft. Infections in recipient of segmental grafts are more likely to resolve with retention of graft function than in those who have infection due to whole pancreas transplantation. PCD can also be performed after surgical exploration for fluid reaccumulation.

Percutaneous aspiration and drainage in complications of renal transplant

Percutaneous procedures can be used as a prelude to or substitute for surgery in the diagnosis and management of perirenal various fluid collections. Patients with declining renal function, fever, mass should be suspected of having peritransplant fluid collections that include : lymphocele, hematoma, urinoma, abscess.

Technique and results

Percutaneous aspiration or drainage are realized with the same techniques than peripancreatic fluid collections. Percutaneous techniques comprise useful adjunctive or definitive therapy.

Symptomatic lymphoceles occur in 1 to 20% of renal recipients ; large collections may deviate and compress the transplanted ureter, causing obstruction or may compress the iliac vein. Needle aspiration and complete percutaneous drainage not only yields the diagnosis but relieves the symptoms immediately. Multiloculated lymphocele collections may require additional punctures. If lymphocele recurs, Betadine (povidone-iodine) sclerosis is often effective in preventing reaccumulation of fluid once the lymphocele cavity is collapsed, without any significant complication rate. Sometimes conservative treatment is not sufficient and surgical exploration is indicated.

Urinary extravasation, though not common, is a serious complication of renal transplantation, and prompt diagnosis is imperative. Vascular insufficiency is the usual cause of ureteral or calyceal fistulas. An urinoma can be drained percutaneously and a percutaneous nephrostomy allows urinary diversion ; diverting the urinary flow enables a fistula to close, or at least, improves the condition of patient for later surgical correction. Sometimes an ureteral internal-external stent or a double J ureteral stent can be used to divert urine and stent the ureter.

Isolated paratransplant abscess is not a common problem but is often associated with other complications such as urinary fistula, lymphocele or hematoma. Percutaneous aspiration can rapidly help to yield the diagnosis. Abscess can be successfully drained percutaneously with the graft in situ.

In Summary

Directed diagnostic aspiration is useful in determining the etiology of fluid collections. The use and safety percutaneous drainage in carefuly selected patients with post-transplant complications allows collection drainage under local anesthesic with a low complication rate, ultimately providing a better surgical candidate if definitive percutaneous treatment is unsuccessful.

ENDOUROLOGIC RESOLUTION OF TRANSPLANT COMPLICATIONS

NIKOLAOS P. PARDALIDIS, M.D.
ARTHUR D. SMITH, M.D.

DEPARTMENT OF UROLOGY
LONG ISLAND JEWISH MEDICAL CENTER
NEW HYDE PARK, NY

INTRODUCTION

The incidence of urologic complications is approximately 10% of all renal transplant patients. These complications may have conseqences such as graft loss and even death and the surgical correction is required. The surgical complications can be divided into: A) Urologic B) Vascular C) Lymphatic and D) extrarenal.[1] More than 90% of urological complications are due to urinary fistulae and ureteric obstruction.[2]

TECHNIQUE OF RENAL ACCESS IN TRANSPLANT PATIENT

The approach to the transplanted kidney depends on the surgical anatomy. Eshghi and Smith[3] described an endourologic approach to transplant kidney; the patient is placed supine with the involved side make slightly oblique with a bolster or sand bag under the hip. Percutaneous nephrostomy is performed after insertion of ureteral catheter and retrograde injection of contrast medium. The stylet is removed, a J-tip guide wire is introduced through the sheath of the 18 gauge needle and manipulated into the ureter. After dilation of the nephrostomy tract to a 34F sheath is left in the renal pelvis and the nephroscope is introduced through it.

EARLY OBSTRUCTION

Early obstruction can be caused mainly by technical errors (inadequate hemostasis of distal ureteral blood vessels.)[4]

J. L. Touraine et al. (eds.), Rejection and Tolerance, 165–173.
© 1994 Kluwer Academic Publishers.

Salvatierra et al[5] reported acute angulation of the
ureteroneocystostomy. Ureteral necrosis usually happens in the
presence of ureteral obstruction and appears within the first six
weeks following transplantation.[6] Acute rejection may produce an
obstruction confusing the clinical picture.[7]

The diagnosis of obstruction in the first 24 hours is manifested
by a sudden drop of urine output. Differential diagnosis can be done
from acute tubular necrosis or hyperacute rejection or thrombosis of
the renal artery or vein. Noninvasive ultrasound, Technetium 99m DTPA
radioisotope renogram study and CT are useful techniques in confirming
the diagnosis of obstruction which may not be obvious in the early
stage. When the diagnosis is in doubt, antegrade nephrostogram study
can be done and the nephrostomy tube could be used for the
decompression of the collecting system.

The management of early obstruction is individualized, however,
cystoscopy and minimal invasive procedures or reoperation are
necessary. Cystoscopy should be performed in order to remove
obstructing blood clots or gently attempt for inserting a catheter
into the ureter.

LATE OBSTRUCTION

Lymphocele can be caused most likely due to leakage of lymph from
recipient lymphatic channels. Obstruction from lymphoceles is not
rare and have been reported to occur in 12-18% after renal
transplantation.[8] Ureteral strictures is another cause of late
obstruction which can usually be found at the ureterovesical junction[9]
and can developed from 3 months to 3 1/2 years after transplantation.
Late ureteral obstruction can be also caused by blood clots,[10] rupture
of an intra-renal abscess[10], perinephric abscess obstructing the
ureter,[11] fungus ball[12].

The diagnosis of the ureteral obstruction in the post-transplant period presents as a gradually deterioriation of the renal function which may mimic progressive hydronephrosis[13,14] or chronic rejection.[14,15] I.V.U. periodically is instrumental provided renal function is adequate and ultrasound is an effective examination when a patient is allergic or has poor renal function.[16] Antegrade pyelography is useful not only in defining the point of obstruction but also in treating infection proximal to the obstruction.

The management of late obstruction depends on the causative factor. In case of lymphocele, multiple aspirations have been successful but recurrence and infection can be occurred.[5] Laparoscopic fenestration between lymphocele and peritoneal cavity is an indication for these cases who have failed to resolve.

Ureteral stenosis can be managed by balloon dilation ureteroplasty or incision of the stricture and placement of an indwelling stent. In cases with severe obstruction when antegrade manipulation has failed revisional surgery is required and a second Politano-Leadbetter ureteroneocystostomy can be performed.[4] Successful percutaneous reanastomosis of a transplanted kidney reported by Korth et al.[17]

URINARY FISTULA

Three to ten percent of the patients following renal transplantation will develop urinary fistula which can be divided into primary or secondary after primary urinary obstruction. Urinary leakage is likely to occur in patients whose the vascularization of the ureter has been damaged during donor nephrectomy.[13] Other causes may be necrosis of the ureter or leakage from the ureter-bladder anastomosis or the cystostomy. The development of fistulae within the first week is most likely to occur due to ureteric necrosis or technical failure and those after that time due to chronic ischemia including rejection.

The diagnosis of the leakage can be done by the presenting features as swelling and pain at the area of the allogragt, oliguria or anuria, fever, hypertension and increased level of creatinine. Noninvasive procedures such as radionuclide scans can be used and may reveal extravasation of the isotope in the pelvis. Ultrasound will show collection around the kidney or dilation if obstruction exists.[19] I.V.U. may be obtained cautiously because renal failure may be precipitated.[20] Retrograde pyelography or cystography should be avoided because of complications or infections but these can be used in order to establishing the diagnosis.

Urinary leakage may originate from the cystostomy suture line or from the ureter bladder anastomosis. Fistulae developing within the first week after transplantation is deemed to be technical failure or due to more chronic ischemia including rejection. Waltzer et al[18] reported immediate repair with a three layer bladder closure and prolonged bladder drainage.

Calyceal fistulas as Palmer et al[21] reported are more often seen in cadaveric grafts with multiple renal arteries. Desai et al[22] managed several complications of urological transplant by use of wide drainage. Self retaining stents are useful; to allow the complication to resolve without further surgical intervention, to stabilize the condition before an open operative repair, to protect the high risk anastomosis of the complication.[23] Hunter et al[24] observed that there is a higher incidence of urinary tract infection in the group of patients when the J stent is left for six weeks or more.

STONES

Renal allograft calculus formation is a relatively uncommon

complication, occurring in less than 1 percent of all transplanted kidneys and only 78 cases of urinary caculi in transplanted kidneys reported before 1985.[25] Predisposing factors are secondary hyperparathyroidism, renal tubular acidosis, papillary necrosis, hypercalciuria, hyperoxaluria, nonabsorbable suture material obstruction and recurrent infection.[26] Urinary stents also has resulted in the formation of renal calculi in transplanted kidneys, since an indwelling stent acts as a foreign body and caused encrustations on the stent and then stone formation. Caldwell and Burns[27] reported 4 patients in whom iatrogenic calculi developed because of indwelling stents were used in 2 to correct urological complications after renal transplantation. The authors referred that the difference in the time required to develop complications might well be a function of stent material that the first was of polyurethrane and the second was of silicone.

TREATMENT

Percutaneous antegrade techniques can be adapted for the removal of renal calculi in transplanted kidneys. The pelvic location of the transplant kidney requires a puncture in the anterior abdominal wall. Dilatation of the nephrostomy tract is required allowing insertion of the sheath of the nephroscope for the inspection of the interior of the collecting system. Eshghi and Smith[3] in 1986 described an approach to a staghorn calculus and infundibular stenosis in a transplanted kidney. Other authors reported a case in which combination ESWL and percutaneous extraction were used to remove multiple calculi from a renal allograft.[26] A flexible nephroscope allows inspection of every part of the kidney. It can be passed down the transplanted ureter into the bladder or into an ileal loop. Stone baskets or small grasping forceps may be passed through this flexible instrument to remove smaller stones.

RENAL ARTERY STENOSIS (RTAS)

RTAs have been reported to occur in 5-25% of renal allograft recipients. The etiology of the narrowing is multifactorial[28] and includes progressive atherosclerotic changes in the receipient artery, faulty suture technique, renal artery trauma, secondary to pulsatile perfusion cannuals or donor surgery perfusion injury, turbulent flow secondary to malpositioning of the kidney, kinking or compression of the renal artery and immunologic factors, which may have an influence on the degree of intimal hyperplasia.

The diagnosis can be performed by elevation of the mean serum creatinine and the mean blood pressure can be confirmed by selective arteriography according to Seldinger's method reduced luminal width by at least 60%.[29] Indications for arteriography include severe and drug resistant hypertension within the first year after transplantation converting inhibitor induced renal failure and persistent graft dysfunction in the absence of rejection on biopsy.

Before the development of interventional radiologic techniques surgical procedures were usually required to correct the arterial lesions. These operations have been associated with a 15% graft loss, a 13% reoperation rate and a 5% mortality rate.[30] Percutaneous transluminal angioplasty (PTA) has been the procedure of choice.[31] In a mean follow-up period of 30 months, hypertension was cured or improved in 83% of the patients with functioning kidneys.[31] In patients with mild or moderate azotemia, the improvement in blood pressure is paralleled by a decrease in blood urea and creatinine.[32]

This event was more evident in patients with atheromatous than fibromuscular disease.[32] Brawn and Ramsay[33] concluded from their results that the improvement rates may be spurious and that the "true benefit of PTA may in fact be the cure rate alone." Others[31] reported that only 2.6% of the patients had post PTA stenosis in excess of 75% (76% of patients pre-PTA). The complications of the procedure include vascular thrombosis, initial flap, arterial perforation by the balloon catheter, pseudoaneurysm and artery dissection.[29]

In conclusion, PTA is a safe and convenient procedure in the renal allograft recipient with renovascular hypertension.

REFERENCES

1. Jirasiritham, Kanjanapanjapol, S, Gojaseni, P. et al: Surgical complication in kidney transplantation: experience in 100 kidney transplants at Rouna Thibodi Hospital. Transpl. Proc. 1992 Vol 24, No 4, 1459-1460.

2. Tan, E.C., Lim, S.M.L., Rauff, A.: Techniques of ureteric reimplantation and its related. Urological Complications. An. Acad. Med. 1991 Vol 20:4, pp 524-525.

3. Eshghi, M., Smith, A.D.: Endourologic approach to transplant kidney. Urol. Dec 1986, pp 504-507.

4. Prout, G.R. Jr, Hume, D.M., Lee, H.M., et al: J. Urol; 97-409, 1967.

5. Salvatierra, O. Jr, Olcoh, C.I., Amend, W.J. Jr et al: J. Urol; 1977 117:421.

6. Williams, G., Birth, A.G., Wilson, R.E. et al: Br. J. Urol; 1970 42:21.

7. Helling, T.S., Thomas, C.Y., Jr, Moore, D.J., Koontz, P.G., Jr.: The surgical approach to obstructive problems of the transplant ureter. Trans Proc. Dec 1982 Vol XIV, No 4, pp751-760.

8. Braun, W.E., Banowsky, L.H., Stratton, R.A., et al: Lymphoceles associated with renal transplantation: report of 15 cases and review of the literature. Am. J. Med., 1974 57:714.

9. Starzl, T.E., Groth, C.G., Putnam, C.W. et al: Ann Surg 1970 172:1.

10. Schweizer, R.T., Bourtus, S.A., Kahn, C.S.:
    J. Urol, 1977 117:125.

11. Zorgornicki, J., Schmidt, P., Kotzaurek, R., Kopsa, H:
    Lancet, Feb, 1973, p. 381.

12. Smith, MJV:
    Transplant Proc 1972 4:651.

13. McLoughlin, M.D.:
    J. Urol; 1977 118:1041.

14. Dunningham, T.H.:
    Urology; 1975 6:363.

15. Zinke, H., Woods, J.E., Hattery, R.R., et al:
    Urology; 1977 9:504.

16. Petrek, J. Tillney, H.L., Smith, E.H., et al: Ultrasound in
    renal transplantation. Ann Surg. 1977 185:441.

17. Korth, K., Kuenkel, M.: Percutaneous reanastomosis of transplant
    ureter. Urol; 1988 Vol. 32.

18. Waltzer, W.C., Zincke, H., Leary, F.J., et al: Urinary tract
    reconstruction in renal transplantation. Urol. Sept 1980,
    Vol XVI No 3 pp 233-241.

19. Zincke, H., Woods, J.E., Leary, F.J. et al: Experience with
    lymphoceles after renal transplantation. Surgery; 1975 77:444.

20. Siegle, R.L. and Lieberman, P: A review of untoward reactions
    to iodinated contract material. J. Urol, 1978 119:581.

21. Palmer, J.M. and Chatterjee, S.N.: Urologic complications in
    renal transplantation. Surg. Clin. N. Am., 1978 58:305.

22. Desai Mc. Roberts, J.W., Hellebusch AA, and Luke R.G.:
    Conservative nonoperative management of ureteral
    fistulas following renal allografts. J. Urol. 1970 112:572.

23. Berger, E.R., Ansell, S.J., Treumann, A.J., Herz, H.J.,
    Rottazi, C.L., Marchoro, L.T.: J. Urol; 124:1980, pp 781-782.

24. Hunter, D.W., Castaneda-Zuniga, W.R., Coleman, C.C.,
    Herrera, M., Amplatz, K.: Percutaneous techniques in the
    management of urological complications in renal transplant
    patients. Radiology, 1985 Vol 148, 407-412.

25. Hulbert, J., Pratap, R., Young, A.T., Hunter, D.W., Castaneda,
    Zunica, W., Amplatz, K., Lange, P.H.: The percutaneous removal
    of calculi from transplanted kidneys. J. Urol. 1985 Vol
    134:324-326.

26. Locke, P.R., Steinbock, G., Salomon, D.R., Bezirdjian, L.,
    Peterson, J., Newman, R.C., Kaude, J. and Finlayson: Combination
    ESWL and percutaneous extraction of calculi in a renal allograft.
    J. Urol, 1988, Vol 139 pp 575-577.

27. Coldwell, T.C., Burns, J.R.: Current operative management of urinary calculi after renal transplantation. J. Urol. 1988 Vol 140:1360-1363.

28. Lacombe, M: Arterial stenosis complicating renal allotransplantation in man: A study of 38 cases. Ann Surg. 1975: 182:283.

29. DeMeyer, M., Pirson, Y., Dautrebend, J. et al: Treatment of renal graft arterial stenosis. Transplantation 1980 Vol 47, 784-788, 5.

30. Grossman, R.A., Dafoe, D.C., Schoenfeld, R.B., et al: Percutaneous transluminal angioplasty treatment of renal transplant artery stenosis. Transplantation 1982, 34:339.

31. Greenstein, S.M., Verstanding, A., McLean, K.G., Dafoe, D.C., Burke, D.R., Merdanze, S.G., Naj, A.: Percutaneous transluminal angioplasty. Transplantation; 1987 Vol 43, 1, p 29.

32. Pickering, T.G, Sos, T.A., Laragh, J.H.: Percutaneous angioplasty in renovascular hypertension. Lancet, Jan 1980, pp. 234-235.

34. Brawn, J and Ramsay, E: Lancet, Dec 1988, p 1313.

DILATION OR OPEN SURGERY IN TREATMENT OF URETERAL STENOSIS

G. BENOIT, R. DERGHAM, P. BLANCHET, H. BENSADOUN, B. CHARPENTIER, A. JARDIN

INTRODUCTION

Ureteral stenosis in kidney transplantation is a relatively frequent complication which requires surgical treatment to preserve renal function. In 1981 Goldstein reviewed 4307 kidney transplantations and estimated the incidence of obstruction at 2.6 %. Kinnaert reported an incidence of ureteral obstruction after kidney transplantation which varied between 2 and 7.5 % (7, 11).

The occurence of ureteral stenosis is influenced by the surgical procedure, and is best prevented by using a short ureter and an extravesical procedure for uretero vesical reimplantation (12, 23, 30).

Ureteral obstruction can be diagnosed by ultrasonography when plasma creatinine levels increase, IVP may also be done and the diagnosis may be confirmed by anterograde pyelography.

Today there are two forms of surgical treatment for ureteral stenosis : open surgical techniques or minimally invasive endourological techniques. The aim of this paper is to report the results of these two different therapeutic techniques.

PATIENTS AND METHODS

Between 1978 and 1992, 1500 kidney transplantations were performed in the department of urology and nephrology in Bicêtre hospital. Urinary tract continuity was reestablished by uretero ureteral anastomosis in 111 patients and the remainder underwent ureterocystostomy with the Politano Leadbetter procedure (14) for 811 cases and the Lich Gregoir procedure for 518 patients (31).

In this paper only cases of ureteral stenosis which required surgical correction are studied. Cases of mild upper urinary tract dilation with normal renal function are excluded.

38 patients developped ureteral stenosis (2.5 %) : 3 patients underwent uretero-ureteral anastomosis (2.7 %). 32 were treated with the Leadbetter procedure (3.9 %) and 3 with the extravesical Gregoir procedure (0.5 %).

Services d'urologie et de néphrologie, Hôpital de Bicêtre, Université Paris-Sud, 78 rue du Général Leclerc, 94270 BICETRE CEDEX FRANCE

J. L. Touraine et al. (eds.), Rejection and Tolerance, 175–182.
© 1994 Kluwer Academic Publishers.

The mean diagnosis time of ureteral stenosis after transplantation was 6.5 month (range 9 days - 5 years). In 9 patients the stenosis was located at the ureteropelvic junction and in 8 patients this obstruction was related to the inverted position of the transplanted kidney in line with our procedure for the right kidney at the beginning of our series of locating the renal pelvis anteriorly.

In 29 patients the stenosis was located at the distal ureter, for 2 patients after uretero ureteral anastomosis, in 24 patients after the Leadbetter procedure and in the 3 remaining patients after the Gregoir procedure. The surgical treatment has been changed over the survey of the study. Before 1986 all patients were treated surgically with a transperitoneal approach and anastomosis of the dilated ureter with the ipsilateral native ureter. Since 1986 patients have been treated by a percutaneous approach. Under general anesthesia we place the patient in a position which allows us to puncture the kidney and carry out a cystoscopy at the same time. The convexity of the kidney is punctured under ultrasonography, with a 22 gauge Chiba needle. An anterograde pyelography is performed and we introduce a guide wire into the ureter. The nephrostomy is dilated with a 14 F dilator and we introduce a cobra stent into the renal pelvis to intubate the ureter and a guide wire is pushed beyond the stenotic area. A cystoscopy can be done if necessary to catch the guide wire and facilitate the progression of the balloon catheter through the stenosis. The stenosis is dilated under fluoroscopic control and a double J stent is left in the ureter.

We used a 7 F diameter double J stent in the 14 first patients and in the 7 remaining patients we used a 10 French double J stent. The stent was left in place for 2 months.

The criteria of success is the disappearance of the stasis and the normalisation of renal function.

RESULTS

75 % of the cases of stenosis occured during the first year post transplantation. 17 patients (10 males and 7 females mean age 33.3 years) were treated by open surgery and the mean creatininemia value was 245 µmol/l. 6 cases of stenosis were located at the uretero pelvic junction, and 11 were located in the distal ureter. In 9 patients the stenotic portion of the ureter was removed, and the transplant ureter was reanastomosed with the native one. In 6 cases, the ureter was reimplanted in the bladder and in 2 patients the ureter was freed from external compression. 2 patients have been reoperated for recurrence of stenosis and 6 patients returned to dialysis, 2 after failure of the operative procedure and 4 due to chronic graft rejection .

The mean hospitalisation time was 10 days. The mean time of follow up was 126 months (range : 84-156 months). 11 of the 17 patients have normal renal function with a blood creatinine level at 1 year of 105 µmol/l, at 5 years 115µmol/l and at 10 years 130 µmol/l.

21 patients (14 males, 7 females, mean age 42 years) have been treated with a minimally invasive technique. The mean blood creatinine level

before the operations was 237 µmol/l. 3 cases of stenosis were located at the pyeloureteral junction, and 18 were located at the ureterovesical anastomosis. In one patient it was impossible to intubate the stenosis with the guide wire under radiological control. This was accomplished percutaneously under direct vision with a flexible ureteroscope pushing the guide wire through the stenotic area and pushing it through the cystoscope. On this way it was possible to dilate the stenosis and to introduce a double J stent.

All the endourological procedures have been carried out using a percutaneous approach and anterograde dilation as it is difficult to locate the ureteral orifice in cases of ureteroneocystostomy. In cases of ureteroureterostomy we can easily locate the ureteral meatus by cystoscopic analysis but it is difficult to pull the guide wire to stiffen it. For this reason the dilations have been done percutaneously.

The mean hospitalisation time was 3 days and the mean follow up time was 66 months (range : 12 to 108 months). We have had 9 failures, 3 because of stenosis at the pyeloureteral junction, one because of internal compression and 5 cases of stenosis at the ureterovesical anastomosis. For these 9 patients one was treated percutaneously and 8 by incisional surgery. 14 of the 21 patients have normal renal function (66 %) with a blood creatinine level at 1 year of 105 µmol/l, at 3 - 5 years 115 µmol/l . We lost one kidney because of surgical failure and 6 kidneys were lost by chronic rejection. Our success rate improved over time the beginning of our study : it was 30 % and is now 70 %. 25 of the 38 patients who developped ureteral stenosis after kidney transplantation have normal renal function. 3 kidneys were lost by obstruction and 10 because of chronic rejection. One patient with a functioning kidney died from pulmonary infection by pneumocystis carini.

DISCUSSION

The incidence of ureteral stenosis can be evaluated in different ways. In a previous article (27) we published an incidence rate of betwen 2,5 and 6,5 % according to the incidence of stenosis requiring surgical intervention and the incidence of radiological stasis of the urinary system.

Mundy reports 9 % of stenosis and 6,4 % of severe stenosis based on 1000 transplantations, Oosteroff reports 3,3 % of severe stenosis with 1038 renal grafts and Salvatiera reports 1,1 % of ureteral stenosis based on 860 transplantations (20, 21, 22, 23). The incidence of stenosis in our series according to the type of anastomosis is identical to that of Canton's (pyeloureteral 1,2 %, Leadbetter 5,2 %, Gregoir 2,8 % (3)). The etiology of these stenosis is related to technical problems. Pyeloureteral junction stenosis occurs when the kidney is transplanted in an inverted position (8, 9) and stenosis is ten times more frequent if the ureter is longer (2). We had few cases of stenosis when we utilised the extra vesical Gregoir procedure for ureterovesical reimplantation (12, 30).

75 % of the cases of stenosis were diagnosed during the first year, similar to Thonalla and Canton, whereas Kinnaert reported an increase in the incidence of stenosis from 4,5 % at one year to 9,5 % at 5 years (3, 11, 28).

Stenosis was diagnosed using echographical analysis which shows dilation of the excretory system associated with an increase in the blood creatinine level. In cases of doubt we used a renal scan with DTPA 99 TC and a lasilx® (furosemide) washout test, which was rarely of any use (9). We have no experience of the Whitaker test (19, 29) , because percutaneous nephrostomy of the graft is a simple way for identifying stenosis and assessing renal function and improvement after derivation (6, 15, 29).

Since 1986 we have used endourologic of treatment which is a simple procedure. Open surgery can be used in cases of failure of percutaneous treatment. This minimally invasive treatment has a low morbidity rate. Farah reported one case of arteriovenous fistula at the point of puncture (4). Reviewing our results, we can anticipate some failure with the percutaneous technique. The percutaneous technique with anterograde dilation should not be used in cases of obstruction of the pyeloureteral junction or in cases of external compression of the ureter. If these two conditions are eliminated we observe a decrease in the failure rate (1). The other factor which improved our results was the utilisation of a 10 French double J stent, kept in place for 2 months. In these latter conditions we have had a 70 % success rate, which is comparable to the results of open surgery. The success rates reported in the literature are comparable to our results. Streem reports a 50 % success rate with 8 cases of stenosis, Farah reports a 53 % success rate with 17 cases, Gansbeke reports a 50 % success rate with 6 cases and Jones reports a 83 % success rate wich 38 cases of stenosis with 36 dilations (4, 5, 10, 25).

CONCLUSION

The treatment of stenosis begins with the preservation of the peripyelic and periureteral fat during organ procurement and by using a short ureter reimplanted in the bladder with an extravesical procedure.

Incisional surgical repair is done by anastomosing the transplanted ureter in the native one, which shows a constant success rate. This incisional operation involves a 10 days hospitalisation. Minimally invasive surgery with shorter hospitalisation shows a comparable success rate, if positive indications are selected : i. e. recent distal ureteral stenosis, we can achieve a 70 % success rate with dilation of the stenosis and by maintaining a 10 F double J stent in place tor 2 monthes. The early diagnosis of stenosis is very important and this requires very close urological observation during the first year after kidney transplantation. Minimally invasive anterograde dilation should be the treatment of first choice, in cases of recent ureteral stenosis.

REFERENCES

1. BENOIT G. ICARD Ph., BENSADOUN H., CHARPENTIER B.,
    MOUKARZEL M., JARDIN A., FRIES D.
    Value of antegrade dilation for late ureter obstruction in renal
    transplant
    Transplant int 1989, 2, 33-35

2. BENOIT G., BENARBIA S., BELLAMY J., CHARPENTIER B.,
    FRIES D.
    Complications urologiques de la transplantation rénale : role de
    la longueur de l'uretère
    Presse Med. 1986, 15, 3, 101-104

3. CANTON F., GELET F., BOUDROUF., MARTIN X., SIMILON B.,
    CADI PO., FAURE JL, DUBERNARD JM.
    Les sténoses urétérales après transplantation rénale.
    J. Urol 1987, 93, 3, 117-121

4. FARAH NB., RODDIE M., LORD RHH., WILLIAMS G.
    Ureteric obstruction in renal transplants : the role of
    percutaneous ballon dilatation
    Nephrol Dial Transplant 1991, 6, 677-681

5. GANSBEKE D.V., MATOS C., GENEVOIS P., PAUWL D.,
    STRUYVEN J. KINNAERT P.
    Percutaneous interventional procedures in the management of
    urologic complications of renal transplantation.
    Transplant. Proc. 1987, 19, 1, 2205

6. GLASS NR., CRUMMY AB., FISCHER DT. VEHLING DT,
    LIEBERMAN R., BELZER FO
    Management of ureteral obstruction after transplantation by
    percutaneous antegrade pyelography and pyeloureterostomy.
    Urol. 1982, 20, 15-19

7. GOLDSTEIN I., CHO SI., OLSSON CA.
    Nephrostomy drainage for renal transplant complications.
    J. Urol 1981, 126, 159-163

8. HUNTER DW., CASTANEDA ZUNIGA WR., COLEMAN CC.,
    HERRERA M., AMPLATZ R.
    Percutaneous techniques in the management of urological
    complications in renal transplant patients.
    Radiol 1983, 148, 407-412

180

9. ICARD P., LUMBROSO J. HIESSE C., CHARPENTIER B.,
    FRIES D., HAMMOUDI Y., JARDIN A., BENOIT G.
    Valeur de la scintigraphie au DTPA après injection de furosemide
    dans le diagnostic d'obstacle en transplantation rénale.
    Ann. Urol 1987, 21, 5, 370-374

10. JONES JW., HUNTER DR., MATAS AJ.
    Successful percutaneous treatment of ureteral stenosis after
    renal transplantation.
    Transpl. Proc 1993, 25, 1, 1993

11. KINNAERT P., HALL M., JANSSEN F. VERCERSTRAETEN P.,
    TOUSSAINT G., GEERTRUYDEN JV.
    Ureteral stenosis after kidney transplantation : true incidence
    and long-term follow up after surgical correction
    J. Urol 1985, 133, 17-20

12. KONNAK JW., HERNIG KR., TURCOLLE JG.,
    External uretero neocystostomy in renal transplantation
    J. Urol 1972, 108, 380

13. KORTH K., KUENKEL M.
    Percutaneous reanastomosis of transplant kidney
    Urol 1988, 32, 1, 25-28

14. LEADBETTER GW., MONACO AP., RUSSEL PS.
    A technique for reconstruction of the urinary tract in renal
    transplantation.
    Surg. Gynec. Obtect. 1966, 123, 839

15. LIEBERMAN RP., CRUMMY AB., GLASS NR., BELZER FO.
    Fine needle antergrade pyelography in the renal transplant.
    J. Urol 1981, 126, 155-158

16. LIEBERMAN RP., GLASS NR, CRUMMY AB., SOLLINGER HW.,
    BELZER FO.
    Non operative percutaneous management of urinary fistulas and
    strictures in renal transplantation
    SGO 1982, 155, 667-672

17. LIST AR., BLOHME I., BRYNGER H., NILSON AE.
    Baloon dilatation for ureteral strictures in graft kidneys. A viable
    alternative to further surgery
    Transplantation 1983, 35, 105

18. LOCKE JK., NORMAN NOE H.
Management of obstruction and resultant complications in
transplant kidney by endoscopic and percutaneous techniques.
Urol. 1987, 30, 1, 43-45

19. MITCHELL A., FELLOW GF., WRIGHT FW., MORRIS PJ
Hydronephrosis in a transplanted kidney
Transplantation 1981, 32, 2, 152-153

20. MUNDY AR., PODESTA ML., BEWICK M., RUDGE CJ.,
ELLIS FG.
The urological complication of 1 000 renal transplants
Brit. J. Urol. 1981, 53, 5, 397-402

21. OOSTERHOF G.O.N., HOITSMA AJ., DEBRUYNE FMJ.
Antegrade percutaneous dilation of ureteral strictures after
kidney transplantation.
Transplant Int. 1989, 2, 36-39

22. OOSTERHOF G.O.N., HOITSMA AJ., WITJES JA.,
DEBRUYNE FMJ.
Diagnosis and treatment of urological complications in kidney
transplantation.
Urol Int. 1992, 49, 99-103

23. SALVATIERRA O., OLCOTT C., AMEND WJ., COCHRUM KC.,
FEDUSKA NJ.,
Urological complications of renal transplantations can be
prevented or controlled.
J Urol 1977, 117, 421-424

24. SCHIFF MJr., ROSENFIELD AT., Mc GUIRE EJ.
The use of percutaneous antegrade renal perfusion in kidney
transplant recipients
J. Urol 1979, 122, 246

25. STREEM SB., NOVICK AC., STEIMMULLER DR., ZELCH MF.,
RISIUS B., GEISMGER MA.
Long term efficacy of ureteral dilation for transplant ureteral
stenosis
J. Urol 1988, 140, 32-35

26. TAYLOR RT.
Inflation dilation for long ureteric stricture
Brit. J. Urol. 1985, 467-468

182

27. THIOUN N., BENOIT G., OSPHAL C., CHARPENTIER B.,
    BENSADOUN H., HIESSE C., MOUKARZEL M., NEYRAT N.,
    BELLAMY J., LANTZ O., JARDIN A., FRIES D.
    Complications urologiques en transplantation rénale à propos de
    1 224 malades.
    Progrès Urol 1991

28. THOMALLA JV., LINGERMAN JE., LEAPMAN SD. FILO RS.
    The manifestation and management of late urological
    complications in renal transplant recipients : use of the
    urological armamentarium
    J. Urol. 1985, 134, 944-948

29. TURNER AG., HOWLETT KA, EBAN R. WILLIAMS GB
    The role of anterograde pyelography in the transplant kidney
    J. Urol 1980, 123, 812-814

30. WASNICK RJ., BUTT KMH., LAUNGANI G., SHIRANI K.,
    HONG JH., ADAMSONS RJ., WATERHOUSE K.
    Evaluation of anterior extravesical ureteroneocystostomy in
    kidney transplantation.
    J. Urol 1981, 126, 306-307

31. WITZEL O.
    Extgraperitoneale ureterocystostomie mit Schrägkanalbildung
    Zentralbl Gynaek 1896, 20, 289

RENAL TRANSPLANT ARTERY STENOSIS (RTAS) : DIAGNOSIS AND TREATMENT

Olivier ROUVIERE 1, Jacques WODEY 2, Gilles GENIN 3, Denis LYONNET 1

1. Service de Radiologie, PAV.P Hôpital E. Herriot   69437 LYON Cx 03
2. Service d'Urologie , Pav.V Hôpital E. Herriot 69437 LYON Cx 03
3. Service de Radiologie Hôpital Croix-Rousse 69004 LYON

INTRODUCTION

Renal transplantation is associated with several complications that lead to significant graft loss, patient morbidity and, occasionally, mortality. Among them, vascular complications occur in up to 30 % of the patients (1). The present report studies the renal transplant artery stenosis (RTAS) which is the most frequent vascular complication in renal transplantation (1, 2).

DEFINITION

Its definition varies from an author to another. Some speak of significant stenosis only when the arterial diameter is reduced of 80 % (3) but hemodynamic turbulences appear as soon as the arterial diameter is reduced of 50 % and this is the figure quoted by most authors (4,5).

EPIDEMIOLOGY

As a result of definition differences, its frequency changes a lot according to authors : 1,5 % to 16 % of transplants (1, 3-13). The survey of more than 8.500 transplants found in the literature gave out an average prevalence of 4,72 %.

MECHANISMS AND RISK FACTORS

There are two types of anastomosis of the graft artery : either end-to-end to the hypogastric artery or end-to-side to the external iliac artery. In both cases stenoses can be divided into three categories according to their position as to the anastomosis (14) :

        - preanastomotic on the recipient artery

        - anastomotic on the suture line

        - postanastomotic on the graft artery itself.

Mechanisms of these stenoses are different according to their position. The rarest stenoses are the preanastomotic ones. They are related either to atherosclerotic disease on the recipient arteries or to surgical clamp injuries on these arteries (5, 14, 15).

J. L. Touraine et al. (eds.), Rejection and Tolerance, 183–193.
© 1994 *Kluwer Academic Publishers.*

Most of the time, the etiology of stenoses which are definitely anastomotic is surgical : tight sutures, incomplete intimal approximation, excessive vessel length, twisting of the vascular pedicle (kinking), large discrepancies between the donor and the recipient arterial size. They can also be related to local reactions to suture material (3, 5, 12, 14, 16, 17). A few cases of anastomotic stenoses related to rejection have been noticed (10, 14).

The main cause of postanastomotic stenoses is acute or chronic rejection. The histologic changes in the stenosed arteries shows subintimal fibrosis and intimal proliferation as in the vascular lesions of rejection, and immunoglobulin and complement nodular deposits have been found in stenosed arterial walls (3, 10-13, 17).
Disturbed hemodynamics beyond anastomoses, especially those beyond end-to-side anastomoses, have also been incriminated (17). At last, surgical injuries of the graft artery can entail postanastomotic strictures : clamp injury, graft perfusion catheter injury, excessive dissection around graft artery leading to the destruction of the vasa vasorum (3, 5).

Suitable knowledge of all these mechanisms enable us to define risk factors of RTAS. Stenoses occur more often in the case of cadaver graft in which rejection reactions are stronger (5, 6, 12, 13). They are more frequent in case of transplantation from a child donnor to an adult recipient or when there are polar arteries : in both cases, surgical difficulties are more important (5, 9). The frequency of stenosis is similar in case of end-to-end anastomosis and in case of end-to-side anastomosis. But stenosis occur predominantly at the anastomosis with end-to-end anastomosis and beyond the anastomosis with end-to-side anastomosis (3, 5).

SIGNS AND SYMPTOMS
RTAS essentially entails severe hypertension, often reluctant to medical treatment, either alone or associated to a moderate renal function impairment (2, 3, 9-12, 14).

However, it is estimated that about 50 % of graft recipients exhibit hypertension and there is a number of other causes of hypertension and/or renal function impairment in them. The main ones are : acute or chronic rejection, ATN, hypertension caused by the native kidneys, reccurence of the original renal disease on the transplant, steroid or cyclosporin-induced hypertension, ureteral obstruction or preexisting essential hypertension (4, 7, 12, 14, 16, 18).

In some cases, an arterial bruit is heard over the transplant. This sign has but little worth as its presence is not necessary. It also can be heard just because of disturbed hemodynamics beyond the anastomosis with no significant stenosis. However, the appearance of such a bruit which did not exist just after the transplantation certainly has a more important diagnostic value (2, 3, 10, 12).

DIAGNOSIS

Today, the screening for RTAS depends on Color Doppler Sonography. It allows to visualize and to quantify the degree of the stenosis especially if it is localized on the main arterial pedicle (14). A recent survey found a sensibility and a specificity rate of 95 % and 92 % for the detection of pedicular complications and of 77 % and 100 % for the detection of intra renal vascular complications (19).

The color doppler sonography is not only a good screening test but also allows to estimate the efficiency of the treatment of the RTAS by radiological dilatation or by surgery.

In all cases, an intra arterial angiography allows the diagnosis of RTAS. It is the most accurate imaging technique for the evaluation of renal artery stenoses. It clearly depicts the three types of stenoses and is considered the gold standard for quantification of degree of stenosis and demonstration of multiple stenoses. It is usually performed with intra arterial digital substraction and a low quantity of contrast media (2, 14).

Even if the graft recipient exhibit hypertension and a significant RTAS, it doesn't mean that the artery stenosis is the only cause of hypertension since there is a number of other causes of hypertension in graft recipients. Some authors advised to perform selective renin evaluation in the graft vein (20) but in most authors' experience, those determinations didn't seem to be helpful. Some patients with severe hypertension corrected by surgery of the stenosis had normal renin values. In the opposite, some patients without hypertension or with chronic rejection can exhibit high renin values (10, 13, 21). Therefore, those determinations are rarely performed. Some authors also advised to perform systematic renal biopsy before treating a RTAS to rule out chronic rejection (3). Indeed, treating a RTAS associated with severe chronic rejection would be useless. However, renal biopsy can be dangerous in hypertensive patients.

WHEN TO SEAK FOR A RTAS ?

The development delay of RTAS varies a lot but it usually appears in the year following the transplantation (median delay : 12 months) (3, 14).

As a number of graft recipients exhibit hypertension, it seems to us that seaking for a RTAS should be reserved for patients with specific hypertensive profils such as newly developped hypertension or marked hypertension resistant to medical therapy associed or not with declining renal function (2, 3, 9-13, 21).

TREATMENT

There are 3 main therapeutic possibilities : either a simple antihypertensive medical treatment, or an invasive therapy (radiological or surgical).

Medical treatment

The efficiency of the medical treatment of RTAS is difficult to estimate because there are only few data about it. Deglise-Favre et al (22) studied 40 RTAS bearing patients, all treated medically with a mean follow-up period of 60 months. During this period, only 7 grafts were lost, 6 from chronic rejection and only one from graft artery thrombosis. The BP and the renal function have been controled in the 33 other patients all along the follow-up period. Others found similar results with, however, less patients (table 1)(1, 12, 23). Beside to arterial thrombosis, the other graft losses were related either to chronic rejection or to hypertension because the patients were not compliant to the treatment.

Thus, the medical treatment can allow a prolonged graft survical. But it's a treatment for life, associating several anti hypertensive drugs and one of the risk is that patients become non compliant to the therapy. The decrease of blood pressure (BP) induced by the treatment may also entail thrombosis of very tight stenoses. So, when the stenosis is very tight, most authors advise an invasive therapy even if BP is controlled by the medical treatment.

Percutaneous transluminal angioplasty (PTA)

PTA have been developped since 1979 (16) but a number of technical improvments have occured since that time. The main difficulties are related to the type (anastomotic stenoses are often fibrous and difficult to dilate), the degree (the catheter can't pass throught some very tight stenoses) or the site of stenoses (the stenoses localized in a curve or involving an end-to-end anastomosis to the hypogastric artery are more difficult to reach).

There are many publications about the results of PTA on RTAS (1, 4, 6-8, 18, 23-28). The table 2 shows the results of the main ones with a total number of 222 PTA. Technical successes were defined as PTA leading to the disapearance of any significant stenosis. The technical success rates are almost the same in all the studies (mean : 79 %). Today, those rates should be better because of technical improvments. The short-term clinical success rates (estimated on the disapearance of stenosis and the control of BP, 1 month later) are also similar for every author and rather good (mean : 81,1 %). However, the middle-term clinical success rates are very different from one author to another. They were evaluated after an average follow-up period of 1 to 3 years. Some authors found very good middle-term success rates (more than 80 %) but others found very low rates (20 to 40 %). These differencies can't be explained by differencies in follow-up and are probably related to the type of stenosis. For example, Roberts et al. dilated a number of anastomotic stenoses to the hypogastric artery which are known to be difficult to dilate (7). The average middle-term success rate was 58,2 % for a mean follow-up period of 2 years.

	Number of patients	Good results	Graft losses	Follow-up (months)	Reference
Deglise-Favre (1991)	40	33	7 (1)	60	22
Jordan (1982)	5	3	2 (1)	ND	1
Whiteside (1982)	5	4	1 (1)	50	23

(ND : Not Determined)

Table 1 : RTAS : Results of medical treatment.

(The figures put in brackets indicate the graft losses directly related to RTAS.)

	Number of patients	Technical success	Clinical success		Reference
			Short-term (1 month)	Middle-term (1 to 3 years)	
Benoît (1991)	49	69,4 %	ND	40,8 %	25
De Meyer (1989)	17	82,4 %	ND	74 %	6
Roberts (1989)	22	ND	ND	22,8 %	7
Greenstein (1987)	39	84,6 %	84,8 %	69,4 %	4
Raynaud (1986)	43	81,4 %	74 %	67 %	26
Mollenkopf (1983)	17	76,5 %	92,3 %	83,3 %	27
Grossman (1982)	17	88,2 %	ND	86,7 %	8
Our data	18	77,8 %	78,9 %	37,5 %	
Total	222	79 %	81,1 %	58,2 %	

(ND : Not Determined)

Table 2 : RTAS : Results of PTA.

	Numbers of patients	Mean serum creatinine			Reference
		Before PTA	After PTA	p	
Raynaud (1986)	32	165	153	NS	26
Mollenkopf (1983)	4	329	130	< .05	27
Grossman (1982)	13	164	147	< .01	8
Whiteside (1982)	4	208	138	< .05	23
Our data	13	283	173	< .05	

(NS : Not Significant)

Table 3 : RTAS : Effects ot PTA on renal function.

	Restenosis	New PTA	Success	Failure	Reference
Benoît (1991)	28,6 %	8	5	3	25
De Meyer (1989)	23,1 %	ND	ND	ND	6
Roberts (1989)	31,8 %	3	0	3	7
Greenstein (1987)	7,7 %	3	0	3	4
Raynaud (1986)	20 %	6	4	2	26
Mollenkopf (1983)	16,4 %	2	2	0	27
Grossman (1982)	0 %	–	–	–	8
Our data	50 %	6	4	2	
Total	21,5 %	28	15	13	

(ND : Not Determined)

Table 4 : RTAS : Restenosis after PTA.

	Number of patients	Middle-term success
Patch angioplasty	61	73,8 %
Resection-reanastomosis (direct)	69	87 %
Resection-reanastomosis (indirect)	21	76,2 %
Crossed reanastomosis (direct or indirect)	58	86,2 %
Venous or arterial bypass	63	74,7 %
Arteriolysis	11	45,5 %
Dacron bypass	5	80 %
Total	288	78,8 %

Table 5 : RTAS : Results of surgical repair.

So, even if the technical success and short-term clinical success rates are very good, there is a results degradation with the time going on.

An accurate evaluation of the effects of PTA on renal function is difficult. Renal function may improve as soon as the day after PTA. In other patients it remains stable. A transient decline in renal function after PTA possibly due to the toxicity of contrast media may occur. One month after, the effects of contrast media have diseappered but rejection may have occured and caused impairment of renal function. One the other hand, some anti hypertensive drugs may be discontinued and renal impairment related to these drugs is diminished. However, most of the time, the drop in serum creatinine level is significant but the number of patients studied is very low (table 3) (8, 23, 26, 27).

Many middle-term PTA failures are related to restenosis. Those restenoses occur between 2 months and 2 years after the PTA. Their prevalence is about 20 %. More than one half of the restenoses reported in the literature could be successfully dilated by a new PTA (table 4) (4, 6-8, 25-27)

There is a wide variety of potential complications of PTA related to the arterial puncture (groin hematoma), the contrast media (ATN) or the catheterism (main or polar artery thrombosis or dissection). The overall morbidity rate is between 5 % and 28 % according to authors (8, 26, 29). In case of arterial thrombosis induced by PTA, some grafts could be saved thanks to immediate intra arterial fibrinolysis throught the dilatation catheter (26). Thus, the average graft loss rate is only 4,8 %. No mortality related to PTA has been noticed.

Vascular surgery

There are many surgical procedures. The most used are resection-reanastomosis techniques : the stenosed aera is resected and reanastomosed either directly or throught a venous autograft. The reanastomosis can be done on the same iliac artery or crossed (done on the other iliac artery of the same side : external iliac artery if it was on the hypogastric artery and vice-versa). In saphenous or arterial bypass, the stenosed aera is only bypassed and not resected. Patch angioplasty is essentially used for anastomotic stenoses. A venous graft is inserted in the arterial wall to increase the arterial diameter. Dacron bypass or arteriolysis (lysis of peri arterial adhesions) are less used procedures (3, 6, 9, 10, 12, 13, 17, 23, 24)

The table 5 shows the review of 288 surgical repairs of RTAS from the literature. The middle-term success rates evaluated on the control of BP, 1 to 3 years after surgery, are similar for all procedures (about 80 %). The only one to show a lower rate is arteriolysis (45 %). This is probably because peri arterial adhesions are rarely the only cause of RTAS.

The renal function is improved in 66 % to 100 % of the patients. The drop in creatinine level is similar to that observed after PTA (6, 17, 24).

The rate of restenosis is less than that observed with PTA (0 % to 15 % according to authors). The appearance delay is the same (2 months to 2 years) (3, 6, 7, 13, 23-25).

The overall surgical morbidity rate is between 5 % to 30 % wich is similar to that observed with PTA. But the mortality is greater (up to 7 %) (23, 25). The review of 272 surgical repairs in the literature also shows a greater graft loss rate (11 %)

In summary...

Surgery seems to be more efficient especially in middle-term studies, with a lower restenosis rate. PTA seems to be less dangerous (without any mortality and with a lower graft loss rate). However, no randomised study have been done to suitably compare these two invasive techniques.

CONCLUSION : which treatment for RTAS?

Medical treatment should always be used and even should be tried alone when the stenosis is not very tight. In case of tight stenoses, an invasive therapy should be proposed.

Some authors prefer surgery because it is more efficient, especially in long-term sudies (30). But the majority think PTA should be tried first because it is less dangerous (no mortality and lower graft losses rate) (4, 6, 8, 23, 26-28).

In case of failure of PTA or restenosis, a surgical repair or a new PTA should be discussed (50 % of the restenoses can be successfully redilated).

Today, a third possibility is appearing : the percutaneous stent. We have placed a stent in one case of recurrent stenosis, incompletely   dilated by PTA. One month later, the clinical results were good. However, more follow-up and further studies are requested to evaluate the efficiency of such a therapy.

The anastomotic stenoses (difficult to dilate) or the stenoses localised in a curve (difficult to recah) should benefit of surgery because of the poor results of PTA in thoses cases (4, 7, 8, 31).

1.   Jordan ML, Cook GT, Cardella CJ : Ten years of experience with vascular complications in renal transplantation. J Urol 1982;128:689-692.
2.   Beachley CB, Pierce JC, Boykin JV, Lee HM : The angiographic evaluation of human renal allotransplants: functional graft deterioration and hypertension. Arch Surg 1976;111:134-142.
3.   Tilney NL, Rocha A, Strom TB, Kirkman RL : Renal artey stenosis in transplant patients. Ann Surq 199;454-460.
4.   Greenstein SM, Verstandig A, McLean GK, Dafoe DC, Burke DR, Meranze SG, Naji A, Grossman RA, Perloff LJ, Barker CF : Percutaneous transluminal angioplasty, the procedure of choice in the hypertensive renal allograft recipient with renal artery stenosis. Transplantation1987;43:29-32.
5.   Stanley P, Malekzadeh M, Diament MJ : Posttransplant renal artery stenosis: angiographic study in 32 children. AJR 1987;148:487-490.
6.   DeMeyer M, Pirson Y, Dautrebande J, Squifflet JP, Alexandre PJ, Van Ypersele de Strihou C :Treatment of renal graft artery stenosis, comparison between surgical bypass and percutaneous transluminal angioplasty. Transplantation 1989;47:784-788.
7.   Roberts JP, Ascher NL, Fryd DS, Hunter DW, Dunn DL, Payne WD, Sutherland DER, Castaneda)Zuniga W, Najarian JS : Transplantation 1989;48:580-583.
8.   Grossman RA, Dafoe DC, Shoenfeld RB, Ring EJ, McLean GK, Oleaga JA, Freiman DB, Naji A, Perloff LJ, Barker CF: Percutaneous transluminal angioplasty treatment of renal transplant artery stenosis. Transplantation 1982;34:339-343.
9.   Munda R, Alexander JW, Miller S, First MR, Fidler JP : Renal allograft artery stenosis. Am J Surg 1977;134:400-403.
10. Dickerman RM, Peters PC, Hull AR, Curry TS, Atkins C, Fry WJ : Surgical correction of posttransplant renovascular hypertension. Ann Surg 1980;192:639-644.
11. Schacht RA, Martin DG, Karalakulasingam R, Wheeler CS, Lansing AM : Renal artery stenosis after renal transplantation. Am J Surg 1976;131:653-657.
12. Doyle TJ, McGregor WR, Fox PS, Maddisson FE, Rodgers RE, Kauffman HM : Homotransplant renal artery stenosis. Surgery 1975;77:53-60.
13. Lacombe M : Arterial stenosis complicating renal allotransplantation in man. Ann Surg 1975;181:283-288.
14. Dodd III GD, Tublin ME, Zajko AB : Imaging of vascular complications associated with renal transplants. AJR 1991;157:449-459.
15. Weigele JB : Iliac artery stenosis causing renal allograft-mediated hypertension: angiographic diagnosis and treatment. AJR 1991;157:513-515.
16. Diamond NG, Casarella WJ, Hardy MA, Appel GB : Dilatation of critical transplant renal artery stenosis by percutaneous transluminal angioplasty. AJR 1979;133:1167-1169.

17. Smith RB, Cosimi AB, Lordon R, Thompson AL, Ehrlich RM : Diagnosis and management of arterial stenosis causing hypertension after succesfulrenal transplantation. J Urol 1976;115:639-642

18. Curry NS, Cochran S, Barbaric ZL, Schabel SI, Pagani JJ, Kangarloo H, Diament M, Gobien RP, Vujic I : Interventional radiologic procedures in the renal transplant. Radiology 1984;152:647-653.

19. Grenier N, Douws C, Morel D, Ferriere JM, Le Guillou M : Detection of vascular complications in renal allograft with color doppler flow imaging. Radiology 1991;178:217-223.

20. Lindfors O, Laasonen L, Fyhrquist F, Kock B, Lindström B : Renal artery stenosis in hypertensive renal transplant recipients. J Urol 1977;118:240-243.

21 Boyer L, Viallet JF : Angioplastie transluminale percutanée des sténoses artérielles rénales. Aulnay-sous-Bois: Guerbet, 1992: 58-62.

22 Deglise-Favre A, Hiesse C, Lantz O, Moukarzel M, Bensadoun H, Benoît G, Charpentier B, Fries D : Sténoses de l'artère du rein greffé: évolution spontanée de 40 cas. Presse Méd. 1991;20:2048-2049.

23 Whiteside CI, Cardella CJ, Yeung H, De Veber GA, Cook GT : The role of percutaneous transluminal dilatation in the treatment of transplant renal artery stenosis. Clin Nephrol 1982;17:55-59.

24. Benoît G, Hiesse C, Icard P, Bensadoun H, Bellamy J, Charpentier B, Jardin A, Fries D : Treatment of renal artery stenosis after renal transplantation. Transplant Proc 1987;19:3600-3601.

25. Benoît G, Moukarzel M, Hiesse C, Bensadoun H, Neyrat N, Charpentier B, Jardin A, Fries D, Bellamy J : Sténoses de l'artère du rein transplanté : place des dilatations endoluminales. Presse Méd. 1991;20:2045-2047.

26. Raynaud A, Dedrossian J, Remy P, Brisset JN, Angel CY, Gaux JC : Percutaneous transluminal angioplasty of renal transplant arterial stenosis. AJR 1986;146:853-857.

27. Mollenkopf F, Matas A, Veith FJ, Sprayregen S, Soberman R, Kuemmel P, Tellis VA, Sniderman K, Sos T, Cheigh JS, Stubenbord W : Percutaneous transluminal angioplasty for transplant renal artery stenosis. Transplant Proc 1983;15:1089-1091.

28. Reisfeld D, Matas AJ, Tellis VA, Sprayragen S, Bakal C, Soberman R, Glicklich D, Veith FJ : Late follow-up of percutaneous transluminal angioplasty for treatment of transplant renal artery stenosis. Transplant Proc 1989;21:1955-1956.

29 Medina M, Butt KMH, Gordon DH, Thanwala S, Solomon N : A complication of percutaneous transluminal angioplasty in the transplanted kidney. Urol Radiol 1981; 3:59-61.

30 Lacombe M : Les sténoses artérielles des reins transplantés : quatre-vingt six cas opérés. Chirurgie 1990;116:848-855.

31. Chandrasoma P, Aberle AM : Anastomotic line renal artery stenosis after transplantation. J Urol 1986;135:1159-1162.

Urinary fistula as a complication of renal transplantation

Albalate P, Molina G, Feitosa LC, Martin X, Dubernard JM.

1 - SUMMARY

1.1 Patients and results

From January 1988 to December 1992, 791 renal transplantations were made by the transplantation department of the Edouard Herriot hospital. Among those, 130 were kidney-panceas transplantations.

The urinary fistula, as a complication of the transplantation, appeared on 23 patients (2.9 %) : 20 fistulas were located at the uretero-vesical anastomosis, 2 at the bladder and 1 at the pelvis.

Among the wole, 4 occured on kidneys with a severed lower polar artery, on 2 patients the anastomosis was carried out on small ans fragile bladders and, in 1 case, the urethra showed sings of serious trauma. The other kidneys were macroscopically normal.

The GREGORY anastomosis was the most frequently used : on 20 patients. On 2 other patients the anastomosis was a LEADBETTER. On 1 other patient the anastomosis was a uretero-ureteral with a clean ureteral.

All fistulas appeared during the first month following the transplantation.

The flow of urine by drainage is the most frequent symptom (10 pantients). Next is pain accompanied by a swell of the operated area (5 patients). Other symtoms were reported but much less frequently.

1.2 Patients and Treatments

On 8 patients, an urgent cystography was the only examination made, and its usage associated with and echography (3 patients) an a scanner (6 patients).

The pyelography by nephrostomic probe was used on 4 patients. Other examinations were made but with less frequency.

The endoscopic treatment, wich consists of a nephrostomia ans the fitting ofa double J probe, was appplied to 10 patients. The basic endoscopy, wtith the fitting of a double J probe was carried out on 3 patients. 4 LEADBETTER and 1 PAQUIN transplantations were made.

1 patient underwent the elargment of the bladder and intestine by the fitting of a nephrostomic probe.

2- INTRODUCTION

The urinary fistula is a serious complication of the renal transplantation. The frequency of the type of complication ranges from 3 to 10 %, although SALVATIERRA (1) reports only 1.7 % in a series of 860 renal transplantations. GOLDSTEIN (2) reports 4.7 % in a series of 4307 transplantations.

J. L. Touraine et al. (eds.), Rejection and Tolerance, 195–198.
© 1994 *Kluwer Academic Publishers. Printed in the Netherlands.*

NOVIC (3) a rate of 3.5 % in series published in 1981 and 1989. But other authors such a TILNEY (4) and FOX (5) report up to 12 %.

Nevertheless, the frequency of urinary fistulas has decreased these last years due to improvements in surgery and to the use of new immuno-suppressive drugs which reduces the doses of steroids. however, the urinary fistula is complication very difficult to eradicate since in most cases its etiopatholigy is related to the vascular deficiency of the excretory path.

This document proposes the sudy of the frequency of the urinary fistulas in our department ant the treatments used.

3- PATIENTS AND METHODS

From january 1988 to December 1992, 791 renal transplantations were made by the transplantation department of the Edouard herriot hospital. Among those, 130 were kidney-pancreas transplantations.

All patient files reporting urinary fistulas as a complication to renal transplantation were studied. The following criteria wereselected : age, characteristics of the removed kidney, presence or not an immediate dieresis, symptomatology, date of appearance of fistulas, the type of examnination made for diagnostic, location of the fistulas ans treatment given.

4- DISCUSSION

The urinary fistula as a complication to renal transplantations occurs during 23 transp^lantations among the 791 made by our department these last 5 years.

This result is 2.9 % lower than SALVATIERRA's (1.7 %) (1) and OOSERHOFF's (7), but higher those published by most authors who rreport rates ranging from 3 to 10 % (8,9,10).

This serious complication, determined by number of global factors (such as uraemia, amenia, hypoproteinemia and immunosuppression) and local factors (vascular deficiency of the urethra) leads to a high morbi-mortality as highlighted by SHIFF (11) who reports rates of 30 % of transplant loss and 25 % of mortality in his own series. SPIGOS (12) reports 34 % of loss and 13 % mortality.

Our series shows that fistulas appeared on 5 patients following urethra vascularisation problems, on 3 patients with small and fragiles bladders. The rest of the fistulas (16 of them-65 %) appeared on macroscopically normalkidneys.

This implies eventual technical errors but most of all the importance og global factors in the pathogen of urinary fistulas

Anyhow, we condider that the lower polar sessels must be absoluted respected ant that the dissection of the ilio-renal must be undertaken very carefully during removal.

20 fistulas (86.9 %) occured on patients treated by anastomosis by the GREGORY technique (the one we use the most), 2 (8.6 %) treated by LEADBETTER technique and 1 (4.3 %) by ureteo-ureteral anastomosis with clean urethra.

95.6 % of the patients showed immediate dieresis although we do not condider this as a significant factor in urinary fistulas. It is not even mentioned by some of the authors we have referred to previously.

All fistulas appeared during the first month following the transplantation although some were early :

7 (30.4 %) during the first 24 hours and 11 (47.8 %) during the first 7 days. Similar figures are produced by CRUZ NAVARRO (14) with even 3 fistulas cases developing 3 months after the operation.

Frome a clinical point of vue, the most frequent event is a flow of urune by drainage (46.4 %). Then comes a swell of the operated area with abdominal pain (5 patients - 21.7 %). Other effects such as scrotal oedema, anuria and a rise of creatrinine were less frequent.

The technique the most frequnatly used for diagnostics was the cystography used on 8 patients (34.7 %).

Then follows the cystography in association with a scanner (6 patients - 26 %) or in association with a echography and an intra-veinal urography (3 patients - 13 %). Also, 4 pyelographies by nephrostomy probe were made (17.3 %). In 2 cases we made an urgent cystoscopy which was enough to make the diagnostic.

These techniques allow, not only to confirm the diagnostic of fistula, but also their location and their expansion. It is not necessary to use all these techniques to do a diagnostic : it is sufficient to use those that will confirm it being at the same time the less agressive as possible.

20 (89.9 %) fistulas were located by the urethra, 2 (8.6 %) by the bladder and 1 (4.3 %) by the pelvis. The treatment was endodcopical for 34.7 % of the patients. In 30.4 % of the cases (7 patients) a LEADBETTER type transplantation was made, in 8.6 % (2 patients) we once again did a GREGORY transplantation and 1 PAQUIN type. For 17.3 % of the patients (4) the reimplantation was pyelo-ureteral with a clean urethra. In once case the receiver had a small and weak bladder : we enlarged the bladder ant the small intestine by fitting a nephrostomy probe.

There is no unique solution to the treatment of urinary fistulas as a complication of renal trasplantation. Some authors advise urology endoscopitechniques at the beginning : nephrostomy percutane and drainage of the urinome, followed by surgical repair if required (15,16,17). Others advise open surgery as the first step (14,18). As for us, we condider that endoscopic surgery is very important in dealing with urinary fistulas, under the condition that the surgery be clearly defined.

Also, we think that in case of suspected fistulas immediate medico-surgery action must be undertaken. When fistulas are large or numerous, we recommend open surgery. for small calicial leaks of obstructive origin, for pyelo-ureteral fistulas with minor necrosis and for small fistulas at the uretero-vesical anastomosis level, we recommend, to begin with, an endoscopic treatment : open surgery would then be used in case of failure.

CONCLUSION

1. urinary fistulas as a complication to renal transplantation appeared on 2.9 % of our patients.

2. Vascular disruptions of the urethra are a predominant factor in the pathogen of this complication.

3. Most fistulas appeared during the first week and all of them within the first month.

4. A medico-surgery attitude must be the response to urinary fistulas thus reducing the morbi-mortality on this serious complication.

5. Endoscopic surgery plays an important role in the treatment of urinary fistulas. Someimes as a definitive treatment and sometimes to improve the renal function and proceed later on to definitive surgery.

BIBLIOGRAPHY

SALVATIERRA O, OLEON C, ET AL. urological complications of renal transplantations can be prevented or controlled. J Urol. 1977;117:421.

GOLDSTEIN I, OLSON C ET AL. Nephrostomy drainage for renal transplant complications. J Urol. 1981;126-159.

NOVICK AC. Surgery of renal transplantations and complications, in vascular problems urologie. Surgery. 1982;233.

TILNEY NL. Surgical considerations of renal transplantations, in surgical care of patient in renal failure. TILNEY NL, Lazarus. JM Philadelphia, Saunders 1982;184.

FOX MD, TOTTECHAN MD. Urinary fistula from segmental infarctions in a transplanted kidney : recovery following surgical repair. J Urol. 1972;44:336.

RIOJA S, GUTIERREZ C. Complicaciones quirurgicas del transplante renal progresors en urologia Cap. 1993; 33:319-329.

OOSTERHOF GO, HOITSMA . Diagnosis and treatment of urological complications in kidney transplantations. Urol. Int. 1992;49:99-103.

BENORT G, THIOUNN N. Les complication urologiques des transplantations. Pace de techniques endo-urologiques. Pressse Med. 1991 nov 27;20.

ISA WA ROBLES JE. Urologic complications in 237 recipients of cadaveric kidney transplantation. Actas. Urol. Espa. 1991 Jul-Aug;15:351-6.

LAUNOIS B, BARDAXOGLOU E. Urologx complications after 333 kidney transplantation chirurgic. 1990;116:283-8, discussion 228-9.

SCHIFF M JR, RODENFIELD AT. Managmen of urinary fistulas after renal transplantation. J. Urol. 1990;155-251.

SPIGOS DG, TAN W ET AL.Dagnosis of urine extravasation after renal transplantation. ASR. 1991;129-409.

NICHOLSON ML, VEITP S ET AL. Urological complication of renal transplantation. Ann R Coll Surg Engl. 1991;73:316.

NAVARRO C MONTANES M ET AL. Fistulas urinarias en el transplante renal. Progresos en urologia. 1993;330-338.

ROMERO T, GUTIERREZ S ET AL. THE endourological treatment of distal ureteral fistula in the kidney transplant. The exclusion or "dry" technic. Arch. Esp. Urol. 1992 May;45:359-62.

CHANTABA A, GOMEZ V. Long Term results of conservatives treatment of ureteral fistulas. Arch. Esp. Urol. 1991 Nov;44:1075-80.

HEFTY THOMAS R. Complications of renal transplantation : The praticing urologists role. AUZA Update Series. 1991X: lesson 8.

GIL-VERNET JM. Cirurgia del transplante renal. 1984;18:175-206.

Endoscopic treatment of vesicoureteric reflux in own kidneys of renal transplant candidates and transplanted kidneys

P. Cloix, X. Martin, A. Gelet, J.M. Dubernard.

Service d'Urologie et Chirurgie de la Transplantation
Hopital E Herriot - Place d'Arsonval 69437 Lyon Cedex
France

INTRODUCTION

Vesico-ureteric reflux (VUR) is a risk factor for the development of acute or chronic urinary tract infections (UTI) in transplant recipients. In the early years of renal transplantation, the treatments commonly described were nephroureterectomy for native kidneys or ureteral reimplantation for kidney transplants. Surgical management was indicated in massive or symptomatic VUR.

The first injections of polytetrafluoroethylene (PTFE) or Teflon paste in the treatment of VUR were realized by Matouschek in 1981 (1). The advantages of this endoscopic treatment are the low rate of morbidity avoiding the difficulties and complications of an open surgical approach and an easy fulfilment with short-lasting anesthesia. Endoscopic treatment of VUR by submucosal

199

J. L. Touraine et al. (eds.), Rejection and Tolerance, 199–210.
© 1994 *Kluwer Academic Publishers.*

injection of Teflon paste is effective in 80 to 95 % of native refluxing ureters (2,3). This technique can also be applied to replanted ureters (4). We report our experience with this technique in VUR in haemodialysis patients waiting for renal transplantation and in transplanted refluxing ureters.

MATERIAL AND METHODS

Between January 1986 and July 1991, 3 groups of patients were investigated. Group 1 consisted of 28 haemodialysis patients (15 males ; mean age 41,5 years, ext 15-63) with VUR waiting for renal transplantation, group 2 consisted of 11 renal transplant patients (8 males ; mean age 38 years-ext 14-60) with endoscopically treated native VUR prior to transplantation, group 3 consisted of 30 patients (16 males ; age 17 to 60-mean 42.0 years) presenting a VUR in the transplanted kidney.

Group 1 and group 2 represent respectively 47 VUR including 19 bilateral VUR and19 VUR including 7 bilateral VUR. Grading of VUR was established according to the international classification (5). The ureters with low grade were injected in cases of controlateral high-grade VUR or when the patient had recurrent UTI. In group 1 there was 5 grades I, 8 grades II, 22 grades III, 8 grades IV and 4 grades V ; in group 2 there was 1 grade I, 7 grades II, 6 grades III, 5 grades IV. In group 3, the reflux was grade II in 9 cases, grade III in 16 cases and grade

recurrent UTI. In group 1 there was 5 grades I, 8 grades II, 22 grades III, 8 grades IV and 4 grades V ; in group 2 there was 1 grade I, 7 grades II, 6 grades III, 5 grades IV. In group 3, the reflux was grade II in 9 cases, grade III in 16 cases and grade IV in 5 cases. The correction of VUR was indicated in group 1 & 2 because of recurrent UTI in 18 cases and high-grade VUR in 10 cases. The VUR was diagnosed by retrograde cystography at the pretransplant medical visit or for patients of group 3, it was diagnosed in 22 patients with reccurent urinary tract infections (UTI) and for renal function deterioration in 6 patients. In 2 cases VUR was suspected because of recurrent pain of the graft. The technique used for reimplantation were the extravesical technique derived from the method of De Campos-Freire (6) in 28 cases and a Leadbetter-Politano replantation in 2 cases (LP).

For the group 1 and 2, mean durations of haemodialysis were respectively 48 months (ext 6-120 mo) and 50 months (ext 2-144 mo). The mean durations between respectively the endoscopic treatment and kidney transplantation (group 2) and kidney transplantation and the endoscopic treatment (group 3) were 13,4 months (ext 2-35 mo) and 3,12 years (ext 0,5-11 years).

The technique used was derived from that described by Puri and O'Donnell (7). The procedure was performed under general anaesthesia. The ureteric orifice was first identified and an endoscopic needle was introduced between the ureter and the detrusor. Polytef paste diluted in glycerin (3/1 vol) was then injected. The mean amont in groups 1 & 2 and group 3 were respectivelly 2,1 ml (ext 1 to 6) and 2.5 ml (ext 1.5 to 10). Identification of the ureteral orifice in groups 1 & 2 was difficult because the detrusor walls became sclerotic and atrophic with long-lived haemodialysis and low urine output. In group 3, needle puncture of the orifice was difficult in 14 cases due to the site of the reimplantation and the orientation of the ureter. The easiest cases being those where reimplantation was on the fixed part of the bladder. The patients were discharged the following day after renal ultrasound was performed to exclude renal dilatation.

Iterative endoscopic treatments were performed in 5 cases in group 1, 3 cases in group 2 and 8 cases in group 3. The standard voiding cystographies was performed post-injection at 1 month systematically and a second injection was done in case of failure. If the VUR was not cured and was classified as high-grade, a nephroureterectomy was performed prior to transplantation in groups 1 & 2. After transplantation, standard voiding cystography was performed.

RESULTS

The mean follow-up periods in groups 1 ; 2 ; 3 were respectivelly 10,4 months (ext 1-72 mo), 30,3 mo (ext 1-53) and 9,6 months (ext 1-60 months). No morbidity related to the technique was observed.

In group1 & 2, complete disappearance of VUR were observed in 51 and 90 %. After only one endoscopic injection, VUR in groups 1 & 2 were cured respectivelly in 42 and 70 %. There was an improvement in 6 cases in group 1: the refluxing ureteral units of various grades were converted to grade I and followed by urinary cultures. In group 3 the reflux was cured in 9 cases (30 %) including the 2 ureters reimplanted according to LP technique. Succesful cases were grade III in 7 cases and grade II in 2 cases. Only one injection was required for these succesful cases. In group 1, mean durations of haemodialysis between succesful cases and failures were respectively 46 and 57 months. Recurrent urinary tract infection leading to death was observed in one patient of group 3.

Failures were treated as follows: in group 1, 9 nephroureterectomies were performed ; in group 3 they were managed by ureteral replantation according to LP technique (4 cases), anastomosis of the renal ureter graft on the native ureter (2 cases), replantation of the renal pelvis graft on the native ureter in one case. Two nephrectomies were performed as chronic rejection was associated with end-stage renal failure. In

25 cases (all groups mixed) no further treatment was indicated and medical treatment of UTI was prescribed whenever necessary.

DISCUSSION

The succes rate obtained in these series 1 ; 2 ; 3 are respectively 51 ; 90 ; 30% with a mean follow-up of 10,4 ; 30,3 and 60 months. Expected group 2, the results are not correlated with those obtained on native ureters (90 %) according to Geiss in a multicenter survey (8). Moreover these results are different from those obtained on reimplanted ureters in non uremic patients (2).

Our policy is to attempt endocopic treatment in infected grade I-II VUR, alteration of renal function and in high degrees of VUR (9). Preservation of the native kidney avoids morbidity and maintain fluid balance, erythropoietin and vitamine D3 production. Open surgery for correction of VUR includes the use of the native ureter when available or iterative replantation in the bladder. This procedure is sometimes difficult, can lead to secondary urological complications such as stenoses and fistulaes and can disturb the transplant. The incidence of UTI episodes in patients with high-grade native VUR is not different from that in patients without native VUR deemed as the treatment of native VUR advisable before transplantation (10).

The bad local conditions with bladder mucosa and detrusor alterations, the difficulties to spot the ureteral orifices in long-lived haemodialysis patients are probably factors affecting success in group 1. In group 2, renal transplantation improves bladder capacity with diuresis and maintains the good results of endoscopic treatment in low and moderate grade VUR. Endoscopic treatment of high grade VUR also in native and transplanted kidneys (groupe 1 & 3) gives poor results (4/16 successes) though in group 2 all high grade VUR have been cured emphasizing increased transplant diuresis.

In group 3, the type of reimplantation leading to anatomical particularities of the ureteral orifice (e.g: extravesical technique) explains that injection of polytef paste between the ureter and detrusor is very difficult. The myotomy performed in extravesical replantation doesn't allow a solid support to the ureter and doesn't allow polytef paste to reinforce the anti-reflux mechanism. This extravesical technique however is used in a number of centers and has been shown to produce minimal rate of stenoses and fistulae (11).

There are three problems with the endoscopic treatment. First, distant migrations of PTFE particles after periurethral injection of Teflon has been well documented in primates (12) and in one patient after treatment of urinary incontinence (13). Second, long-term maintenance of the initial successful results is not well known: pediatric series have reported a recurrence rate of 3 to 6% with a maximun follow-up of one year (14). Staerman et al (15) has reported a recurrence rate of 7,7% in his adult serie with an average follow-up of more than 3 years ; Gabriele et al (16) has not reported recurrences in his serie of endoscopic treatment of VUR following by kidney transplantation. However this drawback is compensated by the possibility of reinjection with good results. Third, the long-terme biocompatibility of Teflon paste still persists.

Polytef paste did not produce any particular complications in this immuno-suppressed population. It is composed of inert particles and provokes an inflamatory granuloma-type reaction. We found this was typical during a histo-pathological examination after a surgical replantation in one of our patients. Polytef paste did not cause any other problems during the surgical correction of reflux after failure of endoscopic treatment. This has also been confirmed by Lacombe (17). The discovery of a new material with a higher biocompatibility and identical physical properties than Teflon paste will make the endoscopic treatment of VUR more acceptable in clinical practice.

Endoscopic subureteric injection of Teflon paste is an attractive method for primary VUR in haemodialysis patients with 64 % success rate and it increases until 90% after kidney transplantation. It avoids the need for nephro-ureterectomy preserving renal hormonal function. Despite the low rate of success of endoscopic treatment of VUR in transplanted kidneys (group 3), it appears to be justified to consider it as the first choice of treatment for symptomatic reflux as repeated open surgery in these cases is associated with significant morbidity (18). This procedure allows a secondary open surgical treatment in case of failure. The morbidity of open surgery in transplant patients is significant (30 % of repeated procedures according to Mundy (19)) and is associated with an high risk of loss of the tranplanted organ.

REFERENCES

1 E Matouschek. Die Behandlung des vesikoureteralen Refluxes durcg transurethrale Einspritzung von Teflonpaste. Urologe A 1981 ; 20: 263-264.

2 CC Schulman, D Pamart , M Hall. (1990). Vesicoureteral reflux in children: endoscopic treatment. Eur Urol ; 17: 314-317.

3 A Gelet, M Salas, X Martin, JL Faure, JM Dubernard. (1988). Vesicoureteric reflux in the adult. Preliminary results of the endoscopic treatment (In french). Presse Med ; 17:373-375.

4 P Cloix, M Dawarha, M Choukair, JL Viguier, A Gelet (1992). Endoscopic treatment of vesicoureteric reflux after ureter reimplantation (excluding renal transplantation) (in french). Progrès en urologie, 2: 66-71.

5 JW Duckett, MF Bellinger. (1982). A plea for standardized grading of vesicoureteral reflux. Eur Urol ; 8: 74-77.

6 De Campos-Freire, GJr. (1974). Extravesical ureteral implantation in kidney transplantation. Urology, 3, 304-308.

7 B O'Donnell, P Puri. (1984). Treatment of vesicoureteric reflux by endoscopic injection of teflon. Br Med J ; 289:7-9.

8 S Geiss, P Alessandrini, G Allouch et al. (1990). Multicenter survey of endoscopic treatment of vesicoureteral reflux in children; Eur Urol ; 17: 328-329.

9 M Salas sironvalle, A Gelet, X Martin, S Gabrielle, JM Clavel, JM Dubernard. Endoscopic treatment of vesicoureteral reflux prior to renal transplantation. Transplant int (1992), 5: 231-233.

10 O Bouchot, B Guillonneau, D cantarovich, M hourmant, L Le Normand, JP Soulillou, JM Buzelin. Vesicoureteral reflux in the renal transplantation candidate. Eur Urol 1991, 20: 26-28.

11 JB Thrasher, DR Temple, EK Spees (1990). Extravesical versus Leadbetter-politano ureteroneocystotomy: a comparaison of urological complications in 320 renal transplants. J Urol, 144, 1105-1109.

12 AA Malizia, HM Reiman, RP Myers, JR Sande, SS Barham, RC Benson, MK Dewanjee, WJ Utz. Migration and granulomatous reaction after periurethral injection of polytef (Teflon). J Am med ass, 251: 3277 (1984).

13 B Vorstman, J Lockhart, KR Kaufman, VA Politano. Polytetrafluoroethylene injection for urinary incontinence in children. J Urology, 1985, 133: 248-250.

14 P Sauvage, S Geiss, C Saussine et al. (1990). Analysis and perspectives of endoscopic reflux in children with a 20-month follow-up. Eur Urol ; 17: 310-313.

15 F Staerman, JM Clavel, X Martin, A gelet. Results of endoscopic treatment of primary vesico-ureteric reflux with a follow-up of 2 to 5 years. Progress in Urology (1991), 1: 37-44.

16 S Gabriele, M Dawhara, JM Marechal, X Martin, A Gelet. Résultats à long terme du traitement endoscopique du reflux chez les hémodialysés en attente de transplantation (in french). Progress in urology (1991), 1: 894-899.

17 A Lacombe. (1990). Ureterovesical reimplantation after failure of endoscopic treatment of reflux by submucosal injection of polytef paste. Eur Urol ; 17: 218-320.

18 P Cloix, A Gelet, O Desmettre, P Cochat, JL Garnier, JM Dubernard, X Martin. Endoscopic treatment of vesicoureteric reflux in transplanted kidneys. British J Urology (1993), in press.

19 AR Mundy, ML Podesta, M Bewick.(1981). The urological complications of 1000 renal transplants. British Journal of Urology, 53, 397-402.

NONSURGICAL TREATMENT OF BILIARY COMPLICATIONS AFTER LIVER TRANSPLANTATION

Ellen M. Ward, M.D.
Mayo Clinic
200 First Street, S.W.
Rochester, MN 55905
(507) 284-2271
Fax (507) 284-2405

Nonsurgical interventions are important methods of treating bile duct complications after liver transplantation. Complication are classified as biliary leaks or biliary obstruction.

Biliary Leaks after Liver Transplantation

Bile duct leaks after liver transplantation are from the T-tube site, the bile duct anastomosis or a nonanastomotic site in the donor bile ducts. Bile leaks occur early, usually within days to a few weeks after transplantation.

T-tube site leaks are common and if small, may resolve spontaneously. They are almost never associated with hepatic artery thrombosis. T-tube links become significant because cyclosporin must be administered intravenously if the leak is treated with external diversion, because bilomas may become infected, and because spontaneous healing may be slow.

211

J. L. Touraine et al. (eds.), Rejection and Tolerance, 211–216.
© 1994 *Kluwer Academic Publishers.*

Endoscopic techniques for T-tube leaks after liver transplantation have become the treatment of choice. Nasobiliary or endoscopic stents with or without sphincterotomy have been used. Recent studies show that endoscopic therapy results in closure of T-tube bile leaks in over 90% of T-tube leaks.[1,2] This is the same closure rate for endoscopic therapy of biliary fistulas as in the non-transplant population.[2] Percutaneous catheter drainage of bilomas may also be necessary.[3] Transhepatic drainage, surgical closure, or conversion to choledochojejunostomy may be necessary in the infrequent case in which endoscopic drainage fails to cure the bile leak.

Recently, we have abandoned the T-tube stent in favor of a straight catheter inserted into the donor cystic duct remnant and anchored with a hemorrhoidal band. We have seen only one bile leak (catheter dislodged) with this technique in approximately 50 grafts in the last year.

Anastomotic bile leaks are sometimes treated with endoscopic or transhepatic techniques. Results are variable because some of these leaks are from donor duct ischemia. If patency of the hepatic artery is established, endoscopic or transhepatic drainage may be useful.

Nonanastomotic bile leaks usually result from bile duct ischemia from hepatic artery thrombosis.[4] Transhepatic biliary drainage of bile ducts and bilomas is helpful to temporize prior to retransplantation, sometimes for several months.[5] In children who may form arterial collaterals, biliary stenting, and biloma drainage may salvage the graft.

Biliary Obstruction After Liver Transplantation

Biliary obstruction after transplantation is usually caused by bile duct strictures. Unusual causes of bile duct obstruction include cystic duct mucoceles, malpositioned stents, ampullary stenosis, and malignancy.

Anastomotic bile duct strictures occur in 2-5% of liver transplants.[6,7] The vast majority of anastomotic strictures are successfully treated with endoscopic or transhepatic balloon dilatation. In our experience balloon dilatation of anastomotic strictures resulted in duct patency in 11 of 12 grafts. Anastomotic revision should be performed only if percutaneous dilatations fail. Hepatic artery patency should be established, since anastomotic strictures are occasionally the dominant cholangiographic finding with hepatic artery thrombosis.

Nonanastomotic bile duct strictures present a much more complex problem. Nonanastomotic strictures are caused by hepatic artery thrombosis or stenosis, prolonged graft ischemia time, ABO blood group donor-recipient incompatibility, chronic ductopenic rejection, or are without known cause.[4,8-10]

We have used percutaneous biliary decompression stenting and balloon dilatation as the primary therapy for nonanastomotic strictures. Exceptions to this include grafts with very diffuse strictures developing within two weeks of transplantation and grafts with poor synthetic function. Early in our experience we stented patients with ductopenic rejection, but no longer attempt this because we were unable to change their clinical course.

We have percutaneously stented and/or dilated nonanastomotic strictures in 37 grafts with nonanastomotic strictures. Etiologies of the strictures included hepatic artery thrombosis or stenosis (8), graft ischemia time $\geq$ 11.5 hours (12), ductopenic rejection (3), and cause unknown (16). Two grafts had more than one possible etiology. 75% of these grafts survived 1-7 years, with 56% having near normal liver function.

Nonanastomotic strictures have required long periods of percutaneous stenting and multiple balloon dilatations. Stent times with 8 to 12 F transhepatic catheters range from 1-27 months (mean 9 months). This is because nonanastomotic strictures develop slowly. Early sludge causes obstruction; firm strictures requiring repeat dilatations often form after several weeks to months. Strictures also may extend more peripherally or new strictures may form weeks to months after initial presentation. Biliary stone and sludge often needs to be removed by baskets or balloons.[11] Because of the slow evolution of nonanastomotic strictures we have not found endoscopic dilatations to be helpful. Endoscopic removal of bile duct sludge occasionally has some benefit.

In conclusion, percutaneous therapy is the treatment of choice for almost all anastomotic and many nonanastomotic post-transplantations bile duct strictures.

References

1. Wolfsen HC, Porayko MK, Hughes RH, Gostowt CJ, Krom RAF, Wiesner FH. Role of endoscopic retrograde cholangiopancreatography after orthotopic liver transplantation. AM J Gastroenterol 1992;87:955-960.

2. Sherman S, Shaked A, Cryer H, Goldstein L, Busuttil R. Endoscopic management of biliary fistulas (BF) complicating liver transplantation (OLT) and other hepatobiliary surgeries (HBS). (Abst.) Gastrointest Endosc 1993;331.

3. Ward EM, Wiesner RH, Hughes RW, Krom RAF. Persistent bile leak after liver transplantation: biloma drainage and endoscopic retrograde cholangiopancreatographic sphincterotomy. Radiol 1991;179:719-720.

4. Zajko AB, Campbell WL, Logsdon GA, et al. Cholangiographic findings in hepatic artery occlusion after liver transplantation. AJR 1987;149:485-489.

5. Kaplan SB, Zajko AB, Koneru B. Hepatic bilomas due to hepatic artery thrombosis in liver transplant recipients: percutaneous drainage and clinical outcome. Radiol 1990;174:1031-1035.

6. Colonna JO, Shaked A, Gomes AS, et al. Biliary strictures complicating liver transplantation. Am Surg 1992;216:344-352.

216

7. Stratta RJ, Wood RP, Langnas AN, et al. Diagnosis and treatment of biliary tract complications after orthotopic liver transplantation. Surgery 1989;106:675-684.

8. Sanchez-Urdazpal L, Gores GJ, Ward EM, et al. Ischemic-type biliary complications after orthotopic liver transplantation. Hepatology 1992;16:49-53.

9. Gugenheim J, Samuel D, Reynes M, Bismuth H. Liver transplantation across ABO blood group barriers. Lancet 1990;336:519-523.

10. Wiesner RH, Ludwig J, Van Hock B, Krom RAF. Current concepts in cell-mediated hepatic allograft rejection leading to ductopenia and liver failure. Hepatology 1991;14:721-729.

11. Ward EM, Kiely MJ, Maus TP, Wiesner RH, Krom RAF. HIlar biliary strictures after liver transplantation: cholangiography and percutaneous treatment. Radiology 1990;177:259-263.

PERIPHERAL T CELL TOLERANCE

Bernard CHARPENTIER, Pascale ALARD, Christian HIESSE,
Olivier LANTZ. Service de Néphrologie, CHU de Bicêtre, 94275
Kremlin Bicêtre and Laboratoire d'Immunologie Cellulaire et de
Transplantation, IRSC-CNRS, 94802 Villejuif - France
Tel : 33.1.45.21.27.22 - Fax : 33.1.45.21.21.16

INTRODUCTION

T-cell tolerance can be defined as specific unresponsiveness of T cells to a nominal antigen or to an alloantigen. In the case of the nominal antigen, the unresponsiveness is expected to be directed towards peptides derived from the protein and associated with self major histocompatibility complex (MHC) molecules. In the case of the alloantigen, the unresponsiveness is expected to be directed to epitopes on the foreign MHC molecule itself as well as to undefined self-peptides associated with foreign MHC molecules. It is also possible that some peptides derived from foreign MHC molecules could be presented by self MHC molecules (1). Physical elimination of self-reactive T cells during their maturation in the thymus is the best-known mechanism for the establishment of self-tolerance, along with a variety of non-deletional mechanisms of tolerance in the thymus and the periphery (2, 3, 4). A detailed knowledge of tolerance induction in mature peripheral T cells is essential for therapeutic intervention, merely to understand and ensure tolerance in organ transplantation. It must be stressed that 3 different situations might bring about some clue on transplantation tolerance, namely in "in vitro" models, in experimental models and finally in the organ transplant human situation. But this last situation is hardly complex, occuring in an immunological status barely "naïve" and associated with other events which might interfere with the establishment and the maintenance of tolerance such as immunosuppressive drugs, as viral infections, blood transfusions.

J. L. Touraine et al. (eds.), Rejection and Tolerance, 217–225.

TOLERANCE TO ALLOGRAFTS IN HUMAN TRANSPLANT RECIPIENTS

In Human, peripheral blood lymphocytes (PBL) of allograft recipients disclose low proliferative and cytotoxic reactivity against the specific donor but not against third-party cells (5, 6). Two main explanations have been suggested to account for this phenomenon : clonal cell deletion of donor reactive cells and suppression of these cells (7, 8).

Recently, the concept of anergy has attracted renewed interest : antigenic stimulation without costimulatory signals leads to an absence of response and to a long-lasting subsequent state of anergy without immunological response after optimal antigenic stimulation. Although there is no widely accepted definition and characterization of anergic cells, one can define anergy as the persistence of antigen-specific cells with a functional T cell receptor as judged by Ca influx after antigenic stimulation without IL-2 secretion or proliferation. However, although this notion is still controversial, in several models of anergy, specific antigen reactive cells (ARC) can display IL2-receptors (CD25) after antigenic stimulation. Especially in self tolerance or in allogenic hyporesponsiveness to Mls after i.v. preimmunization, ARC are present, do not proliferate or secrete IL-2, but display IL2-receptors after activation with the tolerogen or anti-TCR. Thus, anergic cells do not display the effector functions enumerated above but may be not "inert". We have recently shown that both helper and cytotoxic donor-reactive cells are still present in long-term kidney transplant recipients (9), thus eliminating the clonal deletion hypothesis. Therefore, in order to explain allograft acceptance, two non-mutually exclusive hypotheses remain : suppression and/or clonal anergy. In our previous work, the absence of clonal deletion was evidenced by limiting dilution analysis. Since we used strong allostimulation (by LCL) and growth factors, because of this probable supramaximal stimulation it was not possible to test the hypothesis of an anergic state toward donor cells. In a recent study (10), we studied T cells from 8 transplant recipients who displayed a clear hyporesponsiveness after donor cell stimulation, as judged by IL-2 production, proliferation, or cytotoxic activity. We next wondered if the specific alloreactive cells could be activated as shown by an increase in cell size or in the expression of CD25 after allogenic stimulation. Thus, using cytofluorometry, we counted CD25-positive cells after autologous, donor or third-party cell stimulation during the first days of a conventional MLC. Recipients'T cells displayed the same increase in cell size and similar acquisition of CD25 after donor or third party cell stimulation, contrasting with their specific hyporesponsiveness toward donor cell stimulation. These data illustrate the possible involvement of "anergy" in human allogenic tolerance.

There is no realm explanation for the induction and maintenance of this state of anergy. But it has been recently shown that specific allogeneic tolerance to donor tissues can be induced by the transfer of donor lymphohemopoietic cells (11), establishing a state of mixed chimerism. On the other hand cell migration which has been shown after liver transplantation in human, quickly transforms both the graft and the recipient into chimeras and could lead to self perpetuating and presumably linked changes on the host immune response (12). Recent data show that migration of dendritic and lymphoïd cells is associated with graft acceptance rather than rejection, depending on the quality of immunosuppression, the immunological substrate of the organs, donor-recipient histocompatibility and perhaps other factors. This illustrates the fine margin between graft rejection and acceptance.

TOLERANCE IN EXPERIMENTAL MODELS

There are four major mechanisms of T-cell tolerance that have been described : (1) clonal deletion ; (2) clonal anergy : (3) the veto cell phenomenon ; (4) active suppression. These mechanisms have been mainly defined by specific experimental models that have changed over time.

(1) Clonal deletion (13)

In general, there is a substantial evidence for deletion of those immature T-cells that have a T-cell receptor (TCR) with high affinity for self-peptides associated with self MHC molecules expressed on the surface of dendritic/epithelial cells in the thymus. In the normal mouse, evidence for deletion is the reduction of sbusets of mature T-cells in the thymus and in the periphery which express certain $v\beta$ genes which confer reactivity to certain self-MHC class II and Mls antigens. Typical examples are represented by deletion of $v\beta5$ and $v\beta11$ TCR in I.E.[b] mice, and deletion of $v\beta6$ TCR in Mls 1[a] mice. The reduction of the appropriate vβ subset of T cells is also observed when transgenes encording the I.E. antigen are expressed in the thymus of strains that ordinarily do not express I.E.

(2) Clonal anergy (14)

In its strictest sense, clonal anergy in T cells refers to cloned T-cell line that have been rendered unresponsive to the antigen and antigen presenting cells (APC) that ordinarily elicit a response. T cell clones can be rendered anergic for at least several days by exposing the T cells to antigen and fixed APC. In addition, pancreatic β cells expressing foreign I.E.^{b} antigens by virtue of I.E.^{b} transgenes under the control of the insulin promoter render I.E.b reactive T-cell clones anergic. These results suggest that APC lacking certain costimulatory signals can paralyze rather than activate, T-cells. In a broader sense, anergy has also been used to describe the specific unresponsive state of T-cells derived from tolerant mice when no evidence for clonal deletion has been observed, as assessed by the lack of reduction of appropriate vβ expressing subsets of T-cells.

Thus, tolerant transgeneic mice expressing foreign class I or class II MHC transgenes on the β cell or acinar cells of the pancreas, and radiation chimeras tolerant of certain Mls antigens have been described as disclosing evidence of clonal anergy.

Recently, there are two new aspects which have been put forward in the concept of anergy. First, an altered regulation of the IL2 pathway has been proposed as an explanation of the tolerance state observed after blood transfusion in the rat (15). In this case, no true deletion of antigen-reactive cells has been observed, and these allograft recipients do not make active IL2, whereas the expression of the IL2 gene is produced. The cells obtained from these tolerant rats do not respond to IL2 and a decreased expression of α and β chain of the IL2-receptor is observed.

Second, several monoclonal antibodies (mAb) administered either in vivo or in vitro are able to induce a state of immunological tolerance. These mAb include anti CD4 (16), anti vβ + T cells (17), and anti CD3 (18). It must be added that in vitro induction of allo antigen specific hyporesponsiveness in human T lymphocytes can be carried out by blocking interactions of CD 28 with its natural ligand B7/BB1 (19). In this case IL2 and

IFN α mRNA are blocked, and not IL4 mRNA, and this hyporesponsiveness is restored by adding exogenous IL2 to the culture.

(3) The veto cell phenomenon

A poorly defined subset of cells is able to induce in the host a negative signal which has been named the veto phenomenon. In a very convincing publication of Thomas J. et al. (20), it has been shown that veto cells can induce long term kidney allograft tolerance in primates without chronic immunosuppression. In this system, total donor bone marrow cells were fractionated into subpopulations. In "in vitro" proliferation and cytotoxic assays and in vivo studies showed that the suppression was mediated by a small population of bone marrow cells that express a CD2+, CD8+, CD16+, DR-, CD3-, CD8- phenotype. This subpopulation was also able to suppress the acute organ allograft rejection and in vivo and in vitro CTL response, suggesting that a veto mechanism may control the induction phase of allograft tolerance in this model and allowing the development of host immunoregulatory mechanisms necessary for maintaining graft tolerance.

(4) Suppression and suppressor T cells

Although suppressor T cells (TS) have been cloned in only few instances, the existence of a functional cadre of T cells that acts to downregulate the immune response in well documented (8).
Alloreactive suppressor cells were showed in lymph nodes of mice that had been lettraly irradiated, reconstituted with syngenic bone marrow, and given a heart allograft. Ts have since been shown to be present in many allogeneic systems but studies in which their exact nature (lymphocyte a macrophage), CD8+ or CD4+ phenotype, specificity (non specific, antigen-specific, or anti-idiotypic) and sensitivity to irradiation and various drugs was examined have lead to couplicting reports. Very recent data (21) have shown that the maintenance of transplantation tolerance induced in adult mice after short term treatment with nonlytic monoclonal antibodies to CD4 and CD8 was due to the induction of "infectious" transplantation tolerance namely that CD4 + T cells from tolerant mice disabled naive lymphocytes so that they too could not reject the grafts. This process of "infectious tolerance" either is or

very close to a T-cell suppression system and explain why no further immunosuppression was needed to maintain long term transplantation tolerance.

CONCLUSION

In the light of data presented here, it is conceivable that induction of tolerance in human comes of age. Experiments are needed to define more precisely the induction of anergic T cells in transplant recipients as well as the pattern of lymphokine secretion.

AKNOWLEDGEMENTS

This work was supported by grants from ARC, DRC/AP-HP, CNAMTS/INSERM.

REFERENCES

1. BENICHOU G., TAKIZAWA P.A., OLSON C.A., Mc MILLAN M., SERCARZ E.E.
   Donor major histocompatibility complex (MHC) peptides are presented by recipients MHC molecules during graft rejection
   J. Exp. Med., 1992, 175, 305-308

2. STROBER S.
   T-cell tolerance
   Transplant. Proc., 1991, 23, 34-35

3. MILLER J.F.A.P., MORAHAN G.
   Peripheral T cell tolerance
   Annu. Rev. Immunol., 1992, 10, 51-69

4. SACHS D.H.
   Antigen-specific transplantation tolerance
   Clin. Transplantation, 1990, 4, 78-81

5. THOMAS J., THOMAS F., MENDEZ-PICON G., LEE H.
   Immunological monitoring of long-surviving renal transplant recipients
   Surgery, 1977, 81, 125-136

6. CHARPENTIER B., LANG PH., MARTIN B., FRIES D.
   Specific recipient donor unresponsiveness mediated by a suppressor cell
   system in human kidney allograft tolerance
   Transplantation, 1982, 33, 470-476

7. CHARPENTIER B., BACH M.A., LANG Ph., FRIES D.
   Expression of OKT8 antigen and Fc γ receptors by suppressor cells
   mediating specific unresponsiveness between recipient and donor in
   renal allograft tolerant recipient
   Transplantation, 1983, 36, 495-501

8. HUTCHINSON I.V.
   Suppressor T cells in allogenic models
   Transplantation, 1986, 41, 547

9. LANTZ O., ALARD P., BEN ARIBIA M.H. et al.
   Persistance of donor-specific IL2 secreting cells and CTL precursors in
   human kidney transplant recipients evidenced by limiting dilution analysis
   J. Immunol., 1990, 144, 3748-3755

10. ALARD P., LANTZ O., PERROT J.Y., CHAVANEL G., SENIK A.,
    CHARPENTIER B.
    A possible role for specific anergy in immunologic hyporeactivity to donor
    stimulation in human kidney allograft recipients
    Transplantation, 1993, 55, 277-283

11. STARZL T.E., DEMETRIS A.J., MURASE N., ILDSTAD S., RICORDI C.,
    TRUCCO M.
    Cell migration, chimerism and graft acceptance
    Lancet, 1992, 339, 1579-1582

12. ARNOLD B., SCHONRICH G., HAMMERLING G.
    Multiple levels of peripheral tolerance
    Immunol. Today, 1993, 14, 12-14

13. BLACKMAN M., KAPPLER J., MARRACK P.
    The role of the T cell receptor in positive and negative selection of
    developing T cells
    Science, 1990, 248, 1355-1341

14. MUELLER D.L., JENKINS M.K., SCHWARTZ R.H.
    Clonal expansion versus functional clonal inactivation : a costimulatory
    signalling pathway determines the outcome of T cell antigen receptor
    occupancy
    Ann. Rev. Imunol., 1989, 7, 445-480

15. DALLMANN M.J., SHIHO O., PAGE T.H., WOOD K.J., MORRIS P.J.
    Peripheral tolerance to alloantigen results from altered regulation of the
    IL2 pathway
    J. Exp. Med., 1991, 173, 79-87

16. ALTERS S., SHIZURU J.A., ACKERMAN J., GROSSMANN D., SEYDEL
    K.B., FATAMAN C.G.
    Anti-CD4 mediates clonal anergy during transplantation tolerance
    induction
    J. Exp. Med., 1991, 173, 491-494

17. GOSS J.A., PYO R., FLYE M.W., CONNOLLY J.M., HANSEN T.H.
    Major histocompatibility complex-specific prolongation of murine skin
    and cardiac allograft survival after in vivo depletion of Vβ+ T cells
    J. Exp. Med., 1993, 177, 35-44

18. ANASETTI C., TAN P., HANSEN J.A., MARTIN P.J.
    Induction of specific nonresponsiveness in unprimed human T cells by
    anti-CD3 antibody and alloantigen
    J. Exp. Med., 1990, 172, 1691-1700

19. TAN P., ANASETTI C., HANSEN J.A. et al.
    Induction of alloantigen-specific hyporesponsivenes in human T
    lymphocytes by blocking interactions of CD28 with its natural ligand
    B7/BB1
    J. Exp. Med., 1993, 177, 165-173

20. THOMAS J.M., CARVER F.M., CUNNINGHAM P.R.G., OLSON L.C.,
    THOMAS F.T.
    Kidney allograft tolerance in primates without chronic
    immunosuppression. The role of veto cells
    Transplantation, 1991, 51, 198-207

21. SHIXIN Q., COBBOLD S.P., POPE H., ELLIOTT J., KIOUSSIS D.,
    DAVIES J., WALDDMANN H.
    "Infectious" transplantation tolerance
    Science, 1993, 259, 974-976

INDUCTION OF DONOR-SPECIFIC TOLERANCE BY INTRATHYMIC CELLULAR TRANSPLANTATION

George L. Mayo, Andrew M. Posselt, Luis Campos, Barbara C. Deli, Sean P. Mayo, Clyde F. Barker, and Ali Naji

Hospital of the University of Pennsylvania, Department of Surgery, 3400 Spruce Street, 4 Silverstein, Philadelphia, PA 19104, Tele: (215) 662-2066, Fax: (215) 349-5906

INDUCTION OF IMMUNOLOGIC TOLERANCE

The acquisition of immunologic tolerance is primarily achieved by selective deletion of self-reactive T cells within the thymus, whereby the interaction between self-antigen and the T cell receptor at an immature stage in T cell differentiation aborts further development of the cell (1,2). Within the thymus, developing thymocytes are subjected to both positive and negative selection. It is believed that positive selection permits development of thymocytes bearing receptors capable of binding self-MHC and foreign peptide. Negative selection (or tolerance induction), on the other hand, is thought to arrest the maturation of those thymocytes with high affinity for self-MHC (3). Both bone marrow derived antigen presenting cells and thymic epithelial cells have been demonstrated to be involved in tolerance induction within the thymus (4-7).

The ultimate goal of transplantation tolerance is induction of a specific unresponsiveness to donor alloantigens, with retention of full reactivity to all other non-self antigens. This was first established by the experiments of Billingham, Brent and Medawar demonstrating permanent acceptance of allogeneic skin grafts in mice exposed to donor lymphohematopoietic cells during neonatal or perinatal life (8). The cellular basis of the tolerant state in this model is likely to be multifactorial but the prevailing view is that the

227

J. L. Touraine et al. (eds.), Rejection and Tolerance, 227–244.
© 1994 Kluwer Academic Publishers.

unresponsiveness is primarily mediated by the intrathymic deletion or functional inactivation of donor reactive T cells (9-12).

The induction of a comparable state of tolerance in the adult immunocompetent host would be highly attractive but has proven exceedingly difficult to achieve. Most strategies have relied on pretreatment of adult hosts with immunosuppressive agents prior to reconstitution with donor lymphohematopoietic cells. The immunosuppression ensures engraftment of the donor cells by crippling the mature T cells and, in effect, recreates the immunologic naivety of the neonatal model of Billingham, *et al.* (13-17). However, the intensity of the conditioning regimen renders such protocols impractical for clinical utility and therefore attempts to induce transplantation tolerance mandate development of strategies to minimize the risks of the preparative regimens. In the following sections we describe our efforts to assess the feasibility of inducing transplantation tolerance by direct inoculation of donor cells into the thymus of the adult allogeneic recipients.

INTRATHYMIC TRANSPLANTATION OF PANCREATIC ISLETS

We considered the observation by Billingham and Medawar that cells of hematopoietic origin were able to induce tolerance when injected into neonates, but parenchymal cellular populations of liver, testicle, and kidney were unable to promote tolerance. We hypothesized that this might be explained by the consideration that only cells of the hematopoietic origin have the capacity to migrate to and populate the thymic microenvironment where they would be able to influence T cell maturation. This hypothesis was further supported by studies examining the effect of intrathymic inoculation of soluble and cellular antigens on subsequent immune responsiveness of the host. Staples *et al.* found that bovine γ globulin injected into the thymus of sublethally irradiated rats depressed both anti-γ globulin antibody synthesis and DTH responses to the antigen more effectively than when injected into lymph nodes or spleen (18). More recently, Shimonkevitz and Bevan reported that intrathymic injection of allogeneic double negative (CD4-CD8-) prothymocytes (cells previously not thought to have tolerogenic capacities) into lethally irradiated, bone marrow reconstituted mice induced a marked decrease in CTL precursor frequency toward donor alloantigens, suggesting that deletion and/or functional inactivation of alloreactive cells had occurred (19). We sought to examine whether allogeneic cells normally incapable of homing to the thymus, when introduced directly into the thymus could have a similar impact on maturing T cells, possibly causing specific tolerance of their alloantigens.

We initially sought to characterize the thymus as a transplant site for pancreatic islets in recipients rendered chemically diabetic (20). Lewis (RT1^l) or DA (RT1^a) rats were used as islet donors and WF (RT1^u) rats were used as recipients. Freshly isolated islets were inoculated into conventional islet transplant sites (beneath the renal capsule or embolized in the portal vein), into a known immunologically privileged site (the abdominally displaced testicle), or into both lobes of the thymus (Table 1). Transplants to either the liver or the renal subcapsule in non-immunosuppressed WF recipients were promptly rejected. Transplants to the thymus were slightly prolonged, with one of seven grafts surviving indefinitely. We attempted to improve these initial results by adding a single intraperitoneal dose (1 ml) of rabbit anti-rat lymphocyte serum (ALS) at the time of transplantation to the experimental regimen. The addition of ALS slightly prolonged survival of islets transplanted to either the liver or the renal subcapsule. While graft survival was further increased by transplantation to a classic immunologically privileged

Table 1. **Survival of Fresh Lewis Islet Allografts in WF Recipients**

Site of Islet Transplantation	Days of Islet Allograft Survival	
	without ALS	1 ml of ALS
Liver (intraportal)	5, 8, 8, 9 (8)*	6, 22, 29, 35, 36 (29)
Renal subcapsule	9, 9, 10, 13 (9.5)	27, 33, 38, 47, 61, >200x2 (47)
Testicle	- -	50, 50, 76, 110, >200x2 (76)
Thymus	13, 13, 16, 17, 17, 18, >200 (17)	28, 33, 57, >200x10 (>200)

* Median survival time.

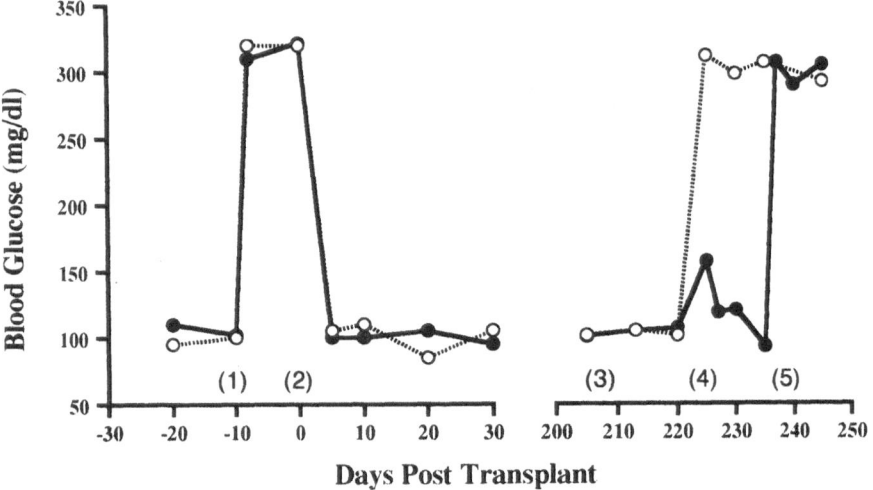

Figure 1. Representative blood glucose profiles of WF rats transplanted with freshly isolated pancreatic islets. (1) Streptozotocin administration. (2) Intrathymic transplantation of fresh Lewis islets with concomitant intraperitoneal administration of ALS (1cc). (3) Second renal subcapsular transplants of either Lewis (●--●) or DA (o--o) islets. (4) Thymectomy. (5) Removal of islet-bearing kidneys.

site (the testicle), most of the islet grafts were rejected between 50 and 110 days. In marked contrast, intrathymic islet allograft survival was vastly superior with the majority of the grafts surviving indefinitely.

Similar results were obtained in spontaneously diabetic BB recipients (21). Diabetic BB rats received either intrathymic or renal subcapsular WF islet grafts. All recipients of intrathymic WF islets maintained normal serum glucose levels for > 120 days, while recipients of renal subcapsular WF grafts became hyperglycemic after 23 and 64 days.

ASSESSMENT OF UNRESPONSIVENESS IN INTRATHYMIC ISLET RECIPIENTS

Given the unique properties of the thymus in the evolution of T cell tolerance, we next explored whether prolonged residence of allogeneic islets in the thymus might induce specific unresponsiveness to extrathymic donor-strain alloantigens. WF rats harboring long term intrathymic Lewis islets failed to reject secondary extrathymic donor strain Lewis islet allografts (Fig. 1). The donor specific nature of this unresponsiveness was confirmed by demonstrating rejection of "third party" DA (Rt1^a) renal subcapsular islet grafts in long term WF recipients of intrathymic Lewis islets. Similarly, BB rats with long term intrathymic Lewis islet allografts received secondary intraportal Lewis islet grafts. All animals remained normoglycemic for > 60 days and remained so following islet-bearing thymectomy to evaluate the function of the secondary intraportal graft.

The composition of pancreatic islets includes not only endocrine elements but also non-endocrine intra-islet antigen presenting cells (APCs). Indeed, it is thought that the latter populations, which include highly immunogenic APCs such as dendritic cells and macrophages, contribute to the immunogenicity of islet allografts (22). To determine which cell population was necessary for inducing the tolerant state observed after intrathymic islet transplantation, we examined the capacity of intrathymic inocula of islets depleted of APCs by in vitro culture to promote survival of secondary donor-strain grafts transplanted beneath the renal capsule (23). WF rats in which long-term (> 120 days) normoglycemia had been achieved by intrathymic transplantation of in vitro cultured Lewis islets in conjunction with a single i.p. dose of ALS received freshly isolated Lewis islets beneath the renal capsule 120 days after thymic inoculation. All animals promptly developed hyperglycemia demonstrating that retransplantation had provoked the rejection of both the primary intrathymic and extrathymic test grafts, and that tolerance induction in this model requires the presence of intra-islet APCs.

INTRATHYMIC ISLET XENOGRAFTS (RAT → MOUSE)

Based upon our initial success utilizing the thymus as a transplant site for pancreatic islet allografts, we investigated the survival of islet xenografts in this organ (24). Islets were isolated from WF (RT1^u) rats and transplanted into the thymus or the renal subcapsule of streptozotocin diabetic C57BL/6 (H-2^b) mice (Table 2). When no immunosuppression was administered, islet xenografts to the thymus did not survive significantly longer than those to the renal subcapsule. The addition of a single dose (0.5 cc) of rabbit anti-mouse thymocyte serum at the time of transplantation significantly prolonged intrathymic islet xenograft survival and 7 of 14 animals remained normoglycemic beyond 100 days. Animals harboring long term intrathymic islet xenografts accepted subsequent extrathymic donor-strain islet xenografts suggesting that the presence of xenogeneic islets in the thymic microenvironment may have promoted unresponsiveness to donor strain xenoantigens.

Table 2. Survival of WF Islet Xenografts in C57/BL6 Mice

Transplant Site	ATS	Graft Survival in Days (MST)*
Renal Subcapsule (RSC)	-	12,12,12,14,20,21,21,26 (17.3)
	+	31,39,43,43,53 (41.8)
Thymus	-	11,12,12,12,13,22,22,39 (17.9)[†]
	+	39,40,57,59,68,70,90,>100x3,>150x4 (>94.5)[§]

*Mean Survival Time
[†]Not significant vs RSC without ATS group
[§]$P < .001$ vs RSC with ATS group

Table 3. **Survival of Lewis Islet Allografts in WF Recipients**

Group	Site of Lewis BMC Inoculation	ALS Treatment	Days of Islet Allograft Survival
1	None	None	9, 9, 10, 13 (9.5)*
2	None	+	8, 9, 14, 15, 18, >173[#] (14.5)
3	Intravenous	+	13, 16, 21, 23, 32, 32 (22)[+]
4	Thymus	+	12, 28, >130x2, >148, >159, >183 (>130)[a]
5	Testicle	+	7, 8, 8, 10 (8)

* Median survival time.   [#] Animal reverted to hyperglycemia after removal of islet-bearing kidney.
[+] $P > .1$ vs. group 2.   [a] $P < .04$ vs. groups 2 or 3.

INDUCTION OF DONOR-SPECIFIC UNRESPONSIVENESS BY

INTRATHYMIC TRANSPLANTATION OF LYMPHOHEMATOPOIETIC CELLS

As described above, the results of our investigations utilizing *in vitro* cultured islets have demonstrated that it is the intra-islet APCs, and not the islet endocrine cells, that lead to the induction of tolerance (23). Specifically, the intrathymic transplantation of pancreatic islet allografts into transiently immunosuppressed rats lead to a state of donor-specific unresponsiveness while the intrathymic transplantation of APC-depleted islets failed to do so. Based upon these experiments, we attempted to extend our observations to evaluate the potential of intrathymic inocula of lymphohematopoietic cells to promote the survival of islet allografts as well as vascularized allografts. We utilized bone marrow cells because of their proven ability to promote neonatal tolerance and hematopoietic chimerism, and the fact that they contain precursors capable of differentiation into cells of macrophage/dendritic cell lineage.

Naive WF rats that were not pretreated with bone marrow cells or ALS rapidly rejected Lewis islet allografts (MST: 9.5 days) (Table 3) (25). The addition of a single i.p. dose of ALS and intrathymic saline 14 days prior to Lewis islet transplantation increased the islet allograft survival but the majority of the grafts were ultimately rejected (MST: 14.5 days). When Lewis bone marrow cells were given intrathymically, 5 of 7 WF recipients remained normoglycemic indefinitely (MST > 130 days). These animals were eventually sacrificed and histologic examination of the islet-bearing kidney revealed well-granulated islets and absence of intra-islet mononuclear cell infiltration.

The thymic specificity of the tolerant state was evaluated in two ways. First, intravenous administration of Lewis bone marrow cells in conjunction with ALS 14 days prior to islet transplantation lead to modest prolongation of Lewis islet allograft survival; however, all allografts eventually underwent rejection within 32 days (MST: 22 days). Second, intratesticular inoculation of Lewis bone marrow cells and i.p. ALS 14 days prior to Lewis islet transplantation was also used. This approach was based upon the fact that the prolonged residence of allogeneic tissue in an immunologically privileged site has been shown to weaken the host's immune responsiveness to subsequent donor-strain allografts transplanted to conventional sites (26). Since the thymic parenchyma is relatively inaccessible to the peripheral immune system, it was possible that the unresponsiveness observed in intrathymically treated rats was due only to the presence of the bone marrow cell inoculum and not due to the unique roles of the thymus in T cell maturation and the induction of self-tolerance. When an intratesticular conditioning inoculum of bone marrow cell was used, all animals rapidly rejected their grafts (MST: 8 days), indicating that the protective influence of the intrathymic bone marrow inoculum on subsequent allografts was unlikely to be explained entirely by its presence in a privileged site. The donor specific nature of the conditioning inoculum was also evaluated. WF animals pretreated with either intrathymic or intravenous Lewis bone marrow cells rejected islet allografts of "third party" DA (RT1^a) donors within 10 days.

We next examined the efficacy of intrathymic inoculation of donor bone marrow cells to promote the survival of vascularized organ allografts. In the high responder combination (DA → Lewis) the normally vigorous response of Lewis rats to DA orthotopic liver allografts was abrogated by the intrathymic inoculation of recipients with donor strain bone marrow cells and a single i.p. dose of ALS (27). The thymic specificity of this approach was verified by the inability of donor-strain cells administered i.v. to promote the survival of liver allografts. Furthermore, the donor specific nature of this approach was verified by the failure of the intrathymic inoculation of WF bone marrow cells to prolong DA liver allograft survival in Lewis rats.

Comparable results was obtained when heterotopic cardiac allografts were used as test graft. Lewis cardiac allografts transplanted to naive WF recipients were rejected promptly (MST: 14 days). Pretreatment of recipients with 1 cc of ALS and intrathymic saline 14 days prior to cardiac transplantation prolonged survival (MST: 24 days), however, all grafts were ultimately rejected. In marked contrast, intrathymic donor Lewis bone marrow cells and ALS prior to transplantation lead to heart graft survival beyond 200 days in 8 out of 9 WF animals. The intravenous administration of donor bone marrow cells with ALS failed to prolong survival of cardiac allografts (MST: 10 days) (28).

MECHANISM OF UNRESPONSIVENESS INDUCED BY INTRATHYMIC CELLULAR TRANSPLANTATION

Islet allografts transplanted intrathymically to nonimmunosuppressed rats with chemically-induced diabetes enjoyed substantially prolonged survival and, if the hosts were briefly immunosuppressed with a single dose of ALS, permanent allograft survival was obtained. Although the precise mechanisms responsible for these findings remain to be elucidated, a partial explanation is suggested by several known morphologic and physiologic characteristics of the organ. Ultrastructural as well as kinetic studies have demonstrated the presence of a blood-thymus barrier surrounding the capillaries in the thymic cortex which prevents extravasation of low molecular weight proteins and radiolabelled cells (29). In addition, although the thymus possesses efferent lymphatics, it lacks an afferent lymphatic supply (30). These details of vascular anatomy may account for the findings of Michie *et al.* that there is little recirculation of mature T lymphocytes through the thymic parenchyma (31). Despite the classification of the thymus as a primary lymphoid organ, it is relatively removed from the immune surveillance which takes place in other tissues, thus explaining the sanctuary it provides for allografts. Though these anatomic and physiological features might account for the survival of allografts implanted into the thymus, they fail to explain the observation that intrathymic islet recipients accept subsequent donor-strain grafts transplanted extrathymically, i.e. are rendered tolerant.

Several mechanisms could account for the unresponsiveness of long-term recipients of intrathymic allogeneic islets to subsequent extrathymic transplants. These include: 1) nonspecific immunosuppression resulting from disruption of thymic function; 2) generation of suppressor/regulatory cells; 3)deletion or inactivation within the thymus of donor reactive T cell populations which could otherwise be expected to destroy extrathymic grafts. Immunofluorescent analysis of lymphocyte subpopulations in the lymph nodes revealed no differences between thymic allograft recipients and naive controls, demonstrating that thymic manipulation had not produced a state of global T cell immunodeficiency.

To determine whether suppression was contributing to the tolerant state, we performed adoptive transfer studies in which 250-300 x 10^6 spleen cells from either non-transplanted WF controls or WF rats harboring established (>200 days) intrathymic Lewis islet allografts were transferred to sublethally irradiated WF hosts. Twenty-four hours later, these animals received islets from Lewis donors beneath the renal capsule. Islet survival in rats given splenocytes from intrathymic recipients was not significantly different from that of the control group and thus provided no evidence for the presence of suppressor cells in tolerant animals.

To assess whether the deletion or functional inactivation of donor reactive T cells lead to the tolerant state mixed lymphocyte cultures (MLC) and limiting dilution analyses (LDA) of donor-specific cytotoxic T lymphocyte precursors (pCTL) were performed using lymphoid cells from long term recipients of intrathymic islets. MLC responses of lymph node cells from islet allograft acceptors to donor-strain and third party stimulator cells were indistinguishable from the responses of naive animals. However, LDA analysis of cervical lymph nodes from these animals showed significantly reduced (40 to 60%) pCTL frequencies to donor-strain alloantigens (Lewis) as compared with untransplanted controls (20). In the same recipients, the pCTL frequencies for DA alloantigens were unchanged. In animals with long term islet or cardiac allograft survival achieved by intrathymic bone marrow cell inoculation, lymph node cells responded normally to third party DA stimulators in a MLC system, however, proliferation of these cells to Lewis stimulators was consistently decreased as compared with responses of unmanipulated controls (25,28). Analysis of pCTL frequencies in recipients bearing established islet or cardiac allografts as a result of pretreatment with intrathymic bone marrow demonstrated significant reductions in pCTL frequencies toward donor (Lewis) alloantigens as compared to the naive host. All animals had similar pCTL frequencies to third party DA alloantigens. Together, these results support the conclusion that the unresponsive state induced by long-term residence of the intrathymic allograft is mediated primarily by intrathymic deletion or inactivation of T cell precursors recognizing alloantigens expressed on the graft.

In several models of specific unresponsiveness achieved by allogeneic bone marrow cell transplantation, tolerance has been shown to correlate with the presence of microchimerism in the thymus and peripheral lymphoid organs of the recipients (32, 33). To determine whether a similar chimeric state had developed in our model, the lymphoid organs of WF rats that had received intrathymic Lewis bone marrow cells (without subsequent islet grafts) were examined at various times after inoculation by immunofluorescence and immunohistochemistry utilizing a murine monoclonal antibody specific for Lewis class I alloantigens. By FACS analysis, chimerism was detected in the thymus for only 4-5 days after intrathymic transfer and not observed in the lymph nodes of these animals at any time after intrathymic injection. However, immunohistochemistry routinely demonstrated the presence of donor strain cells scattered throughout the thymus in animals inoculated with Lewis bone marrow 2 to 45 days earlier. Similarly, in animals which had accepted Lewis islet grafts after conditioning with intrathymic Lewis bone marrow, donor-strain cells were found in the thymus when it was examined 140-170 days after inoculation, although the number of cells was markedly reduced as compared to organs examined at earlier time points. In contrast, donor-strain cells were not detected in the thymus or lymph nodes of animals given intravenous bone marrow cells. Thus, it appears that the thymic microenvironment can support the long-term survival of implanted hematopoietic cells and is capable of protecting them (or their descendants) from elimination by immune mechanisms.

Several recent studies have also confirmed the feasibility of promoting prolonged survival of skin, cardiac, and renal allografts in adult rodents following intrathymic inoculation of donor spleen or glomerular (containing APCs) cells (34-39). The induction of unresponsiveness requires transient reduction of peripheral mature T cells at the time of the intrathymic transplantation of the conditioning inoculum. The requisite tolerogenic component of the conditioning inoculum appears to be cells of the macrophage/dendritic cell lineage, populations known to have a critical role in the development of T cell tolerance in the thymus. The plausible mechanism for the unresponsiveness following the intrathymic transplantation of donor antigen presenting cells is the efficacy of these populations to establish thymic microchimerism leading to the deletion and/or functional inactivation of alloreactive T cell clones. Protocols based upon the intrathymic model of tolerance induction may have widespread clinical applicability, with the potential for successful transplantation in the absence of chronic immunosuppression.

REFERENCES

1.   Goodnow CC, Crosbie J, Jorgensen H, Brink RA, Basten A: Induction of self-tolerance in mature peripheral B cells. Nature, 1989; 342:385-391.

2.   Ramsdell F, Fowlkes BJ: Clonal deletion versus clonal anergy: the role of the thymus in inducing self tolerance. Science, 1990; 248:1342-1348.

3.   Kappler JW, Roehm N, Marrack P: T cell tolerance by clonal elimination in the thymus. Cell, 1987; 49:273-280.

4.   Lo D, Ron Y, Sprent J: Induction of MHC-restricted specificity and tolerance in the thymus. Immunol. Res., 1986; 5:212-221.

5.   Suzuki G, Kawase Y, Hirokawa K: Tolerance induction in the organ-cultured thymus lobes upon contact with allogeneic thymus lobes.   Eur. J. Immunol., 1989; 19:1525-1530.

6.   Ramsdell F, Lantz T, Fowlkes BJ: A nondeletional mechanism of thymic self tolerance. Science, 1989; 246:1038-1041.

7.   Salaun J, Bandeira A, Khazaal I, Calman F, Coltey M, Coutinho A, LeDouarin NM: Thymic epithelium tolerizes for histocompatibility antigens. Science, 1990; 247:1471-1474.

8.   Billingham RE, Brent L, Medawar PB: 'Actively acquired tolerance' of foreign cells. Nature (Lond.) 1953; 172:603-606.

9.   MacDonald HR, Pedrazzini T, Schneider R, Louis JA, Zinkernagel RM, Hengartner H: Intrathymic elimination of Mls^a-reactive (Vb6 +) cells during neonatal tolerance induction to Mls^a-encoded antigens. J. Exp. Med., 1988; 167:2005-2010.

10.   Streilein JW: Neonatal tolerance of H-2 alloantigens. Procuring graft acceptance the "old-fashioned" way. Transplantation, 1991; 52:1-10.

11.   Wood PJ, Strome PG, Streilein JW: Characterization of cytotoxic cells in mice rendered neonatally tolerant of MHC alloantigens: evidence for repertoire modification. J. Immunol., 1987; 138:3661-3668.

12.   Gowas JL, McGregor DD, Cowen DM: The role of small lymphocytes in the rejection of homografts of skin. In: The immunologically competent cell. Ciba Found. Study group 10. Wostenholme GE, O'Conner M, eds. Churchill, London, 1963; p. 20.

13. Monaco AP: Studies in rodents on the use of polyclonal anti-lymphocyte serum and donor specific bone marrow to induce specific unresponsiveness to skin allografts. Transpl. Proc., 1991; 23:2061-2067.

14. Mayumi H, Good RA: Long-lasting skin allograft tolerance in adult mice induced across fully allogeneic (multimajor H-2 plus multiminor histocompatibility) antigens by a tolerance-inducing method using cyclophosphamide. J. Exp. Med., 1989; 169: 213-238.

15. Eto M, Mayumi H, Tomita Y, Yoshikai Y, Nishimura Y, Nomoto K: The requirement of intrathymic mixed chimerism and clonal deletion for a long-lasting skin allograft tolerance in cyclophosphamide-induced tolerance. Eur. J. Immunol., 1990; 20: 2005-2013.

16. Cobbold SP, Martin G, Qin S, Waldmann H: Monoclonal antibodies promote marrow engraftment and tissue graft tolerance. Nature, 1986; 323: 164-166.

17. Ilstad ST, Sachs D: Reconstitution with syngeneic plus allogeneic or syngeneic bone marrow leads to specific acceptance of allografts or xenografts. Nature, 1984; 307:170-172.

18. Staples PJ, Gery I, Waksman BH: Role of the thymus in tolerance. III. Tolerance to bovine γ globulin after direct injection of antigen into the shielded thymus of irradiated rats. J. Exp. Med., 1966; 124: 127-139.

19. Shimonkevitz RP, Bevan MJ: Split tolerance induced by the intrathymic adoptive transfer of thymocyte stem cells. J. Exp. Med.,1988; 168: 143-156.

20. Posselt AM, Barker CF, Tomaszewski JE, Markmann JF, Choti MA, Naji A: Induction of Donor-Specific Unresponsiveness by Intrathymic Islet Transplantation. Science, 1990; 249: 1293-1295.

21. Posselt AM, Naji A, Roark JH, Markmann JF and Barker CF: Intrathymic Islet Transplantation in the Spontaneously Diabetic BB Rat. Annals of Surgery, 1991; 214(4) 363-373.

22. Lafferty KJ, Prowse SJ, Simeonovic CJ: Immunobiology of tissue transplantation: a return to the passenger leukocyte concept. Ann. Rev. Immunol., 1983; 1:143-173.

23. Campos L, Posselt AM, Mayo GL, Pete K, Deli BC, Barker CF, Naji A: Intrathymic Transplantation of Non-Immunogenic Islet Allografts Fails To Promote Induction of Donor-Specific Unresponsiveness. Transplantation (In Press).

24. Mayo GL, Posselt AM, Campos L, Barker CF, Naji A: Intrathymic Transplantation Promotes Survival of Islet Xenografts (Rat → Mouse). Transpl. Proc. (In Press).

25. Posselt AM, Odorico JS, Barker CF, Naji A: Promotion of Pancreatic Islet Allograft Survival by Intrathymic Transplantation of Bone Marrow. Diabetes, 1992; 41:771-775.

26. Barker CF, Billingham RE: Immunologically privileged sites. In: Kunkel HG, Dixon FJ, eds. Advances in immunology: Vol.25, New York, Academic Press, 1977.

27. Campos L, Alfrey EJ, Posselt AM, Odorico JS, Barker CF, Naji A: Prolonged Survival of Rat Orthotopic Liver Allografts After Intrathymic Inoculation of Donor-Strain Cells. Transplantation, 1993; 55:866-870.

28. Odorico JS, Barker CF, Posselt AM, Naji A: Induction of donor-specific tolerance to rat cardiac allografts by intrathymic inoculation of bone marrow. Surgery, 1992; 112:370-377.

29. Raviola E, Karnovsky MJ: Evidence for a blood-thymus barrier using electron-opaque tracers. J. Exp. Med., 1972; 136:466-.

30. Weiss L, ed.: The blood cells and hematopoietic tissues. McGraw-Hill, 1977; pp. 503-522.

31. Michie SA, Kirkpatrick EA, Rouse RV: Rare peripheral T cells migrate to and persist in normal mouse thymus. J. Exp. Med., 1988; 168:1929-1934.

32. Streilein JW, Strome PG, Wood PJ: Failure of in vitro assays to predict accurately the existence of neonatally-induced H-2 tolerance. Transplantation, 1989; 48:630-634.

33. Morrissey PJ, Sharrow SO, Kohno Y, Brozofsky JA, Singer A: Correlation of intrathymic tolerance with intrathymic chimerism in neonatally tolerized mice. Transplantation, 1985; 40:68.

34. Remuzzi G, Rammi M, Limberti O, et al: Kidney graft survival in rats without immunosuppression after intrathymic glomerular transplantation. Lancet, 1991; 337:750.

35. Ohzako H, Monaco AP: Induction of specific unresponsiveness (tolerance) to skin allografts by intrathymic donor-specific splenocyte injection in antilymphocyte serum treated mice. Transplantation, 1992; 10:90.

36. Goss J, Nakafusa Y, Flye W: Intrathymic injection of donor alloantigens induces donor-specific vascularized allograft tolerance without immunosuppression. Ann. Surg, 1992; 216:409.

37. Oluwole SF, Chowdhury NC, Fawwaz R, et al: Induction of specific unresponsiveness to rat cardiac allografts by pretreatment with intrathymic donor major histocompatibility complex class I antigens. Transplant Proc., 1993; 25:299.

38. Krokos NV, Brons IGM, Sriwatanawongsa V, et al: Intrathymic injection of donor antigen-presenting cells prolongs heart graft survival. Transplant Proc., 1993; 25:303.

39. Odorico JS, Posselt AM, Naji A, et al: Promotion of rat cardiac allograft survival by intrathymic inoculation of donor splenocytes. Transplantation, 1993; 55:1104.

USE OF ANTI-CD4 MONOCLONAL ANTIBODIES FOR TOLERANCE INDUCTION

Kathryn J. Wood

Nuffield Department of Surgery, University of Oxford, John Radcliffe Hospital, Oxford OX3 9DU England

INTRODUCTION

Polyclonal antibody preparations, anti-lymphocyte globulin (ALG or ALS) and anti-thymocyte globulin (ATG) have been used successfully as anti-rejection agents for many years (1). Monoclonal antibodies (mabs) targeting a number cell surface molecules on either T cells, most notably, CD4 (e.g.. (2-6)), CD25 (IL-2R) and CD11a/CD18 (LFA-1) (7-10), or the cells of the organ graft, CD54 (ICAM-1) (8) have also been shown to be capable of prolonging graft survival. The ability of antibodies, either polyclonal or monoclonal to create an environment for the induction of tolerance to alloantigen is currently under investigation.

When a T cell encounters any antigen it can make 3 choices, it can ignore the antigen and therefore will be unaffected as a result of the encounter; it can become activated or it can switch off and therefore be unresponsive to subsequent stimulation by the same antigen, a process that will lead to tolerance. The response to antigen can therefore be modified in either a positive or a negative fashion dependent on a number of parameters including for example, the status of the recipient, the route of antigen delivery, the form of the antigen, or the timing between the first and second antigen exposure. The administration of alloantigen to an adult subject may therefore modify the way in which the immune system responds to those antigens when they are encountered for the second time. The first encounter with alloantigen may be at the time of transplantation, in other words the organ graft itself, but can also occur if potential transplant recipients are exposed to alloantigen in a controlled manner before transplantation, for example as a result of blood transfusion. Anti-CD4 mabs can be used to manipulate the environment in which the antigen encounter takes place, thereby promoting inactivation rather than activation of alloreactive T cells. The strategies adopted by research groups working in this area fall into one of two broad categories, those that

245

J. L. Touraine et al. (eds.), Rejection and Tolerance, 245–254.
© 1994 Kluwer Academic Publishers.

aim to use anti-CD4 mab therapy to induce tolerance or unresponsiveness to alloantigen in the long term after transplantation and those with the much more difficult aim of inducing specific unresponsiveness to donor alloantigens at the time of transplantation. This review will focus on selected examples of strategies using anti-CD4 mabs to induce tolerance to alloantigen.

TOLERANCE IN THE LONG TERM AFTER TRANSPLANTATION

Anti-CD4 mabs have been shown to facilitate the induction of tolerance to alloantigens in variety of experimental models (e.g.. (2-6)). Depletion of the target cells is not always essential for tolerance to be induced, blockade of the function of the CD4 molecule may be sufficient in some circumstances (11-14). My own research group has shown that tolerance to alloantigens expressed by cardiac allografts can be induced in the long term, ie 50-100 days after transplantation, when recipient are treated in the peri-operative period with either depleting or non-depleting anti-CD4 mabs (14, 15). Although both types of mab are effective, the treatment protocol used has to be designed to take into account the molecular properties of the mab involved. For example, using a depleting anti-CD4 mab YTS 191, (the kind gift of Professor Herman Waldmann (2)), tolerance to alloantigen can be achieved following treatment with only 50μg of mab the day before and the day of transplantation (15); no further immunosuppression is required. In contrast, this same protocol was totally ineffective when a non-depleting anti-CD4 mab, KT6 (the kind gift of Dr Kyuhei Tomonari), was used. To achieve prolonged cardiac allograft survival using this anti-CD4 mab, KT6 had to be administered both at the time of transplantation and on the 12th post-operative day (14).

Anti-CD4 mab therapy administered at the time of transplantation creates an environment for the induction of tolerance to donor alloantigens in the long term, but in the early post-operative period the immunosuppressive effects induced by treatment with the anti-CD4 mabs lack antigen specificity. For example, when C3H. He (H-2^k) mice are treated with the depleting anti-CD4 mab YTS 191 as described above, the animals are immunocompromised for approximately 21 days following antibody treatment (16). During this time, the survival of cardiac allografts from a number of different strains of mice show prolonged survival. However, as the time after transplantation increases tolerance to the alloantigens of the organ donor is induced. The induction of tolerance does not occur as a single event, instead tolerance induction appears to be a dynamic process that continues to evolve for at least the first 100 days after transplantation in this mouse model (15, 17). For example, by 50 days after transplantation recipients of a C57BL/10 (H-2^b) heart graft can be shown to be tolerant of C57 alloantigens provided that the mice are challenged with a second C57 heart graft. If the mice are challenged at this time point with a C57 skin graft, the grafts are rejected. Thus in the early phases of induction, tolerance appears to be tissue specific. As the post-transplant period progresses, ie >100 days after transplantation, recipients also exhibit tolerance to donor antigens expressed by other types of tissue including skin.

The experimental studies using anti-CD4 mabs in vivo, including data obtained in primates (12, 13) look promising. Trials designed to evaluate the efficacy of an anti-CD4 mab, OKT4A, in clinical renal transplantation are currently in progress (18). It should be noted however, that the mab therapy is being added to an existing immunosuppressive protocol involving other agents. In all of the promising experimental studies reported, anti-CD4 mabs have been used as the sole immunosuppressive agent. While it is ethically very difficult to exclude proven agents, such as cyclosporin from a clinical protocol, the possibility that these agents may diminish or abrogate the tolerance inducing potential of the anti-CD4 mab under investigation should not be overlooked.

TOLERANCE AT THE TIME OF TRANSPLANTATION.

The administration of alloantigen in the form of one or more blood transfusions before transplantation has been shown in experimental models (e.g.. (19-21)) and the clinic (e.g.. (22, 23)) to improve graft outcome. This phenomenon is known as the blood transfusion effect. However, in recent years, whilst experimental data have continued to support this approach as a means of modifying the immune response to alloantigen before transplantation, the beneficial effect of transfusions on graft prolongation in clinical transplantation has been less marked, and in some centres has disappeared altogether (24-26). This combined with the introduction of heamopoeitin and the risks of infection associated with the use of blood products have resulted in a change in transfusion policy at some centres, particularly in the USA. If antigen pretreatment is to continue alternative strategies are required.

A number of studies have shown that the efficacy of pretreatment with donor antigen can be improved if antigen treatment is combined with another immunosuppressive agent, for example ALS. This approach has been shown to be successful when ALS is used in combination with donor antigen at the time of transplantation. Monaco and his colleagues designed a strategy for the induction of tolerance to skin grafts in mice that involved combining ALS therapy with bone marrow from the organ donor (27). The rationale for this protocol was that ALS would eliminate host leukocytes at the time of transplantation, thereby reverting the recipient's immune system to a more immature state which had been shown by Medawar and his co-workers to favour the induction of unresponsiveness. This strategy has subsequently been developed successfully in higher animal models, including primates, and is currently being evaluated in clinical renal transplantation (28-30). Clearly the use of donor antigen in conjunction with other immunologically non-specific immunosuppressive agents will not result in the induction of unresponsiveness to donor alloantigens in the short term. However, it is hoped that the requirement for immunosuppressive drug therapy to maintain the survival of the kidney graft will diminish as tolerance develops. Preliminary data from the trial are encouraging, but longer follow-up times are required before a full assessment of efficacy can be made (30, 31).

It may be possible to use mabs instead of ALS in this type of approach for the induction of tolerance to alloantigen. Two different groups have shown that it is possible to induce tolerance to soluble protein antigens by treating recipients with the antigen at the same time as treatment with an anti-CD4 mab (32, 33). My own laboratory has adapted these approaches for use in transplantation. We have shown that by administering donor antigen in combination with anti-CD4 mab before transplantation unresponsiveness to a subsequent cardiac allograft can induced that is both immunologically specific at the time of transplantation and effective in the long term (16). In this case, recipients are pretreated with donor antigen, in the form of a blood transfusion together with anti-CD4 mab before transplantation. Recipients are then rested until the nonspecific effects of the anti-CD4 mab therapy have decayed and immunocompetence to all other, but not donor alloantigens, has recovered. Thus when the heart graft is transplanted, they are specifically unresponsiveness to the alloantigens of the organ donor.

MECHANISMS OF TOLERANCE INDUCTION
Above I have described just a few of the strategies that are currently being explored for the induction of tolerance to alloantigen in adults using anti-CD4 mabs. The mechanisms responsible for the induction and maintenance of peripheral tolerance to alloantigen are still being investigated, particularly at the molecular level, and continue to be hotly debated. Four, non-mutually exclusive hypotheses have been proposed to explain the induction of peripheral tolerance. These are in broad terms, deletion, anergy, ignorance and suppression. What is clear from all studies is that tolerance induction is a dynamic process and any or all of these mechanisms may be operating at different stages of the induction process and maintenance process. What is also clear is the confusion generated by different definitions for the terms are used to describe what may be the same phenomena!

The mechanism responsible for the induction and maintenance of tolerance following anti-CD4 mab therapy are complex. As mentioned above, the induction of tolerance in anti-CD4 treated recipients is a dynamic process. A number of studies have shown that anergic T cells are present in anti-CD4 treated mice with long term surviving allografts (34, 35). Anergic T cells are usually identified because although they are present in a tolerant animal they are unable to respond when stimulated through their antigen receptor with either antigen or a mab specific for the TCR they express. In some models anergy has also been shown to be associated with a down regulation of cell surface expression of TCR and accessory molecules such as CD8 (36, 37).

The cytokine environment may also play a role in influencing the outcome when T cells encounter antigen. It has been suggested that the cytokines, IL-4 and IL-10 that are produced by T_H2 cells, may be associated with the development of unresponsiveness (38, 39) or alternatively that a low or defective production of the T_H1 cytokines, IL-2 and interferon-γ (IFNγ) might be responsible (40-42). Clearly the two situations may be related. Certainly, many studies have shown that there is a difference between the pattern and kinetics of cytokine expression in rejecting and tolerant recipients (e.g., (41, 42)). However, convincing evidence that the development of a T_H2-like environment is the critical factor for the induction of tolerance to alloantigen is still awaited, so far only causal associations have been implied. Clear evidence supporting these ideas will likely only be obtained from studies which attempt to manipulate the cytokine environment in vivo. So far little has been done in this area, but studies using for example antibodies to IFN-γ, an important T_H1 cytokine, have proved ineffective to date at both inhibiting graft rejection and inducing tolerance (43).

In many transplant models, it is possible to adoptively transfer cells from animals bearing long term surviving allografts to a fresh syngeneic recipient and show that these are able to modify the rejection response to a fresh graft (44). It is important to note that suppressor cells are most frequently described in the maintenance phase of graft survival, usually 50 or more days after transplantation in rodent models. Mice bearing long term surviving grafts as a result of anti-CD4 mab therapy are no exception. Thus it may be that the mechanisms responsible for tolerance induction converge in the longer term after transplantation. Although it remains possible to demonstrate the phenomenon of suppression, the idea that suppressor cells control unresponsiveness has largely fallen into disrepute because even with advances in technology, it has proved very difficult to isolate and characterise cells with suppressor activity. In the recent literature suppressor or regulatory cells seem to be enjoying a revival of interest and it may not be too long before speculation regarding their existence is finally put to rest.

Another phenomenon which can be considered as fitting into the same category as suppression is that of infectious tolerance. Again demonstrable in recipient bearing long term surviving allografts, where the transfer of naive syngeneic lymphocytes to the recipient will not induce graft rejection (e.g.. (5, 45)). Recent elegant experiments from Waldmann and his colleagues have shown that in mice rendered tolerant to skin grafts by treatment with anti-CD4 and anti-CD8 mabs, a CD4+ population of cells in the tolerant host is responsible for switching off the naive cells (46). Interestingly, the naive cells must be resident in the tolerant host for 14 days before they lose the capacity to reject a fresh graft. Experiments of this type may help elucidate the molecular properties of the cells responsible for maintaining tolerance to alloantigen in the long term.

CONCLUSIONS

Anti-CD4 mabs are powerful immunosuppressive agents in vivo. Experimental studies suggest that these agents may not only induce long term graft survival, but may also facilitate the induction of tolerance to alloantigens.

REFERENCES

1.　　Starzl TE. Heterologous antilymphocyte globulin. New England Journal of Medicine 1968;279:700.

2.　　Cobbold SP, Jayasuriya A, Nash A, Prospero TD, Waldmann H. Therapy with monoclonal antibodies by elimination of T-cell subsets in vivo. Nature 1984;312:548-551.

3.　　Cobbold S, Waldmann H. Skin allograft rejection by L3T4+ and LYT-2+ T cell subsets. Transplantation 1986;41:634-639.

4.　　Madsen JC, Peugh WN, Wood KJ, Morris PJ. The effect of anti-L3T4 monoclonal antibody on first-set rejection of murine cardiac allografts. Transplantation 1987;44(6):849-852.

5.　　Shizuru JA, Gregory AK, Chao CT-B, Fathman CG. Islet allograft survival after a single course of treatment of recipient with antibody to L3T4. Science 1987;237:278-280.

6.　　Shizuru JA, Seybel KB, Flavin TF, Wu AP, Kong CC, Hoyt EG, Fujimoto N, Billingham ME, Starnes VA, Fathman CG. Induction of donor-specific unresponsiveness to cardiac allografts in rats by pretransplant anti-CD4 monoclonal antibody therapy. Transplantation 1990;50:366 - 373.

7.　　Benjamin RJ, Qin S, Wise MP, Cobbold SP, Waldmann H. Mechanisms of monoclonal antibody-facilitated tolerance induction: a possible role for the CD4 (L3T4) and CD11a (LFA-1) molecules in self-non-self discrimination. European Journal of Immunology 1988;18:1079 -1088.

8.   Isobe M, Yagita H, Okumura K, Ihara A. Specific acceptance of cardiac allografts after treatment with antibodies to ICAM-1 and LFA-1. Science 1992;255:1125 - 1127.

9.   Nakakura EK, McCabe SM, Zheng B, Shorthouse RA, Scheiner TM, Blank G, Jardieu PM, Morris RE. Potent and effective prolongation by anti-LFA-1 monoclonal antibody monotherapy of non-primarily vascularized heart allograft survival in mice without T cell depletion. Transplantation 1993;55:412 - 417.

10.   Talento A, Nguyen M, Blake T, Sirotina A, Fioravanti C, Burkholder D, Gibson R, Sigal NH, Springer MS, Koo GC. A single administration of LFA-1 antibody confers prolonged allograft survival. Transplantation 1993;55:418 - 422.

11.   Qin S, Wise M, Cobbold SP, Leong L, Kong Y-CM, Parnes JR, Waldmann H. Induction of tolerance in peripheral T cells with monoclonal antibodies. European Journal of Immunology 1990;20:2737 - 2745.

12.   Cosimi AB, Delmonico FL, Wright KJ, Wee. S-L, Preffer FI, Jolliffe LK, Colvin RB. Prolonged survival of nonhuman primate renal allograft recipients treated with only anti-CD4 monoclonal antibody. Surgery 1990;108:406 - 413.

13.   Cosimi A, Delmonico F, Wright J, Wee S, Preffer F, Jolliffe L, Bedle M, Colvin R. OKT4A monoclonal antibody immunosuppression of Cynomolgus renal allograft recipients. Transplantation Proceedings 1991;23:501 - 503.

14.   Darby CR, Morris PJ, Wood KJ. Evidence that long-term cardiac allograft survival induced by anti-CD4 monoclonal antibody does not require depletion of CD4$^+$ T cells. Transplantation 1992;54:483 - 490.

15.   Pearson TC, Darby C, Bushell AR, West L, Morris PJ, Wood KJ. The assessment of transplantation tolerance induced by anti-CD4 monoclonal antibody in the murine model. Transplantation 1993;55:361 - 367.

16.   Pearson TC, Madsen JC, Larsen C, Morris PJ, Wood KJ. Induction of transplantation tolerance in the adult using donor antigen and anti-CD4 monoclonal antibody. Transplantation 1992;54:475 - 483.

17.   Pearson TC, Bushell AR, Darby CR, West LJ, Morris PJ, Wood KJ. Lymphocyte changes associated with prolongation of cardiac allograft survival in adult mice using anti-CD4 monoclonal antibody. Clinical and Experimental Immunology 1993;92:in press.

18.   Norman DJ, Bennett WM, Cobanoglu A, Hershberger R, Hosenpud JD, Meyer MM, Misiti J, Ott G, Ratkovec R, Shihab F, Vitow C, Barry JM. Use of OKT4A (a murine monoclonal anti-CD4 antibody) in human organ transplantation: Initial clinical experience. Transplantation Proceedings 1993;25:802 - 803.

19.   Fabre JW, Morris PJ. The effect of donor strain blood pretreatment on renal allograft rejection in rats. Transplantation 1972;14:608 - 617.

20.   Wood KJ, Morris PJ. The blood transfusion effect: Suppression of renal allograft rejection in the rat using purified blood components. Transplantation Proceedings 1985;17:2419 - 2420.

21.   Wood KJ, Evins J, Morris PJ. Suppression of renal allograft rejection in the rat by class I antigen on purified erythrocytes. Transplantation 1985;39:56 - 62.

22.   Morris PJ, Ting A, Stocker JW. Leucocyte antigens in renal transplantation. The paradox of blood transfusion in renal transplantation. Medical Journal of Australia 1968;2:1088 - 1090.

23.   Opelz G, Sengar DPS, Mickey MR, Terasaki PI. Effect of blood transfusions on subsequent kidney transplants. Transplantation Proceedings 1973;5:253 - 259.

24.   Opelz G. Blood transfusions and renal transplantation. In: Morris PJ, ed. Kidney Transplantation. Principles and Practice. 3rd ed. Philadelphia: W.B. Sanders Company`, 1988: 417-438.

25.   Opelz G. The role of HLA matching and blood transfusions in the cyclosporine era. Transplantation Proceedings 1991;21:609 - 612.

26.   Ahmed Z, Terasaki PI. Effect of transfusions. In: Terasaki PIaC J.M., ed. Clinical Transplants 1991. Los Angeles: UCLA Tissue Typing Laboratory, 1991: 305 - 312.

27.   Wood ML, Monaco AP. Suppressor cells in specific unresponsiveness to skin allografts in ALS-treated, marrow-injected mice. Transplantation 1980;29:196-200.

28.   Thomas FT, Carver FM, Foil MB. Long-term incompatible kidney survival in outbred higher primates without chronic immunosuppression. Annals of Surgery 1983;198:370.

29.   Thomas JM, Carver M, Cunningham P. Promotion of incompatible allograft acceptance in rhesus monkeys given posttransplant anti-thymocyte globulin and donor bone marrow. I. In vivo parameters and immunohistologic evidence suggesting microchimerism. Transplantation 1987;43:332 - 338.

30.   Barber WH. Induction of tolerance to human renal allografts with bone marrow and antilymphocyte globulin. Transplantation Reviews. 1990;4:68 - 78.

31.   Barber WH, Mankin JA, Laskow DA, Deierhoi MH, Julian BA, Curtis JJ, Diethelm AG. Long-term results of a controlled prospective study with transfusion of donor-specific bone marrow in 57 cadaveric renal allograft recipients. Transplantation 1991;51:70 - 75.

32.   Wofsy D. Mayes DC, Woodcock J, Seaman WE. Inhibition of humoral immunity in vivo by monoclonal antibody to L3T4: Studies with soluble antigens in intact mice. Journal of Immunology 1985;135(3):1698-1701.

33.   Benjamin RJ, Waldmann H. Induction of tolerance by monoclonal antibody therapy. Nature 1986;320:449-451.

34.   Alters SE, Shizuru JA, Ackerman J, Grossman D, Seydel KB, Fathman CG. Anti-CD4 mediates clonal anergy during transplantation tolerance induction. Journal of Experimental Medicine 1991;173:491 - 494.

35.   Qin S, Cobbold S, Benjamin R, Waldmann H. Induction of classical transplantation tolerance in the adult. Journal of Experimental Medicine 1989;169:779-794.

36.   Kisielow P, Bluthmann H, Staerz UD, Steinmetz M, von Boehmer H. Tolerance in T-cell-receptor transgenic mice involves deletion of nonmature $CD4^+8^+$ thymocytes. Nature 1988;333:742-746.

37.   Arnold B, Schonrich G, Hammerling GJ. Multiple levels of peripheral tolerance. Immunology Today 1993;14:12 - 14.

38.   Takeuchi T, Lowry RP, Konieczny B. Heart allografts in murine systems - The differential activation of TH2-like effector cells in peripheral tolerance. Transplantation 1992;53:1281 - 1294.

39.   Papp I, Wieder KJ, Sablinski T, O'Connell PJ, Milford EL, Strom TB, Jw K-W. Evidence for functional heterogeneity of rat CD4+ T cells in vivo. Differential expression of IL-2 and IL-4 mRNA in recipients of cardiac allografts. J Immunol 1992;148(5):1308-14.

40.   Mohler KM, Streilein JW. Lymphokine production by MLR-reactive reaction lymphocytes obtained from normal mice and mice rendered tolerant of Class II MHC antigens. Transplantation 1989;47(4):625-633.

41.   Dallman MJ, Shiho O, Page TH, Wood KJ, Morris PJ. Peripheral tolerance to alloantigen results from altered regulation of the interleukin-2 pathway. Journal of Experimental Medicine 1991;173:79 - 87.

42.   Bugeon L, Cuturi M-C, Hallet J, Paineau J, Chabannes D, Soulillou J-P. Peripheral tolerance of an allograft in adult rats - characterisation by low interleukin-2 and interferon-γ mRNA levels and by strong accumulation of major histocompatibility complex transcripts within the graft. Transplantation 1992;54:219 - 225.

43.   Paineau J, Priestley C, Bergh J, Tengblad A, Hallgren R. Effect of recombinant interferon-γ and interleukin-2 and of a monoclonal antibody against interferon gamma on the rat immune response against heart allografts. J. Heart-Lung Transplant. 1991;10(3):424 - 30.

44.   Hutchinson IV. Suppressor T cells in allogeneic models. Transplantation 1986;41:547 - 555.

45.   Billingham RE, Brent L, Medawar PB. Quantitative studies on tissue transplantation immunity. III. Actively acquired tolerance. Philosophical transactions of the Royal Society (London). Series B 1956;239:357 - 412.

46.   Qin S, Cobbold SP, Pope H, Elliott J, Kioussis D, Davies J, Waldmann H. Infectious transplantation tolerance. Science 1993;259:974 - 977.

Clonal deletion and clonal anergy mediated by antibodies to the human CD4 protein

S. Fournel[1], C. Vincent[1], P. Morel[1], A. Fathmi[1], J. Wijdenes[2]
and J.P. Revillard[1]

[1] Laboratoire d'Immunologie - INSERM U. 80, Pavillon P, Hôpital E. Herriot - 69437 Lyon Cédex 03, France

[2] Innothérapie Laboratoires - BP 1937 25030 Besançon Cédex, France

Monoclonal antibodies (mAbs) to the CD4 protein are potent immunosuppressive agents which were shown to induce long term survival of skin, heart and pancreatic islet allografts in murine models and to delay the rejection of skin and kidney allografts in monkeys (1). Treatment with anti-CD4 antibodies was also reported to prevent the progression of several spontaneous auto-immune diseases in mice (e.g. diabetes in the NOD mouse, lupus-like disease of NZB/NZW, BxSB and MLR/lpr strains). One remarkable effect of anti-CD4 antibodies is their capacity to induce long term tolerance to their own antigens and to foreign antigens presented during their administration (2-5). For all these reasons, numerous preliminary clinical trials have been initiated with murine or chimeric anti-CD4 antibodies in auto-immune or chronic inflammatory diseases such as psoriasis, inflammatory bowel diseases, multiple sclerosis, rheumatoid arthritis, vasculitis or polychondritis (6,7). Although nearly all these trials were not placebo-controled, some beneficial clinical effects were suggested and the side effects were reported to be minimal. However, in several recent trials, a very short course of humanized anti-CD4 antibodies was shown to induce long lasting profond CD4+ lymphocyte depletion, especially in patients who were treated with low doses of methotrexate or corticosteroids. Such side effect carries a risk of severe iatrogenic immunodeficiency which should not be acceptable in most clinical situations. Furthermore in some reports, CD4+ lymphocyte depletion was not associated with clinical improvement. Conversely, several murine mAbs were shown to induce clinical remissions without depleting circulating CD4+ cells. The efficacy of these non-depleting treatments have been extensively demonstrated in animal models (2, 8-10) but their mechanisms of action are still poorly understood. We therefore re-examined the effect of anti-CD4 mAbs on *in vitro* responses of normal peripheral blood lymphocytes to

255

J. L. Touraine et al. (eds.), Rejection and Tolerance, 255–264.
© 1994 *Kluwer Academic Publishers.*

various stimuli, including allogeneic B cells in mixed lymphocyte cultures (MLC) and the superantigen staphylococcal enterotoxin B (SEB).

Anti-CD4 mAb therapy in rheumatoid arthritis and psoriasis

We performed a first clinical trial in rheumatoid arthritis with BL4, mouse IgG2a mAb prepared in our laboratory (11). The objective was to determine the daily dose of antibody required to achieve saturation of all CD4 molecules on peripheral T cells, owing to the fact that, *in vitro*, nearly all anti-CD4 mAbs were reported to inhibit primary MLC only at saturating concentrations, whatever their subclass and fine epitope specificity (12). Furthermore, all beneficial effects reported in animal models of allografts and auto-immune diseases had been achieved at dosages far higher than those used in previous clinical trials. Six patients with severe rheumatoid arthritis were treated. A daily dose of 40 mg (0.8 mg/kg/d) was sufficient to achieve saturation (11) and down regulation of CD4 surface expression (13). CD4+ lymphocyte counts in peripheral blood dropped during BL4 infusion but returned to pre-treatment values three days after completion of a 10 day-treatment (11). Delayed hypersensitivity reactions to recall antigens were depressed and clinical indices of disease activity were markedly improved in the six patients during one or two months following treatment.

The second phase I/II trial was performed in three patients with severe psoriasis who were treated during one week with BB14/BF5, a murine anti-CD4 IgG1 mAb (14). Doses were 0.2 mg/kg/d in one patient and 0.4 to 0.8 mg/kg/d in the two others. Clinical improvement, with major reduction of Psoriasis Area Severity Index, was manifest within a few days of treatment and continued for 2 to 3 weeks. Lesional skin samples demonstrated (1) gradual improvement in parakeratosis, papillomatosis and acanthosis, (2) decreased expression of ICAM-1 and HLA-DR by keratinocytes, (3) an increase in CD1a+ Langerhans cell number, (4) partial decrase in epidermal T cell infiltrate, but (5) no significant change in the dermal infiltrate, especially no decrease of dermal CD4+ lymphocytes. Peripheral blood CD4+ cell counts were within the normal range immediately after completion of antibody treatment, while immunohistochemical markers of keratinocyte alterations were progressively disappearing. This study showed that a brief course of anti-CD4 mAb at relatively low doses initiated major changes in the skin lesions, which continued to improve in the absence of antibody. This effect suggested that anti-CD4 mAb had not only blocked cytokine synthesis by activated CD4+ cells in the dermis, but had possibly modulated activation signals generated through the CD3/TCR complex in such a way that the activated T cells involved in the generation of tissue lesions were selectively made anergic and/or deleted.

Inhibition of *in vitro* proliferative T cell responses by anti-CD4mAbs

Studies of *in vitro* effects of anti-CD4 mAbs on T cell proliferative responses yielded highly divergent results which may be accounted for by differences in antibody epitope specificity, subclass and nature of cell suspensions (peripheral blood mononuclear cells or lymphocytes, purified CD4+ lymphocytes or T cell clones). In most reports, anti-CD4 mAbs did not modify responses to phytohemagglutinin (PHA) and concanavalin A (Con A) (12,15-17), but partially reduced the responses to anti-CD3 antibodies (16-19), phorbol esters (16,17) and allogeneic cells in MLC (12,15,17,20). Similarly activation of purified T cells or CD4+ cell lines by specific antigens were reported to be decreased by anti-CD4 mAbs or their F(ab')$_2$ fragments (15,19).

Our own studies were performed with peripheral blood mononuclear cells partially depleted from monocytes by treatment with L-leucine methylester or by blood defibrination and adherence, yielding mononuclear cell suspensions containing 1.4 ± 0.8 percent monocytes as identified by flow cytometry after staining with an anti-CD14 mAb. The results in table I demonstrate a moderate but significant inhibition of ^{3}H-thymidine incorporation stimulated by SEB, Pokeweed mitogen (PWM), PHA and by the anti-CD3 antibody OKT3 in solid phase. Interestingly inhibition was not reproducibly observed when the experiments were performed with cell suspensions containing about 10 % of monocytes (not shown).

Induction of apoptosis

Newell and coworkers first reported that cross-linking of surface CD4 molecules followed by stimulation with anti-TCR monoclonal antibody of mouse spleen T cells induced cell apoptosis whereas the same treatment followed by activation by anti-CD3 antibody resulted in cell proliferation (21). Although the difference in the signalling pathways triggered by these two mAbs which recognized different epitopes of the TCR/CD3 complex was not clear, this study suggested that prior ligation of surface CD4 molecules could modify peripheral mature T cells in such a way that a TCR-mediated

Table 1. Inhibition of proliferative responses to T cell mitogens by B-F5
(anti-CD4 mouse IgG1) [1]

Stimulant	n	Anti-CD4 mAb [2]		Inhibition (%)	p value [3]
		-	+		
0	19	2.2 ± 0.5	1.1 ± 0.2	37	NS
MLC	21	32.4 ± 23.7	10.4 ± 8.9	68	p < 0.05
SEB (50 ng/ml)	16	24.0 ± 3.1	15.7 ± 2.8	34	p < 0.05
PWM (1 µg/ml)	14	11.1 ± 1.6	8.0 ± 6.8	28	p < 0.05
PHA (20 µg/ml)	16	46.2 ± 6.3	37.1 ± 4.7	25	p < 0.05
ConA (10 µg/ml)	5	35.7 ± 8.7	21.7 ± 3.3	39	NS
OKT3 (liquid phase)	7	10.1 ± 2.5	9.9 ± 2.6	2	NS
OKT3 (solid phase)	13	46.3 ± 5.3	27.2 ± 4.7	41	p < 0.05
PMA (50 ng/ml)	5	11.8 ± 2.9	13.1 ± 3.5	-11	NS
PMA + iono (50ng/ml + 1µg/ml)	5	34.0 ± 5.8	26.8 ± 6.5	21	NS

[1] *peripheral blood mononuclear cells (monocytes 1.4 ± 0.8 percent) ;*
[2] ^3HT-*dpm mean ± SE ;*
[3] *student's t test on paired values. NS : not significant*

Table 2. Primary MLR. Effect of various antibodies

	IgG class	BL60[1]	
		-	+
RPMI medium	-	0.85[2]	20.0
normal mouse IgG	polyclonal	0.69	16.7
832ALB (a1-m)	IgG1	1.05	19.4
BE104 (b2-m)	IgG2a	1.42	20.1
BL2 (DR)	IgG2b	4.09	12.5
AFOL1 (LFA1, CD11a)		0.54	1.8
B-F5 (CD4)	IgG1	0.41	2.82
B-F5 pulse 3h		0.60	6.1
B-F5 F(ab')2		0.91	4.6
BL4 (CD4)	IgG2a	0.41	5.5
13B8.2 (CD4)	IgG1	1.08	11.0

[1] *mitomycin-treated BL60 cells (Burkitt's lymphoma cell line)*
[2] *dpm x 10^{-3} at day 6*

activating signal would trigger cell death. This could represent an *in vitro* model of peripheral T cell tolerance by clonal deletion. More recently, Banda and coworkers reported experiments of cross-linking of CD4 proteins by either anti-CD4 mAbs or by HIV gp120 and anti-gp120 antibodies (22), followed by activation by anti-TCR antibodies. Under such experimental conditions, a proportion of CD4+ T cells underwent apoptosis. In those experiments apoptosis only occurred when cross-linking of CD4 was performed prior to that of TCR, suggesting again that ligation of CD4 had converted a TCR-mediated activation signal into programmed cell death.

Knowing that superantigens can induce clonal deletion of immature T cells when presented in the thymus but, instead, polyclonal activation of mature T cells, we used the superantigen SEB to study whether prior ligation of CD4 could induce apoptosis of the subset of SEB-responding CD4+ cells. The results show a significant increase of apoptotic cells, as determined by nuclear condensation and/or fragmentation after staining with Hoechst 33342 (23); Such effect was achieved at antibody concentration as low as 0.1 µg/ml, that is 100 times lower than concentrations required to saturate all CD4+ molecules.

Induction of clonal anergy

Peripheral blood lymphocytes were co-cultured with mitomycin-treated Burkitt's lymphoma cell lines (BL60, Raji, Daudi) and their proliferative response was measured by ^{3}H-thymidine incorporation after 6 days of primary culture in presence or absence of anti-CD4 mAbs. In this model, anti-CD4 mAbs and their F(ab')$_2$ fragments induced a dose-dependent inhibition of proliferation, even if present during the first 3h of culture, or if added at various time intervals after initiation of the culture. A similar effect was observed with an anti-CD11a antibody and anti-HLA-DR antibody, but not with subclass control antibodies of other specificities (table 2).

Inhibition of MLC in this model was associated with a complete suppression of IL-2 and IFNγ synthesis (as demonstrated by Northern blot analysis of mRNA in the cell pellet and determination of cytokines by ELISA in culture supernatants). In parallel VLA-1 expression was markedly decreased as well as the percentage of CD4+ blasts identified by their light scattering properties by flow cytometry. In contrast the surface expression of CD25 was not decreased (table 3). Therefore anti-CD4-treated cells

Table 3. Inhibition of primary MLR by anti-CD4 mAb

Treatment		^{3}H-T	CD25	IL-2	blasts		IFNγ	VLA-1
day 1		dpmx10^{-3}	%	ng/ml	CD4+	CD4-	U/ml	%
-	-	0.8	2.8	0.00	1.9	2.0	1.36	1.6
B-F5	-	0.4	3.0	0.00	1.6	1.8	0.1	1.6
-	BL60-m	28.0	19.9	0.39	14.3	33.3	12.7	15.2
B-F5	BL60-m	12.1	17.7	0.00	8.9	26.9	3.0	5.3

Table 4. Induction of clonal anergy by primary MLR in the
presence of the anti-CD4 mAb BF5

treatment			dpm x 10^{-3} (1)		
d1		d10	d 6	d 12	d 17
-	BL60	-	22.8	6.6	5.3
B-F5	BL60	-	2.9	4.8	4.4
-	BL60	BL60	-	43.2	7.6
B-F5	BL60	BL60	-	14.4	7.7
-	BL60	Raji	-	34.2	70.7
B-F5	BL60	Raji	-	24.8	72.4

(1) Peripheral blood lymphocytes were stimulated by mitomycin-treated BL60 cells with or without B-F5 mAb during 6 days, then resuspended in normal medium and re-stimulated at day 10 with BL60 or Raji cells.

presented a typical dissociation between a normal expression of IL-2 receptor α chain and a lack of IL-2 synthesis. Such profile has been reported in anergic T cells (24). In order to study whether a primary culture in presence of anti-CD4 mAb not only blocked the primary response of CD4[+] lymphocytes, but rendered them refractory to a subsequent stimulation in absence of antibody, cells were re-stimulated at day 10 with the same stimulator or third party cells and ^{3}H-thymidine incorporation was evaluated at days 12 (secondary response) and 17 (primary response). A typical experiment is presented in table 4, showing that exposure to anti-CD4 mAb during the primary culture blocked a further response to the same stimulator but did not impair the primary response to a third party cell line. Interestingly this specific unresponsiveness to allogeneic cells could not be achieved if cells were exposed to rIL-2 or to an anti-CD28 IgM mAb along with anti-CD4 during the primary culture.

Discussion

The present studies demonstrate that anti-CD4 mAbs may modify the activation of human peripheral blood T cells by superantigens or allogeneic stimulating B lymphoblasts. However the outcome in these two models was different. Part of SEB-stimulated T cells were shown to undergo apoptosis after prior ligation of their CD4 molecules by anti-CD4 mAbs or F(ab')2 fragments. Neither antibody nor SEB added separately could induce significant apoptosis over background levels, indicating the need for coordinated signals through CD4 and TCR. This model has some similarities with those of Newell *et al*.(21) and Banda *et al.* (22) who used anti-TCR mAbs instead of superantigens, but differs from them by at least two features : 1/ with SEB, cross-linking of CD4 by two layers of antibodies is not necessary, and apoptosis can be induced by low amounts of anti-CD4 mAbs of different isotypes (IgG1 or IgG2a) or even with F(ab')2 fragments. Under these conditions capping of CD4 proteins and down regulation of surface expression are limited to a very small proportion of cell surface CD4 proteins. 2/ Induction of apoptosis by SEB does not occur when the percentage of monocytes is raised from 1% to 5-10 %, suggesting that monocytes generate survival and co-activation signals. One possible candidate is B7/CD28 interaction (25). Although the fusion protein CTLA4 Ig does not block the proliferative response to SEB by itself (26) it might synergise with anti-CD4 mAbs to induce apoptosis. Experiments along this line are presently in progress.

In the MLC model there was no evidence of apoptosis but the percentage of activated T cells may be too low to detect apoptotic cells. Conversely there was a clear evidence of clonal unresponsiveness and typical features of anergized T cells (CD25+, no IL-2 expression). So far a similar *in vitro* induction of anergy in mature T cells has only be reported with anti-CD3 antibodies (27) and with CTLA4 Ig (28), but this situation is very close to that achieved by non depleting anti-CD4 mAbs *in vivo* (2). It is expected that these and other *in vitro* models will help to clarify the mechanisms whereby anti-CD4 antibodies may induce clonal deletion and clonal anergy in mature T cells in order to provide, together with antigen, a powerful tool of specific immuno-intervention in transplantation and auto-immune diseases.

REFERENCES

1.   Waldmann H. Manipulation of T-cell responses with monoclonal antibodies. Ann Rev Immunol 1989;7:407-44

2.   Qin S, Cobbold S, Tighe H, Benjamin R, Waldmann H.. CD4 monoclonal antibody pairs for immosuppression and tolerance induction. Eur J Immunol 1987;17:1159-61

3.   Wood KJ, Pearson TC, Darby C, Morris PJ. CD4: a potential target molecule for immunosuppressive therapy and tolerance induction. Transplant Rev 1991;5:150-64

4.   Shizuru JA, Alters SE, Fathman. Anti-CD4 monoclonal antibodies in therapy: creation of nonclassical tolerance in the adult. Immunol Rev 1992;129:105-30

5.   Cobbold SP, Qin S, Leong LYW, Martin G, Waldmann H. Reprogramming immune system for peripheral tolerance with CD4 and CD8 monoclonal antibodies. Immunol Rev 1992;129:165-201

6.   Herve P, Racadot E, Wendling D, Rumbach L, Tiberghien P, Cahn JY, Flesch M, Wijdenes J. Use of monoclonal antibodies in vivo as a therapeutic strategy for alloimmune or autoimmune reactivity: the Besançon experience. Immunol Rev 1992;129:31-55

7.   Riethmuller G, Rieber EP, Kiefersauer S, Prinz J, Van Der Lubbe P, Meiser B, Breedveld F, Eisenburg J, Krüger K, Deusch K, Sanders M, Reiter C. From antilymphocyte serum to therapeutic monoclonal antibodies: first experiences with a chimeric CD4 antibody in the treatment of autoimmune disease. Immunol Rev 1992;129:81-104

8.   Jonker M, Nooij FJM, Steinhof G. Effects of CD4 and CD8 specific monoclonal antibodies in vitro and in vivo on T cells and their relation to the allograft response in Rhesus monkeys. Transplant Proc 1987;19:4308-14

9. Carteron NL, Wofsy D, Seaman WE. Induction of immune tolerance during administration of monoclonal antibody to L3T4 does not depend on depletion of L3T4[+] cells. J Immunol 1988;140:713-16

10. Cosimi AB, Delmonico FL, Wright JK, Wee SL, Preffer FI, Bedle M, Colvin RB. OKT4A monoclonal antibody immunosuppression of cynomolgus renal allograft recipients. Transplant Proc 1991;23:501-03

11. Goldberg D, Morel P, Chatenoud L, Boitard C, Menkes CJ, Bertoye PH, Revillard JP, Bach JF. Clinical and biological effects of anti-CD4 antibody administration in rheumatoid arthritis patients. J Autoimmunity 1991;4:617-30

12. Merkenschlager M, Buck D, Beverley PCL, Sattentau QJ. Functional epitope analysis of the human CD4 molecule. The MHC class II-dependent activation of resting T cells is inhibited by monoclonal antibodies to CD4 regardless whether or not they recognize epitopes involved in the binding of MHC class II or HIV gp120. J Immunol 1990;145:2839-45

13. Morel P, Vincent C, Wijdenes J, Revillard JP. Down-regulation of lymphocyte CD4 antigen expression by administration of anti-CD4 monoclonal antibody. Clin Immunol Immunopath 1992; 64: 248-53

14. Morel P, Revillard JP, Nicolas JF, Wijdenes J, Rizova H, Thivolet J. Anti-CD4 monoclonal antibody therapy in severe psoriasis. J Autoimmunity 1992;5:465-77

15. Engleman EG, Benike CJ, Metzler C, Gatenby PA, Evans RL. Blocking of human T lymphocyte functions by anti-Leu2 and anti-Leu3 antibodies: differential inhibition of proliferation and suppression. J Immunol 1983;130:2623-28

16. Schrezenmeier H, Fleischer B. A regulatory role for the CD4 and CD8 molecules in T cell activation. J Immunol 1988;141:398-403

17. Carrera AC, Sanchez-Madrid F, Lopez-Botet M, Bernabeu C, De Landazuri MO. Involvement of the CD4 molecule in a post-activation event on T cell proliferation. Eur J Immunol 1987;17:179-86

18. Bank I, Chess L. Pertubation of the T4 molecule transmits a negative signal to T cells. J Exp Med 1985;162:1294-303

19. Merkenschlager M, Altmann DM, Ikeda H. T cell alloresponses against HLA-DQ and -DR products involve multiple epitopes on the CD4 molecule. Distinct mechanisms contribute to the inhibition of HLA class II-dependent and -independent T cell responses by antibodies to CD4. J Immunol 1990;145:3181-87

20. Engleman EG, Benike CJ, Glickman E, Evans RL. Antibodies to membrane structures that distinguish suppressor/cytotoxic and helper T lymphocyte subpopulations block the mixed leucocyte reaction in man. J Exp Med 1981;153:193-98

21. Newell MK, Haughn LH, Maroun CR, Julius MH. Death of mature T-cells by separate ligation of CD4 and the T-cell receptor for antigen. Nature 1990;347:286-89

22. Banda NK, Bernier J, Kuraha DK, Kurrle R, Haigwood N, Sekaly RP, Finkel TH. Crosslinking CD4 by human immunodeficiency virus gp120 primes T cells for activation-induced apoptosis. J Exp Med 1992;176:1099-106

23. Fournel S, Morel P, Revillard JP, Lizard G, Bonnefoy-Berard. Inhibition of human T cell response to staphylococcal enterotoxin B by prior ligation of surface CD4 molecules. Cellular Immunol 1993;150: in press

24. Schwartz RH. A cell culture model for T lymphocyte clonal anergy. Science 1990;248:1349-56

25. Goldbach-Mansky R, King PD, Taylor AP, Dupont Bo. A co-stimulatory role for CD28 in the activation of CD4+ T lymphocytes by staphylococcal enterotoxin B. International Immunol 1992;4:1351-60

26. Damle NK, Klussman K, Leytze G, Linsley PS. Proliferation of human T lymphocytes induced with superantigen is not dependent on costimulation by the CD28 counter-receptor. 1993;150:726-35

27. Anasetti C, Tan P, Hansen A, Martin PJ. Induction of specific nonresponsiveness in unprimed human T cells by anti-CD3 antibody and alloantigen. J Exp Med 1990;172:1691-700

28. Tan P, Anasetti C, Hansen JA, Melrose J, Brunvand M, Bradshaw J, Ledbetter JA, Linsley PS. Induction of alloantigen-specific hyporesponsiveness in human T lymphocytes by blocking interaction of CD28 with its natural ligand B7/BB1. J Exp Med 1993;177:165-73

TOLERANCE TO ALLOANTIGENS AND RECOGNITION FOR "ALLO + X" INDUCED IN HUMANS BY FETAL STEM CELL TRANSPLANTATION

TOURAINE J-L., RONCAROLO M.G., PLOTNICKY H.,BACCHETTA R., SPITS H., GEBUHRER L. & BETUEL H.

Pr. Jean-Louis Touraine, Department of Transplantation and Clinical Immunology, INSERM U80 & UCBL, Pavillon P, Hôpital Edouard Herriot, 69437 Lyon cedex 03, France.

INTRODUCTION

Transplantation of normal hemopoietic stem cells from the fetal liver can cure a number of diseases in experimental animals as well as in humans. Because of immune immaturity of the human fetus during the first trimester of gestation, fetal liver cells of 8-12 weeks post-fertilization are devoid of any T lymphocyte ; therefore they do not induce graft-versus-host disease (GvHD) after transplantation into an allogeneic host, despite full mismatch [1]. Prevention of rejection of these transplanted stem cells can be ensured by immunodeficiency disease of the host, by immunosuppressive treatment or by immune immaturity of the host when the transplant is performed into a fetal patient [2]. The stem cells from the fetal donor progressively differentiate into T lymphocytes within the environment of host antigens, and give rise to mature T cells exerting their functional activities and restoring immune defenses to the patient [3]. In most cases, the fetal donor and the patient host are fully mismatched at the class I and the class II loci of the major histocompatibility complex (MHC). T lymphocytes deriving from the donor stem cells are therefore confronted with HLA-different host cells (monocytes-macrophages, B lymphocytes, NK cells, target cells of various kinds, etc) after they have matured in this HLA-different host

J. L. Touraine et al. (eds.), Rejection and Tolerance, 265–277.

environment. This situation provides us with a unique model to study recognition of "self" and "allo" by helper and cytotoxic T cells, as well as the acquisition of tolerance during T cell ontogeny. Positive and negative selection processes are further demonstrated to be separate phenomena, likely to be induced by distinct cell categories.

PATIENTS

Since October 1974, 63 patients have been treated in our institution by fetal liver and thymus transplantation for severe immunodeficiency diseases or inborn errors of metabolism, with a success rate of 64% and a follow-up over 7 years in half of them. After immunological reconstitution, the formerly immunodeficient patients become healthy, and they live a normal life ; most of them do not take any additional therapy ; some of them however, who developed reconstitution of cell-mediated immunity, still have relatively low immunoglobulin levels and they receive immunoglobulin substitution. These patients have demonstrated virtually normal immune defenses *in vivo* against micro-organisms, including viruses. In most patients, a few years after transplantation, no unusual infection occurred and the spontaneous recovery from the frequent viral infections of childhood has been perfectly normal. Antibody production to these micro-organisms has been normal in many of the patients, *in vivo*.

MATERIALS AND METHODS

Peripheral blood lymphocytes have been obtained from the first patient (PS) who received fetal liver and thymus cells from 2 fetal donors more than 16 years ago. T lymphocytes were shown to derive from the first (10-20%) as well as the second (80-90%) donor. B lymphocytes, monocytes and NK cells were all shown to be of host type. There was a complete mismatch at the A, B, C and DR loci of the HLA regions, between host, donor 1 and donor 2 [4]. Other patients more recently treated have also been studied [5], with confirmatory results. The laboratory methods used for these investigations have been previously reported [3-8].

"ALLO + X" RECOGNITION BY HELPER T CELLS

Normal titers of anti-tetanus toxoid (TT) antibodies were produced by patient PS after *in vivo* immunization with TT. *In vitro* anti-TT antibodies were also shown to be normally synthetized by peripheral blood lymphocytes of this patient, despite HLA mismatch between T cells on the one hand, B cells and monocytes on the other hand [6].

Following a booster injection of TT into the patient, lymphocytes were separated from a blood sample, then stimulated *in vitro* with TT, and T cell clones specific for TT were prepared. Some of these clones were shown to derive from the first transplant, the others from the second one. An extensive analysis of T cell reactivity to TT presented by a spectrum of antigen-presenting cells (APC) exhibiting a variety of HLA phenotypes was carried out [7]. The results can be summarized as follows : (a) APC from the host were effective in inducing reactivity of all T cell clones to TT ; (b) some T cell clones reacted with TT presented by maternal APC, others by paternal APC ; (c) using a large variety of APC of extra-familial origin, it was shown that TT could be presented either by HLA-DR4 or by HLA-DR5 which served as element of restriction although neither was present on the T cells (HLA-DR4 and 5 were the specificity of the host, one being inherited from the mother, the other from the father) ; (d) a few clones had a more promiscuous pattern of reactivity and could react with TT presented by virtually all HLA DR+ APC tested, but no clone was reactive solely to TT presented by donor-type APC (the specificities DR1 and 8, or DR3 and 9, characteristic of both stem cell donors and therefore of the 2 types of T cell clones, could never serve as restriction elements in these experiments) ; (e) the reactivity of T cell clones to APC+TT was blocked by anti-HLA-DR monoclonal antibodies.

Helper T cells from chimeric patients therefore appear to recognize the antigenic peptide when presented in the groove of an MHC molecule of the host (in which stem cells differentiated into T cells) and not of the donor (although donor MHC was expressed by these T cells).

"ALLO + X" RECOGNITION BY CYTOTOXIC T CELLS

The cytotoxic capacity of peripheral blood T lymphocytes from patient PS was studied against Esptein-Barr virus (EBV)-infected target cells. PS had previously developed an asymptomatic EBV infection resulting both in seroconversion and in anti-EBV cell-mediated immunity.

Following appropriate expansion and activation, the patient T lymphocytes were shown to lyse specifically certain target cells, among the many different cell lines investigated [8]. Host and host-HLA-matched B lymphoblastoid cells, infected with EBV, were shown to be recognized and lysed by these T cells, whereas donor-HLA-matched cells were not. This lysis was significantly reduced by anti-class I or anti-class II antibodies. Lymphocytes from the father or from the mother were only killed when EBV-infected.

Host HLA antigens were thus demonstrated to serve as restricting determinants for the anti-viral cytotoxic T cells. In HLA-mismatched chimeric patients, therefore, "Allo + X" recognition, instead of the usual "Self + X" recognition, also appeared to target the activity of cytotoxic T cells (figure 1), as it does that of helper T cells.

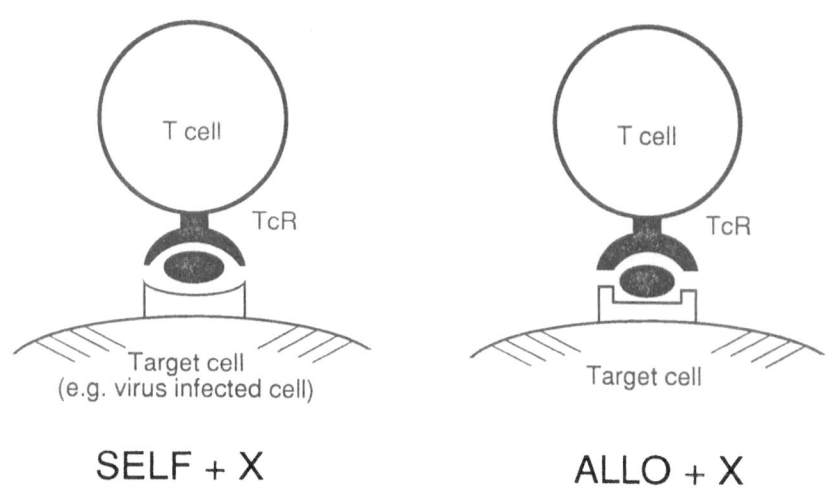

Figure 1 : Two distinct varieties of T lymphocytes differentiating in the thymus, one with the "self + X" recognition structures (left), the other with "Allo + X" recognition structures (right).

TcR is T cell receptor for antigen.

HOST-REACTIVE T CELLS

Not only host-reactive T cell clones were not deleted from the repertoire of these patients, but they were found in high frequency among peripheral blood lymphocytes : when preparing T cell clones specific for tetanus toxoid, we obtained 15 out of 50 clones that directly recognized host HLA antigens [7]. These clones had been isolated either after stimulation with EBV+ lymphoblastoid cell lines from the patient [7] or after polyclonal activation with PHA or anti-CD2 antibodies [5]. There were CD8+ and CD4+ T cell clones with cytotoxic and/or proliferative properties [4]. CD4+ T cells recognized class II HLA antigens on the patient cells.

CD8+ T cells recognized class I HLA antigens on the patient cells. They also reacted with HLA antigens on peripheral blood lymphocytes and PHA-lymphoblasts from either the mother or the father.

The frequency of CD8+ host-reactive cells in patient PS was comparable to that of allo-reactive cells whereas T cells specific for the HLA antigens of the first and the second donors appeared to be deleted [5].

Lymphokine production by host-reactive T cells from chimeric patients was characterized by high amounts of γ-IFN and, following activation, GM-CSF, IL5 and IL2 ; interestingly, no IL4 was ever produced, irrespective of the mode of activation [5].

A very significantly increased production of IL10 by cells from these chimeric patients has been observed and postulated to play a part in immunological tolerance to alloantigens [9]. This finding is in accordance with experimental data in mice [10].

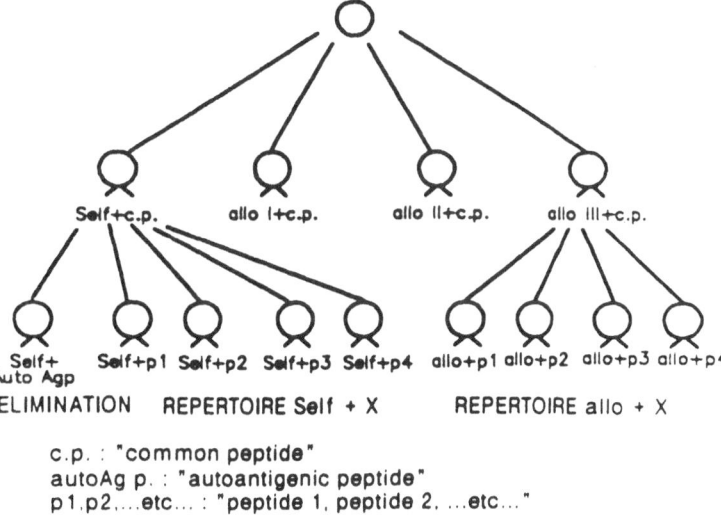

c.p. : "common peptide"
autoAg p. : "autoantigenic peptide"
p1,p2,....etc... : "peptide 1, peptide 2, ...etc..."

Figure 2 : Development ans selection of a large variety of T lymphocytes with distinct recognition structures, during the differentiation process from the stem cell after the migration to the thymus.

In the figure, c.p. is 'common peptide' ; auto Ag is 'autoantigenic peptide' ; p1... p4 are 'peptide 1... peptide 4'.

POSITIVE AND NEGATIVE SELECTIONS

In our patients, positive selection occurred in the context of host determinants. It is therefore likely that donor stem cells matured within the host thymus where "education" and positive selection of lymphoid cells were mainly governed by host epithelial cells.

Thymocytes differentiating from donor stem cells might have first acquired recognition structures for the various histocompatibility antigens, possibly associated with a common peptide (figure 2). In normal individuals, only those

T cells with recognition for self histocompatibility antigens would be induced to proliferate and develop a second degree of diversity at the level of the T cell receptor, leading to "self + X" recognition. By contrast, in chimeric patients, a given set of other histocompatibility molecules is continuously presented to the developing T cell within the thymus. Those T cells with recognition for the given allo-determinants would then be solicited, would proliferate and develop the gene rearrangment leading to the expression of T cell receptors which recognize the various antigens in the context of these allogeneic molecules [11].

As far as negative selection is concerned, following fetal stem cell transplantation, donor-reactive – but not host-reactive – cells are deleted from the T cell repertoire [5]. Clonal deletion would be responsible for tolerance to antigens of the donors, clonal anergy for tolerance to host antigens. "Auto-reactive" T cell clones might be deleted upon interaction with stem cell-derived macrophages or dendritic cells [4], as also suggested by animal experiments [12-16].

In brief, progenitor T cells deriving from the transplant(s) would mature in the host thymus containing (a) positively selecting epithelial cells (of host origin), and (b) deleting cells provided by the donor(s) and homing in the recipient thymus at the same time as prothymocytes. These influences of host and donor cells on the T lineage, during the differentiation of T cells from donor stem cells, result in mature T lymphocytes with exogenous and endogenous peptidic recognition restricted by recipient MHC and with immunological tolerance to antigens of donor 1, of donor 2, and of recipient (figure 3).

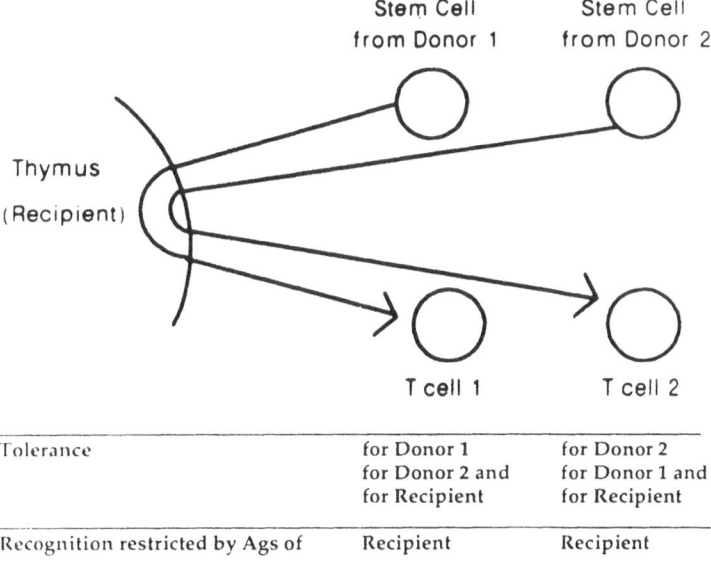

		Stem Cell from Donor 1	Stem Cell from Donor 2
Tolerance		for Donor 1 for Donor 2 and for Recipient	for Donor 2 for Donor 1 and for Recipient
Recognition restricted by Ags of		Recipient	Recipient

Figure 3 : Differentiation of T lymphocytes from stem cells of donors 1 and 2, within the host thymus, in contact with host and donor cells, resulting in cells with peptidic antigen recognition restricted by host MHC and with tolerance to host antigens and to both donors antigens.

CONCLUSION

Fetal livers of less than 13 weeks following fertilization only contain immature cells which do not induce GvHD when transplanted to allogeneic host. Despite HLA mismatch with the recipient, these cells can give rise to fully immunocompetent T lymphocytes with helper and cytotoxic functions. Host cells impose positive selection and donor cells impose negative selection during T cell maturation in these chimeric patients.

To further facilitate tolerance of the recipient to donor cells, especially in patients without the most complete forms of immunodeficiency diseases, fetal liver cell transplants can be performed during the early phase of fetal development, immediately after prenatal diagnosis [2, 11]. In such circumstances, immune immaturity of donor cells prevents GvHD and immune immaturity of host cells prevents rejection of the transplant. One fetal patient with β_0 major thalassemia has thus been engrafted with allogeneic fetal liver cells while she was 12 weeks post fertilization [11]. She is the first human with successful engraftment of allogeneic stem

cells resulting neither from immunosuppressive and myeloablative conditioning nor from congenital immunodeficiency disease. Efficient transplantation and stable tolerance have been obtained in this patient, as they had in the classical experiments carried out in the newborn mouse [17]. Such results are due to the very immature state of the thymus and the thymus-dependent immune system at the time of transplantation, i.e. at birth in the murine species and at the end of the first trimester of fetal development in the human species.

REFERENCES

1   Touraine J-L. Bone marrow and fetal liver transplantation in immunodeficiencies and inborn errors of metabolism : Lack of significant restriction of T-cell function in long-term chimeras despite HLA-mismatch. Immunol Rev 1983 ; 71 : 103-121.

2   Touraine J-L, Raudrant D, Royo C, Rebaud A, Roncarolo M G, Souillet G, Philippe N, Touraine F, Betuel H. *In utero* transplantation of stem cells in bare lymphocyte syndrome. Lancet, 1989 ; i : 1382.

3   Touraine J-L, Roncarolo M G, Royo C, Touraine F. Fetal tissue transplantation, bone marrow transplantation and prospective gene therapy in severe immunodeficiencies and enzyme deficiencies. Thymus 1987 ; 10 : 75-87.

4   Spits H, Touraine J-L, Yssel H, de Vries J E , Roncarolo M G. Presence of host-reactive and MHC-restricted T-cells in a transplanted severe combined immunodeficient (SCID) patient suggest positive selection and absence of clonal deletion. Immunol Rev 1990 ; 116 : 101-116.

5   Bacchetta R, Vandekerckhove B A E, Touraine J-L, Bigler M, Martino S, Gebuhrer L, de Vries J E, Spits H, Roncarolo M G. Chimerism and tolerance to host and donor in severe combined immunodeficiencies transplanted with fetal liver stem cells. J Clin Invest 1993 ; 91 : 1067-1078.

6   Roncarolo M G, Touraine J-L, Banchereau J. Cooperation between major histocompatibility complex mismatched mononuclear cells from a human chimera in the production of antigen-specific antibody. J Clin Invest 1986 ; 77 : 673-680.

7   Roncarolo MG, Yssel H, Touraine J-L, Bacchetta R, Gebuhrer L, de Vries J E, Spits H. Antigen recognition by MHC-incompatible cells of a human mismatched chimera. J Exp Med 1988 ; 168 : 2139-2152.

8   Plotnicky H, Touraine J-L. Cytotoxic T-cells from a human chimera induce regression of EBV-infected allogeneic host cells. Int Immunol (submitted).

9   Bacchetta R, Bigler M, Touraine J-L, de Waal Malefyt R, de Vries J E, Roncarolo M G. High levels of IL-10 production with tolerance in a SCID patient transplanted with fetal stem cells. J Exp Med. (in press).

10   Donckier V, Abramowicz D, Durez P, Gerard C, Velu T, Goldman M. La tolérance néonatale aux alloantigènes s'accompagne d'une activation des lymphocytes TH2 et de la production d'interleukine 10. Abstract présenté à la réunion annuelle de la Société Française de Transplantation, Paris, 4-5 décembre 1992.

11   Touraine J-L. Transplantation of fetal haemopoietic and lymphopoietic cells in humans, with special reference to *in utero* transplantation. In : R.G. Edwards ed. Fetal Tissue Transplants in Medicine, , publ. Cambridge University Press, Cambridge U.K., chapter 6, 1992 : 155-176.

12   Vandekerckhove B A E, Namikawa R, Bacchetta R, Roncarolo MG. Human hematopoietic cells and thymic epithelial cells induce tolerance via different mechanisms in the SCID-hu mouse thymus. J Exp Med 1992 ; 175: 1033-1043.

13   Heeg K, Wagner H. Analysis of immunological tolerance to major histocompatibility complex antigens. I. High frequencies of tolerogen-specific cytotoxic T lymphocyte precursors in mice neonatally tolerized to class I major histocompatibility complex antigens. Eur J Immunol 1985 ; 15: 25-30.

14   Flajnik M F, Du Pasquier L, Cohen N. Immune responses of thymus/lymphocyte embryonic chimeras : Studies on tolerance and major histocompatibility complex restriction in *Xenopus*. Eur J Immunol 1985 ; 15: 540-547.

15   Houssaint E, Torano A, Ivanyi J. Split tolerance induced by grafting chick embryo thymic epithelium allografted to embryonic recipients. J Immunol 1986 ; 136 : 3155-3159.

16   Von Boehmer H, Schubiger K. Thymocytes appear to ignore class I major histocompatibility complex antigens expressed on thymus epithelial cells. Eur J Immunol 1984 ; 14 : 1048-1052.

17   Billingham R E, Brent L, Medawar P B. Actively acquired tolerance of foreign cells. Nature 1953 ; 172 : 603-606.

ROLE OF IL-10 IN TRANSPLANTATION TOLERANCE

Maria-Grazia Roncarolo, Rosa Bacchetta, Jean-Louis Touraine[#], Rene de Waal Malefyt, and Jan E. de Vries, DNAX Research Institute of Cellular and Molecular Biology, 901 California Avenue, Palo Alto, CA USA 94304, FAX: 415-496-1200, Telephone: 415-496-1274. [#]INSERM U80, Hopital E. Herriot, 69374 Lyon, FRANCE.

Introduction

Transplantation of allogeneic hematopoietic stem cells in man can cure a variety of diseases including primary immunodeficiencies, metabolic diseases, hematological disorders and malignancies [see for review 1]. Graft versus host disease (GVHD), however, continues to be the major clinical problem, with a mortality rate as high as 50% [2]. Although the precise effector mechanisms of the GVHD are not clear, it is well established that three prerequisite are necessary for the development of the disease: a histocompatibility antigen difference between the donor and recipient, a source of donor immunocompetent cells, and the inability of the host to reject the graft. There are, however, cases in which transplantation of HLA mismatched cells in a non immunocompetent recipient is not followed by GVHD but, on the contrary, it results in full tolerance between host and donor cells. One of such an example are children with Severe Combined Immunodeficiency (SCID) successfully transplanted with HLA mismatched fetal liver stem cells. In these patients no signs of GVHD

279

J. L. Touraine et al. (eds.), Rejection and Tolerance, 279–290.

have been observed despite the HLA incompatibility between the donor and the host cells and the *in vitro* isolation of donor derived T cells with strong anti-host reactivity [3,4]. The activity of these T cells, which are not deleted from the repertoire, should be suppressed *in vivo* in order to maintain the homeostasis.

Interleukin 10 (IL-10) is a potent suppressor factor for T cell proliferation and has anti inflammatory effects [see for review 5, 6 and 7]. In the present study we analyzed endogenous IL-10 production in SCID patients transplanted with fetal liver stem cells. It is shown that high levels of endogenous IL-10 production may account for the maintenance of transplantation tolerance and the prevention of GVHD in these patients.

Characterization and production of IL-10

Murine IL-10 (mIL-10), which is produced by T helper 2 (Th2) cells, has been discovered because of its capacity to inhibit cytokine synthesis, particularly of IFN-γ, by T helper 1 (Th1) cells [see for review 5,6, and 7]. Human IL-10 (hIL-10) was cloned from a cDNA library established from a CD4+ human T cell clone by cross-hybridization using the mouse IL-10 probe. Human IL-10 has a molecular size of 18 kDa and the IL-10 gene is mapped on chromosome 1. Human IL-10 shares a high degree of homology not only with the mIL-10 but also with a previously uncharacterized sequence in the open reading frame in the Epstein Barr Virus genome BCRF1. This BCRF1 product has been designated viral IL-10 (vIL-10). IL-10 is produced by a variety of cells, including T lymphocytes and monocytes. Interestingly, in contrast to mIL-10, which is a Th2 product, human IL-10 is produced by Th0, Th1 and Th2 cells, but the levels of IL-10 production by Th2 cells are generally somewhat higher than those produced by the Th0 or Th1 subsets [8].

Effects of IL-10 on T cells and monocytes

Like all other cytokines IL-10 is pleiotropic. Among its various biological activities, hIL-10 has an anti-proliferative effect on T cells. Proliferation of peripheral blood T cells in response to exogenous antigens (Ag) or mitogens is strongly suppressed by hIL-10 or vIL-10 when monocytes are used as antigen presenting cells (APC) [9]. In addition, both h- and v-IL-10 strongly inhibit the antigen specific proliferation of human Th0, Th1 and Th2 cell clones. This inhibition is due to a reduced Ag-presenting capacity of the monocytes, which is associated with a strong downregulation of the class II HLA antigens constitutively expressed on these cells. IL-10 also suppresses the proliferative and cytotoxic responses toward alloantigens generated in primary mixed leukocyte cultures (MLC). Such inhibition is also observed when purified CD3+ T cells are used as responder and purified allogeneic monocytes, or B cells as stimulator cells. Increased proliferation of the responder T cells is obtained when primary MLCs are carried out in the presence of neutralizing anti-IL-10 mAbs, indicating that endogenous IL-10 secreted in primary MLC accounts for suppression of proliferative responses in these cultures [10].

In addition to the anti-proliferative effects of h- and vIL-10 mediated trough APC, IL-10 was found to have direct effects on T cell proliferation. These direct effects are caused by specific suppression of IL-2 gene expression and IL-2 production by the T cells, whereas the production of other cytokines such as IFN-γ, IL-4 and GM-CSF is not affected [11]. Furthermore, IL-10 also inhibits the production of pro-inflammatory cytokines (TNF-α, IL1α, IL1β, IL-6, IL-8) and hematopoietic growth factors (G-CSF, GM-CSF) by activated monocytes. In contrast, the production of the IL-1 receptor antagonist, which has been shown to have anti-inflammatory activity, is upregulated by IL-10. Modulation of these cytokine production by monocytes occurs at the transcription level [12].

IL-10 and transplantation tolerance

We investigated the role of IL-10 in maintaining tolerance in SCID patients reconstituted with fetal liver cells derived from HLA mismatched donors. These patients are split chimeras in whom the T cells are of donor-, and the B cells and monocytes are of host-origin. Despite the incompatibility of the donor derived T cells and the host cells, tolerance towards the donor and the host was established after transplantation, as proven by the absence of GVHD and the presence of a specific unresponsiveness of donor derived T cells to host HLA antigens in a primary MLC [13]. However, extensive studies performed with T cell clones established from two different transplanted patients, showed that donor derived T cells which recognize host HLA antigens were not deleted from the repertoire [4,13]. Both CD4+ and CD8+ T cells, specific for the host class II and class I HLA antigens respectively, could be isolated with high frequencies from the peripheral blood of these patients several years after transplantation (Table 1). In general, the CD4+ cell displayed a low proliferative capacity and produced low levels of IL-2 after specific stimulation with host HLA antigens. In contrast, high levels of IL-10 production were detected, particularly in patient RV (Figure 1). These high levels of IL-10 synthesis were only observed after stimulation via the TcR, and were specific for host-reactive T cell clones. Alloreactive T cell clones isolated from the same patient produced significant lower levels of IL-10, which were in the normal range and comparable to those detected in the supernatants of alloreactive T cell clones isolated from normal donors. Kinetic studies have indicated that T cell clones produce IL-10 late after activation and no differences in kinetics were observed between T cell clones belonging to the Th0, Th1 or Th2 subsets [8]. In contrast, host-reactive T cell clones produced IL-10 very early after activation. In addition, blocking experiments using neutralizing anti-IL-10 mAbs showed that this endogenously produced IL-10 was able to suppress the proliferation of these T cell clones in an autocrine fashion.

Consistent with the high IL-10 production *in vitro*, high levels of IL-10 were also observed *in vivo* by comparative PCR analysis of freshly isolated peripheral blood mononuclear cells from the two patients. Cell fractionation experiments indicated that in addition to the donor derived T cells, purified monocytes of host origin expressed high levels of IL-10 mRNA in the absence of any activation. This high expression of IL-10 mRNA was never observed with freshly isolated T cells or monocytes from normal donors. These data indicate that high levels of IL-10, produced by both host monocytes and donor derived T cells, are

Table 1: Proliferative and cytotoxic responses of donor-derived T cell clones from patient SP to host-derived EBV transformed B cell line (SPS)

T cell clones	Phenotype	Poliferation c.p.m. x 10⁻³	Cytotoxicity % lysis	HLA specificity
SP-A3	CD4⁺	80.3	25	DR4
SP-B18	CD4⁺	8.5	32	DR4
SP-B23	CD4⁺	83.2	35	DR4
SP-B24	CD4⁺	15.0	0	DR5
SP-B33	CD4⁺	78.0	0	DR4
SP-B37	CD4⁺	12.7	0	DR4
SP-A8	CD8⁺	5.3	27	class I
SP-A10	CD8⁺	12.3	37	B47
SP-B30	CD8⁺	14.4	28	class I
SP-C5	CD8⁺	8.2	63	A3
SP-C6	CD8⁺	7.9	50	class I
SP-C12	CD8⁺	5.0	40	class I
SP-D47	CD8⁺	8.3	51	B14
SP-D68	CD8⁺	12.9	60	A3

_-2 and IL-10 production by host-reactive T cell clones from patient RV following antigen-specific or polyclonal stimulation

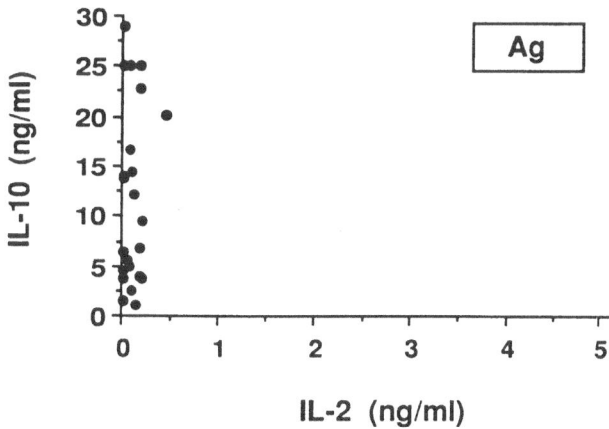

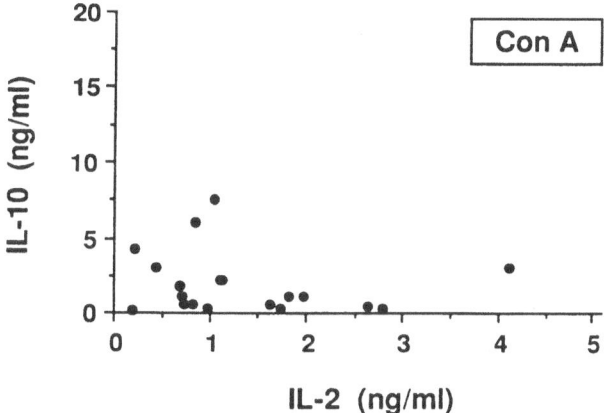

present *in vivo* in these patients. This notion is supported by the observation that class II HLA expression on the monocytes of one of these patients was significantly lower compared to that on monocytes isolated from normal donors. In addition, class II HLA expression on the patient's monocytes was partially restored by short term incubation of these cells in the presence of neutralizing anti-IL-10 mAbs, supporting the notion that endogenous IL-10 indeed is responsible for the reduced class II HLA expression of these cells *in vivo*.

Collectively, these data indicate that endogenous IL-10 production may play an important role not only in establishing and maintaining transplantation tolerance, but also in preventing GVHD. Although the mechanism of induction of endogenous IL-10 production in these patients remains to be determined, one possible explanation could be that the specific recognition by donor-derived T cells of the HLA antigens expressed on the host monocytes, results in high levels of IL-10 production. These continuous interactions would lead to a mutual activation and IL-10 production by these cells. Locally produced IL-10 could account for the prevention of T cell activation, IL-2 production and major expansion of host-reactive T cells.

Concluding remarks

Despite significant progress made in the last ten years, GVHD remains the major barrier to effective allogeneic transplantation [2,14]. This disease is due to an immune response of donor T cells toward host tissues. Although donor T cells present in the transplanted cell suspension play a major role in this immune reaction, it is clear that pro-inflammatory cytokines produced by the T cells itself as well as by the accessory cells contribute to the induction and maintenance of this process. Animal studies have indicated that blocking of IL-1 and TNF-α production can significantly improve the outcome of the disease [15]. Therefore, because of its inhibitory effects on the production of pro-inflammatory cytokines and its inhibition and/or prevention of T cell activation and proliferation, exogenous or endogenous IL-10 may be useful to prevent, or reduce, GVHD.

DNAX Research Institute of Molecular and Cellular Biology is supported by Schering-Plough Corporation.

References

1.   Storb R, Thomas ED. Transplantation of Bone Marrow. In: Samter M, Talmage DW, Frank MM, Austen KF, Claman HN, editors. Immunological Diseases. Boston: Little, Brown and Company, Inc. 1988: 467-495.

2.   Parkman R. Human Graft-versus-host disease. Immunodef Rev 1991;2:253-64.

3.   Touraine JL, Roncarolo MG, Royo C, Touraine F. Fetal tissue transplantation, bone marrow transplantation and prospective gene therapy in severe immunodeficiencies and enzyme deficiencies. Thymus 1987;10:75-87.

4.   Roncarolo MG, Yssel H, Touraine JL, Betuel H, de Vries JE, Spits H. Autoreactive T cell clones specific for class I and class II HLA antigens isolated from a human chimera. J Exp Med 1988;167:1523-34.

5.   Moore K, O'Garra A, de Waal Malefyt R, Vieira P, Mosmann TR. Interleukin 10. Ann Rev Immunol 1993;11:165-90.

6.   Howard M, O'Garra A, Ishida H, de Waal Malefyt R, de Vries JE. Biological properties of interleukin 10. J Clin Immunol 1992;12:239-47.

7.   de Waal Malefyt R, Yssel H, Roncarolo MG, Spits H, de Vries JE. 1992. Interleukin-10. Curr Opin Immunol 1992;4:314-20.

8.   Yssel H, de Waal Malefyt R, Roncarolo MG, Abrams JS, Lahesmaa R, Spits H, de Vries JE. 1992. IL-10 is produced by subsets of human CD4+ T cell clones and peripheral blood T cells. J Immunol 1992;149:2378-84.

9. de Waal Malefyt R, Haanen J, Spits H, Roncarolo MG, te Velde A, Figdor C, Johnson K, Kastelein R, Yssel H, de Vries JE. Interleukin 10 (IL-10) and viral IL-10 strongly reduce antigen-specific human T cell proliferation by diminishing the antigen-presenting capacity of monocytes via down-regulation of class II major histocompatibility complex expression. J Exp Med 1991;174:915-24.

10. Bejarano MT, de Waal Malefyt R, Abrams JS, Bigler M, Bacchetta R, de Vries JE, Roncarolo MG. Interleukin 10 inhibits allogeneic proliferative and cytotoxic T cell responses generated in primary mixed lymphocyte cultures. Int Immunol 1992;4:1389-97.

11. de Waal Malefyt R, Yssel H, de Vries JE. Direct effects of IL-10 on a subset of human CD4+ T-cells clones and T cells: specific inhibition of IL-2 production and proliferation. J Immunol 1993; in press.

12. de Waal Malefyt R, Abrams J, Bennett B, Figdor C, de Vries JE. Interleukin 10 (IL-10) inhibits cytokine synthesis by human monocytes: an autoregulatory role of IL-10 produced by monocytes. J Exp Med 1991;174:1209-20.

13. Bacchetta R, Vandekerckhove BAE, Touraine JL, Bigler M, Martino S, Gebuhrer L, de Vries JE, Spits H, Roncarolo MG. Chimerism and tolerance to host and donor in severe combined immunodeficiencies transplanted with fetal liver stem cells. J Clin Invest 1993;91:1067-78.

14. Ferrara JLM, Deeg HJ. Graft-versus-host disease. N Engl J Med 1991;324:667-74.

15. Antin JH, Ferrara JL. Cytokine dysregulation and acute graft-versus-host disease. Blood 1992;80:2964-68.

VETO CELLS AND THE INDUCTION OF TRANSPLANT TOLERANCE IN PRIMATES

Authors: Judith M. Thomas, Kathryn M. Verbanac, John P. Smith, F. Melinda Carver, Jane Kasten-Jolly, Ulrike M. Gross, Lorita M. Rebellato, Carl E. Haisch and Francis T. Thomas

Address: Judith M. Thomas, East Carolina University School of Medicine, Department of Surgery, Division of Transplantation, Brody Building room 4S-16, Greenville, NC 27858. Telephone (919) 816-2625; FAX (919) 816-3542.

Introduction: Long term success of clinical allotransplantation is still limited by persistent donor directed immunologic rejection. Although nonspecific maintenance immunosuppressive drug therapies are currently in use to prevent graft rejection, these therapies are not entirely effective and the chronic use of immuno-suppressive drugs frequently is accompanied by debilitating complications. Transplantation tolerance has been achieved in many animal models but there are few clinically applicable treatment strategies that induce specific immunologic unresponsiveness to donor antigens without chronic immunosuppressive drugs.

To investigate immunobiologic mechanisms underlying tolerance induction and to facilitate preclinical application of tolerance strategies, we have developed a kidney allograft tolerance model in rhesus monkeys [1,2]. We use the term tolerance here to designate functional long term graft acceptance without chronic immunosuppressive drugs. Our studies in nonhuman primates have utilized a basic treatment strategy of posttransplant (postTx) rabbit antithymocyte globulin (RATG) and donor bone marrow cell (BMC) infusion, as adapted from a murine allograft tolerance model [3]. The infusion of unfractionated donor BMC, particularly a BMC subset, into rhesus kidney transplant (KTx) recipients given only a 5 day course of RATG promotes long term kidney allograft acceptance [1,2,4,5]. We found that donor BMC infusion specifically inhibited the generation of donor-directed CTL and we have postulated that this was due to a *veto* effect [4,5].

J. L. Touraine et al. (eds.), Rejection and Tolerance, 291–323.

The veto concept of allograft tolerance: The veto hypothesis has also been considered in other models of CTL unresponsiveness and graft tolerance induced by donor BMC, lymphoid cells or DST in T cell deficient rodents [6-10] and in the specific inactivation of CTLp after DST in humans [11-13]. The veto concept, originated by Miller, is a functional designation for a mechanism by which donor antigen presenting cells (APC) function as veto cells by specifically inactivating rather than stimulating host CTLp clones that recognize class I or class I-associated antigens present on the veto cell [14-20]. Unique to this model of specific allogeneic unresponsiveness, the antigen specificity and restriction is dictated entirely by the allogeneic veto cell, and the veto effect on CTLp inactivation *in vitro* occurs in the presence of cells and factors that normally induce CTLp activation. Like conventional APC, cells exhibiting veto activity are bone-marrow derived and have been found in tissues associated with T cell maturation.

The veto effect has been associated with clonal inactivation of antigen-specific CTLp by functional deletion [8,15,21-26]. The inactivation can result from anergy [6,24] or clonal deletion [21,23,24]. CTLp appear to be highly susceptible to veto effects, particularly and, in some cases exclusively, the helper-independent [26-28] and high affinity, donor-directed CTLp population(s) [6]. Recent studies have shown that BM-derived cells can also inactivate antigen-specific Th cells which recognize them [21,29-33], although little is known about the mechanism of inhibition. The overall relevance of the veto effect to transplant tolerance has been recently reviewed by our group [34-36] and general observations on the veto effect have been reviewed by others [17,19,37].

Host milieu in tolerance induction: There is persuasive evidence in inbred rodents and also in large outbred species that allograft tolerance can be induced in MHC mismatched adult recipients, provided that recipient peripheral T cells are depleted with either anti-T lymphocyte antibody [1,38-43] or irradiation [44-48] or both [49-51]. This is consistent with the hypothesis that presentation of donor BMC in a T cell-deficient environment favors tolerance, although questions remain concerning the unique contribution of each of these components. The immaturity of responding T cells may also be critical for tolerance signals [52-56]

RATG, a cornerstone of our KTx model, has potent immunosuppressive activity in monkeys and humans and remains a key component of clinical prophylactic and rescue immunosuppressive strategies [57-61]. RATG has broad reactivity against leukocyte antigens [62], acutely depletes circulating T lymphocytes [61] and enhances suppressor cell activity [63]. The sustained distinctive immunological milieu created by RATG appears to be critical to the BMC-mediated induction of tolerance in rhesus monkeys.

A subpopulation of allogeneic BMC mediates the veto effect in vitro and in vivo: In order to investigate the mechanism of rhesus BMC-induced unresponsiveness, we developed an MLR-induced CML assay system in which the addition of freshly isolated allo BMC to the MLR cultures in the presence of exogenous IL2 inhibited donor specific CTL responses in a dose dependent manner [5]. Furthermore, the specificity of inactivation for CTL responses to stimulator cells from the BMC donor was confirmed in three-cell experiments [65] in which bystander effects on CTL responses to unrelated stimulator cells were minimal, even in the same culture wells. Using a Mab-depletion negative selection method with immunomagnetic beads, *in vitro* studies showed that CTLp inhibition depended on the presence of a phenotypically distinct BMC population [5]. BMC that exhibit veto activity in MLR-induced CML are $CD1^+$, $CD2^+$, $CD8^+$, $CD16^+$, $DR^{-/dim}$, $CD3^{-/dim}$ and do not express CD4, CD7, CD11b, CD20, CD28, CD38, CD45RA, CD58 or TCRβ.

To investigate the hypothesis that a donor BMC subset might also promote allograft acceptance *in vivo*, donor BMC were depleted of defined subpopulations prior to infusion into RATG treated recipients. Veto activity *in vitro* and promotion of graft acceptance *in vivo* was more consistently achieved by removal of the DR^{bright} cells from allo BMC. Allograft survival could be regularly prolonged to a median 4-5 months survival following infusion of either intact donor BMC or $DR^{-/dim}$ donor BMC ($p < 0.001$ and $p < 0.00001$ vs RATG only controls)[65]. However, the $DR^{-/dim}$ donor BMC subpopulation had a superior effect in promoting allograft acceptance, resulting in an 84% increase in median GST compared to intact donor BMC (p < 0.05). Graft acceptance extended to one year in 11% of recipients given intact donor BMC and in 23% of recipients given DR$^{-/dim}$ donor BMC.

Depletion of DR^{bright} cells represents a ~30% purification of the active BMC population, which may partially account for the advantage. However, outbred, unrelated rhesus monkeys are strong responders to alloantigen, and a more likely explanation is that depletion of DR^{bright} cells removes highly immunogenic APC subsets that antagonize tolerogenic signals delivered by BMC veto cells. Low doses of DR$^{-/dim}$ BMC appeared to be more effective in tolerance induction, perhaps because the veto population is small, and large numbers of bystander cells in donor BM carry a risk of sensitization to class I without apparent benefit. Consistent with the monkey findings, class II expression on BMC has been implicated in resistance to tolerogenic effects of donor BMC in neonatal mice [66] and also to resistance to veto effects on CTLp [32].

Limiting dilution analysis (LDA) of PBL taken from rhesus KTx recipients after infusion of DR$^{-/dim}$ donor BMC exhibited specific clonal inactivation of donor-directed CTLp [65,67]. In contrast, recipients given either no donor BMC, irradiated BMC [65], or BMC that was depleted of CD8 cells [68], failed to show reduction in donor-reactive CTLp or development of KTx tolerance. In each of these groups, there was no significant reduction in CTLp *f* against third party stimulators/targets. These studies verified the donor-directed specificity of CTLp unresponsiveness, consistent with a BMC-mediated veto effect. In addition, the loss of veto activity after CD8 depletion is in agreement with work by others [37,69] which suggest an important role for CD8 in veto effects.

In further agreement with *in vitro* findings, allo BMC depleted of CD2$^+$ or CD16$^+$ cells have also failed to promote KTx tolerance indicating that the tolerance-promoting allo BMC population is contained in these subpopulations [5,68]. Recent *in vitro* studies also indicate heterogeneous expression of CD5. FACS analysis of defined veto associated markers on BMC indicates that veto activity is mediated by a small BMC population (<5%). We are presently investigating whether this population represents a single or multiple lineage.

A precursor BMC population is involved in the suppressive effect of allogeneic BMC in vitro and in vivo: In both the *in vitro* veto assay system with normal allogeneic responders and in the LDA studies of CTLp in transplant recipients, the inhibitory effect of allo BMC is consistent with a precursor cell. *In vitro*, veto activity was eliminated if fresh BMC were either irradiated (1500 cGy) or pretreated with mitomycin, suggesting that fresh BMC contain a precursor of the cell that mediates the veto effect [65,70]. Similarly, *in vivo* studies showed that the effect of donor BMC in reducing donor-directed CTLp frequency (*f*) and in promoting KTx acceptance was lost, if recipients were treated with the antimetabolite drugs Azathioprine [71] or Cyclophosphamide or if the BMC were irradiated immediately before infusion [65,71]. In addition to implicating a precursor cell, these studies indicated that conventional antimetabolite immunosuppressive agents failed to promote tolerance induction by allo BMC in monkeys.

The veto effect and the maintenance of tolerance: We have proposed that a veto effect of donor BMC on donor-directed CTLp is key to the induction phase of KTx tolerance in outbred rhesus monkeys [4,5]. In contrast to recipients treated with RATG and donor BMC, non-BMC treated RATG controls maintained donor-reactive CTLp *f* [65], generated CTL effectors [5], and develop acute cellular rejection within 3-7 weeks [65]. The specific BMC-mediated reduction in donor-reactive CTLp, however, is not complete and is not permanent. The significance of the remaining CTLp is unclear, but they may represent the low affinity, helper dependent alloreactive clones that have been proposed to have limited in vivo relevance [72]. Recovery of CTLp to preTx levels occurs between 2.5-4.5 months after transplantation [65]. Approximately 50% of KTx recipients given RATG & donor BMC undergo rejection within this time frame, but the relationship of CTLp recovery to the instability of tolerance is unclear since mature CTLs were not detected by CML. The recovery of donor-directed CTLp frequencies to normal levels, in the absence of mature CTL effectors in stable, long-term survivors [73] suggests that systemic inactivation of those CTLp clones that are able to directly recognize native alloantigen is critical only for induction but not for the maintenance of allograft tolerance.

A persuasive explanation for the return to normal CTLp *f* in the absence of mature CTL effectors is that the predominance of donor-directed CTL fades when donor APC presenting native alloantigen have left the graft and are presumably eliminated systemically by host NK cells that recognize the absence of self [74]. Without costimulating signals from allogeneic APC, donor-reactive CTLp might recover their clonal frequency but should remain dormant. CTLp that happen to be sequestered early within the graft parenchyma [75,76] may be anergized there or deleted locally by BMC-derived chimeric cells that home to the graft site, as suggested in our earlier studies [4,77]. We next investigated several possible mechanisms of CTLp inactivation in the context of experimental findings in the rhesus model.

Cell-cell contact is required for BMC-induced inactivation of CTL: Retention of relative specificity in CML suppression within three-cell experiments suggested a close cell-cell interaction in the suppressive mechanism. This was addressed in Transwell cultures in which allo BMC were separated from the MLR culture by a semipermeable membrane. Results showed no CTL inhibition unless the BMC and responders were on the same side of the membrane, indicating a requirement for BMC-responder contact or a paracrine effect of BMC [65]. Since excess exogenous IL2 is routinely added to veto assays, IL2 consumption could be excluded from the inhibitory mechanism. Furthermore, kinetic studies indicated that BMC inhibited CTL generation at an early stage, also eliminating cold target blockade as a mechanism [65].

BMC that mediate veto activity are resistant to pretreatment with L-leucyl-leucine methyl ester (leu-leu-OMe): Although the phenotyping data are consistent with a restricted lineage of veto BMC, they do not define a homogeneous population. The $DR^{-/dim}$, $CD3^{-/dim}$, $CD2^+$ $CD8^+$, $CD16^+$ expression suggested a NK/LAK population, and both NK [78] and LAK cells [10,79] have been implicated as effectors of veto activity in mice. Since rhesus NK and LAK cells express CD45RA and CD38 [80,81], and veto BMC do not, the role of NK/LAK cells in this system was uncertain. NK,

LAKp, CTLp, monocytes and macrophages contain the lysosomal enzyme dipeptidyl dipeptidase I (DPPI) and are killed by the lysosomotrophic agent L-leu-leu-OMe [82,83]. Leu-leu-OMe at low concentrations ($<200\ \mu$M) does not impair stem cell progenitors in humans or monkeys but can exert toxic effects on committed myeloid, erythroid and monocyte precursors [84]. We thus used Leu-leu-OMe as a tool to further define the rhesus BMC subpopulation(s) which mediates veto activity.

We found that pretreatment of rhesus DR$^{-/dim}$ BMC with 50-200 μM Leu-leu-OMe had no significant effect on in vitro veto activity [65]. In control assays, MLR responding Th cells, which also lack DPPI, were not inhibited by leu-leu-OMe, but LAKp and NK activities were significantly inhibited. These data indicate that BMC veto cells were deficient in DPPI and argue against NK, LAK, CTLp, macrophages or monocytes as mediators of the veto effect. Recent evidence indicates that donor BMC which mediate veto activity and promote tolerance in irradiated mice are also resistant to leu-leu-OMe [48,85].

Veto activity may be mediated by BMC dendritic precursor cells: Associations between reported properties of dendritic cell (DC) precursors and monkey veto BMC support a hypothesis that allo BMC dendritic cells may mediate the veto effect: (1) Blood DC lack DPPI and are resistant to leu-leu-OMe, which has been used to purify these cells from contaminating monocytes, macrophages, NK and LAK cells [86]; (2) Like monkey veto BMC, some DC are sensitive to high dose, but not low dose UVb treatment [65]; (3) BM-derived CD8$^+$ DC have been implicated in tolerance [87]; (4) There are phenotypic similarities between veto BMC and DC. Murine and human DC precursors [86,88] have low expression of class II MHC that is upregulated after maturation [88,89]. Futhermore, both veto BMC and DC have been shown to express CD1, CD2, CD8, and CD45, but lack CD45RA expression [87,90,91]. The low affinity Fc IgG receptor CD16, however, has not yet been reported on DC. Whether CD16 represents a second regulatory population or is a property of monkey DC is yet unclear. CD16 is a myeloid marker, and recent evidence has revealed the presence of another myeloid marker, CD33, on human blood DC [86]. Furthermore,

CD16 is present on some monkey thymic DC (J.M. Thomas, unpublished observations. (5) Finally, TGFβ, which has been implicated in the rhesus veto mechanism, has been shown to be expressed on DC [92].

The veto mechanism of CTLp inactivation: The role of CD8 and transforming growth factor-beta (TGF-β): The finding that the veto BMC is leu-leu-OMe-resistant indicated that veto-induced suppression in this model was not mediated by direct cytolysis. Our data from the Transwell cultures and the three-cell experiments suggested that the veto mechanism did not involve a profuse release of nonspecific immunoregulatory cytokines [65]. Recent data, however, suggests that the veto mechanism may be mediated, at least in part, by paracrine or focal TGF-β expression or release, regulated through the veto cell CD8 — responder cell class I ligand interaction [68]. These studies provide support for the role of CD8 as an immunoregulatory molecule in the veto effect of monkey BMC, a concept initially proposed by Miller's and Tykocinski's studies in mouse and human veto models, respectively [37,69].

The hypothesis that TGF-β could be involved in the veto effect on CTLp was stimulated by several immunosuppressive properties that are shared by veto cells. TGF-β, like veto BMC, inhibits MLR-induced CML in the presence of IL2, acting at an early stage in CTL maturation [68,93-95]. We detected TGF-β only in MLR/CML cultures containing DR$^{-/dim}$ BMC or L-leu-leu-OMe-treated BMC and, most significantly, BMC-mediated suppression in MLR/CML cultures was relieved by anti-TGF-β antibody [68]. We found that responder pretreatment with anti-class I or BMC pretreatment with anti-CD8 appeared to regulate veto activity and treatment of DR$^{-/dim}$ BMC with anti-CD8 mAbs elicited TGF-β secretion. The levels of active TGF-β in culture supernatants were low ($\sim$ 30-130 pg/ml), consistent with a paracrine effect in the veto mechanism.

We suggest that the allospecificity of BMC-directed CTLp inhibition may be a function of close T cell — veto cell interaction, such that the nonspecific immunosuppressive factor TGF-β would be available at biologically effective concentrations only within the microenvironment of intimate T cell — BMC conjugates. We are investigating the precise effects of TGF-β on CTLp, with special attention to reported TGF-β effects. TGF-β may induce apoptosis on CTLp [96-98] or, alternatively, may induce CTLp anergy by inhibiting perforin gene expression or BLT esterase activity [95] or by causing cell cycle arrest in the pre-replicative G1 phase [99-101].

Alloantibody, DR sharing, and the stability of allo-BMC induced KTx tolerance: Since the mechanism of allograft rejection is primarily T cell-mediated, strategies for inducing allograft tolerance have appropriately targeted CTLs. However, the deleterious effects of postTx alloantibodies on graft survival cannot be ignored [102-106]. The role of alloantibody in allograft rejection appears to depend on the type of allograft, the immunologic status of the recipient and the donor-recipient immunological disparity [107-110]. Donor-specific cytotoxic antibody has been associated clinically with kidney rejection [105,111-114], however it has not always been established whether antibody is a cause or a consequence of graft injury. In a rat model, DST has been shown to suppress anti donor IgG production [103]. In our KTx model, we have tested recipient serum in RATG controls and those given DR$^{-/dim}$ donor BMC for presence and titer of IgG antidonor antibody by antibody dependent cellular cytotoxicity (ADCC), complement dependent cytotoxicity, and FACS cross-matches at various times after KTx [104]. Results showed that infusion of DR$^{-/dim}$ BMC specifically inhibited antidonor class I IgG antibody responses in the first two months ($p < 0.05$). However, untreated controls and BMC-treated recipients were still capable of responding to RATG with appropriate IgG titers. The suppression of antidonor IgG antibody by DR$^{-/dim}$ BMC was not permanent; most recipients (77%) eventually developed serum antibody. Moreover, the appearance of serum antibody showed a significant, predictive correlation with the temporal development of KTx rejection. These findings can be interpreted through the veto concept, with a veto effect of donor BMC on Th cells. This concept is consistent with recent mouse studies that have shown veto effects on Th cells [21,28,30]. In support of this theory, preliminary experiments indicate that rhesus DR$^{-/dim}$ allo BMC can inhibit Th mediated MLR responses. Our observations that low density BMC, which are effective at CTLp inactivation, fail to suppress early antidonor antibody responses [104] suggest that the subpopulation that "vetoes" the CTLp differs from that which suppresses alloantibody. However, we have not yet determined whether interacting donor BMC populations are involved in the suppression of antidonor IgG responses in rhesus monkeys.

Retrospective typing for MHC disparities in recipient-donor combinations have suggested that stable tolerance requires one DR haplotype sharing. All recipient-donor combination exhibited strong one-way MLR responses, but typing for class II DR showed differences in DR haplotype sharing. We used a combination of methods for class II DR typing, including serological typing with human reagents, restriction fragment length polymorphism (RFLP) analysis and rhesus monkey sequence specific primer (SSP)-PCR analysis using allele-specific sequences of DRβ genes [115]. Of those recipientswho rejected in < 3.5 months, 100% of donors (6/6) shared 0 DR antigens with the recipient. In contrast, among those surviving 4 months to > 1 year, 90% (9/10) shared 1 DR antigen, and 1 shared 2 DR antigens. Thus the sharing of 1 DR haplotypehad a significant positive effect in facilitating tolerance induction by donor DR$^{-/dim}$ BMC. DR one haplotye sharing has also been shown to have a beneficial effect on DST in human transplantation. This mechanism has not been elucidated, however both van Rood [11] and van Twuyver [117] have recently postulated a veto effect may be responsible.

The suppressive effect of DR$^{-/dim}$ BMC on cytotoxic IgG antidonor antibody mirrored the graft tolerance-promoting effect and showed a similar association with one DR haplotype sharing. The recipients making early antidonor IgG responses were those with 0 DR matches. The specificity of the antidonor IgG in 0 DR matched recipients is currently under study, but preliminary data indicate many early antibodies are class I directed. A remarkably similar effect of DR sharing on DST effects on class I antibodies in humans has been noted [11,13,116,117]. Thus, a clear consequence of class II DR one haplotype matching was to suppress cytotoxic anti-class I IgG antibody production. Anti-class I cytotoxic antibodies are potentially more deleterious than those directed to class II, because of the widespread distribution of class I on endothelium and limited distribution of class II during immunological quiescence. Alloantibody responses in this model may be caused by T independent B cell responses or by a Th1/Th2 cytokine imbalance of donor-reactive clones. Alternatively, the processing of donor MHC molecules by host cells and presentation of donor allo MHC peptides on self-restricted host MHC class II molecules could open an indirect avenue for a different phase of effector activity mediated through host APC/T helper/B cell interactions. We suggest that this latter mechanism likely mediates late rejection in this model, and that 1 DR haplotype sharing extends the range of donor BMC veto effects to the indirect APC pathway.

Recent studies suggest that presentation of donor MHC peptides by host APC may be a common event during in vivo alloresponses [118-120]. This indirect pathway of allopeptide presentation may be the most relevant in chronic rejection because the graft is less likely to stimulate direct recognition after migration of passenger leukocytes [119]. This was recently supported by adoptive transfer studies in which CD4$^+$ T cells activated by the direct pathway initiated acute rejection of normal allografts, but not of passenger leukocyte-depleted grafts [121]. Thus, the T cell population involved in early rejection may be different from those in late rejection.

Relationship of Chimerism to Graft Tolerance in RATG & BM-treated Models: Chimerism has become almost synonymous with the mechanism of transplant tolerance, but *per se*, chimerism reveals little about the cellular process by which unresponsiveness is either induced or maintained. There are many degrees of chimerism, from macrochimerism seen in therapeutic full replacement BM transplantation, to the midichimerism seen in mixed allogeneic BMC irradiation tolerance models [9,122,123], to microchimerism [4,49,65,124-128]. While some studies have shown a direct correlation between tolerance and the presence and/or degree of chimerism [9,53,122,123,129], others indicate conversely that mice with neonatal-induced chimerism can reject donor allografts [130].

A functional role of chimerism in maintaining tolerance has been suggested by experiments in rodents in which deliberate elimination of chimeric cells resulted in loss of tolerance [53,122-124,129,131]. Together these data suggest that the maintenance of tolerance is dependent on the persistence of radiation sensitive cell(s) of donor origin. The inability of normal syngeneic lymphocytes to break tolerance is entirely consistent with a veto function of chimeric cells. Early studies showed tolerance could be adoptively transferred with lymphoid cells [132] and was originally attributed to T suppressor cells [133,134]. However, as efforts to identify T suppressor cells failed, alternative explanations for the adoptive transfer phenomenon have arisen, including the infectious tolerance concept of Waldmann [135] and a veto effect mediated by chimeric populations within the transferred cells [15,38,124-127,136].

We have carried out preliminary studies on chimerism in various models of donor BMC-induced allograft tolerance in RATG-treated monkey KTx recipients, using two PCR methods, sequence-specific conformational polymorphism (SSCP) [137,138] and SSP [115], which take advantage of the high degree of polymorphism within the MHC DRβ genes. In the RATG and DR$^{-/dim}$ donor BMC KTx model with graft prolongation from 87-635 days, all recipients studied exhibited temporary PBL microchimerism, the decline of which predicted rejection. However, despite rejection, chimerism remained in the BM, skin and liver. FACS studies using allele-specific anti-class II mAbs indicated chimeric cells mainly expressed CD8. Together with in vitro functional data, this suggests that a small population of CD8$^+$ chimeric cells may be responsible for the veto effect on CTLp in the induction of specific KTx tolerance.

A question unresolved in most chimerism studies is whether the chimeric cells derive from the tolerizing BMC or from the tolerized graft. We have begun to confront this issue with two experimental strategies. In one set of experiments, we transduced cultured DR$^{-/dim}$ donor BMC with pHSG*neo* recombinant retrovirus [139] prior to infusion. This method provided a permanent DNA marker on the BMC to define the derivation of chimeric populations. In the two recipients who received transduced BMC, graft survival was prolonged and PBL chimerism was detected. Interestingly, *neo*$^+$ BMC homed preferentially to skin & LN, which further supports the hypothesis that a BMC dendritic cell precursor may mediate veto effects.

To expedite analysis of BMC-derived chimerism issues, we

have developed another experimental model using transgenic C3H mice as BMC donors and normal C3H mice as skin donors to B6AF1 recipients [140] in a Wood/Monaco ALS treatment model [141]. The transgene in these BMC donor mice, the rat myosin heavy chain gene, was not expressed in BMC, so the presence of the transgene could not affect survival of the BMC. We found that donor BMC-derived chimerism persisted in PBL, skin and LN for 2 weeks; however, after 4 weeks, chimerism persisted only in recipient skin, even beyond rejection. In both mouse and monkey chimerism studies in RATG-treated recipients, the emerging pattern suggests that PBL rather than tissue chimerism is correlated with unresponsiveness.

Synergistic effects of posttransplant LI in promoting stable tolerance: Our earlier studies made it apparent that conventional antimetabolite immunosuppressive drugs failed to promote allograft tolerance induction by allo BMC in monkeys. We thus developed a strategy for stable tolerance by supplementing RATG and donor BMC with postTx lymphoid irradiation (LI) [51,142]. LI is an effective immunosuppressive technique that activates natural suppressor cells and establishes a favorable immunological milieu for tolerance induction, in the absence of chronic immunosuppressive drug therapy [143-145]. LI has the advantage of targeting noncirculating cells not depleted by RATG, thus providing more complete lymphoid depletion. In addition, LI is delivered through narrow ports that can be designed to shield and spare host bone marrow.

Although postTx LI by itself is not immunosuppressive [51,146,147], we developed a strategy using judicious application of postTx, low dose fractionated LI, after RATG-induced peripheral T cell depletion but before infusion of the radiosensitive $DR^{-/dim}$ BMC. This supplementation of LI to the RATG, $DR^{-/dim}$ BMC protocol led to a more uniform and stable KTx tolerance [51]. Our initial report indicated a 60% one year actuarial graft survival by administering a total dose of 500-625 cGy to splenectomized recipients given RATG and $DR^{-/dim}$ $CD3^{-/dim}$ donor BMC [51]. Expanded results in the animals given the full combination treatment indicate an actual 63% (5/8) GST beyond 300 days, with three animals surviving >1000 days (manuscript in preparation). Only two recipients that died from complications of irradiation exposure due to protocol aberrations were excluded in this analysis. These results are far superior to those splenectomized recipients given only RATG and postTx LI or those given only RATG and $DR^{-/dim}$ $CD3^-$ donor BMC [51].

A significant observation in the PT-LI series was the requirement for CD3 depletion of the donor $DR^{-/dim}$ BMC to obtain a beneficial effect with PT-LI [142]. Without CD3 depletion, graft survival results with $DR^{-/dim}$ BMC were not significantly increased by supplemental PT-LI. DR matching was not a factor since there was no difference in DR incompatibilities between these groups. In the recipient group supplemented by PT-LI and splenectomy, microchimerism in PBL and other tissues (including bone marrow, heart, liver, skin and proximal lymph node) was still observed at the time of necropsy. PBL chimerism was both more prominent and more stable in the group given $DR^{-/dim}$ BMC containing $CD3^+$ cells, thus, a likely hypothesis for KTx failure in this group is subclinical or chronic GVH reaction.

Immunological monitoring studies revealed unique immunosuppressive effects in recipients given RATG, LI and CD3-depleted $DR^{-/dim}$ BMC [51]. PostTx LI was found to delay the monkey IgG alloantibody responses, as detected by ADCC, although the onset of anti-RATG responses were similar in LI and non-LI-treated animals. The actual mechanism of the synergy in this highly effective combination treatment of RATG, postTx LI and $DR^{-/dim}$ $CD3^-$ donor BMC in this transplant model, remains to be elucidated, but this strategy holds great promise for clinical application.

In conclusion, we have demonstrated the feasibility of tolerance induction in outbred primates without the use of chronic immunosuppressive drugs. Our studies showed that infusion of donor BMC into RATG-treated recipients resulted in CTLp functional deletion with subsequent long term kidney allograft survival. We propose that this occurs by a veto mechanism. CTLp inactivation was dependent on intimate CTLp—veto cell contact, and our data suggested a paracrine role of TGF-β in CTLp inactivation. Phenotypic analysis indicated that veto activity is associated with a $DR^{-/dim}$, $CD3^-$, $CD2^+$, $CD8^+$, and $CD16^+$ subpopulation which may represent a population of dendritic precursors. Chimerism studies showed that the persistence of donor BMC-derived cells in PBL of KTx recipients was associated with graft survival in this primate model. Donor BMC infusion was found to suppress the early appearance of alloantibody which correlates with graft rejection. Retrospective MHC typing analysis showed that 1 DR haplotype sharing significantly delayed the onset of antidonor antibody production and chronic rejection. This has led us to postulate that the 1 DR sharing affords the persisting donor BMC-derived cells the means of functionally depleting antidonor Th clones responsible for providing help for the antidonor antibody responses. Finally, adjunctive postTx LI affords exceptional KTx survival and represents a promising strategy for tolerance induction in human transplantation.

Acknowledgements:

We acknowledge Dr. Stephen Vore and Dr. Bill Pryor for veterinary support and Mr. Dennis Purvis for monkey care.

References:

1. Thomas J, Carver M, Foil B, Haisch C, Thomas F. Renal allograft tolerance induced with ATG and donor bone marrow in outbred rhesus monkeys. Transplantation 1983; 36:104.

2. Thomas FT, Carver FM, Foil B, et al. Long-term incompatible kidney survival in outbred higher primates without chronic immunosuppression. Ann Surg 1983; 198(3):370-375.

3. Wood ML, Monaco AP, Gozzo JJ. Use of homozygous allogeneic bone marrow for induction of tolerance with antilymphocyte serum: Dose and timing. Transplant Proc 1971; 3:676.

4. Thomas J, Carver M, Cunningham P, Park K, Gonder J. Promotion of incompatible allograft acceptance in rhesus monkeys given posttransplant antithymocyte globulin and donor bone marrow: I. In vivo parameters and immuno-histologic evidence suggesting microchimerism. Transplantation 1987; 43(3):332-338.

5. Thomas JM, Carver FM, Cunningham PRG, Olson LC, Thomas FT. Kidney allograft tolerance in primates without chronic immunosuppression: The role of veto cells. Transplantation 1991; 51(1):198-207.

6. Heeg K, Wagner H. Induction of peripheral tolerance to class I major histocompatibility complex (MHC) alloantigens in adult mice: Transfused class I MHC-incompatible splenocytes veto clonal responses of antigen-reactive Lyt-2 + T cells. J Exp Med 1990; 172(3):719-728.

7. Rammensee HG, Fink PJ, Bevan MJ. The veto concept: An economic system for maintaining self-tolerance of cytotoxic T lymphocytes. Transplant Proc 1985; 17(1):689-692.

8. Wood ML, Orosz CG, Gottschalk R, Monaco AP. The effect of injection of donor bone marrow on the frequency of

donor-reactive CTL in antilymphocyte serum-treated, grafted mice. Transplantation 1992; 54:656-671.

9. Ildstad ST, Wren SM, Oh E, Hronakes ML. Mixed allogeneic reconstitution (A+B ---> A) to induce donor-specific transplantation tolerance. Transplantation 1991; 51(6):1262-1267.

10. Azuma E, Kaplan J. Role of lymphokine-activated killer cells as mediators of veto and natural suppression. J Immunol 1988; 141(8):2601-2606.

11. van Rood JJ, Claas FHJ. The influence of allogeneic cells on the human T and B Cell repertoire. Science 1990; 248:1388-1393.

12. Lagaaij EL, Ruigrok MB, van Rood JJ, et al. Blood transfusion induced changes in cell-mediated lympholysis: To immunize or not to immunize. J Immunol 1991; 147(10):3348-3352.

13. van Twuyver E, Mooijaart RJD, Ten Berge IJM, et al. Pretransplantation blood transfusion revisited. N Eng J Med 1991; 325:1210-1213.

14. Muraoka S, Miller RG. Cells in bone marrow and in T cell colonies grown from bone marrow can suppress generation of cytotoxic T lymphocytes directed against their self antigens. J Exp Med 1980; 152:54-71.

15. Martin DR, Miller RG. In vivo administration of histo-incompatible lymphocytes leads to rapid functional deletion of cytotoxic T lymphocyte precursors. J Exp Med 1989; 170(3):679-690.

16. Rammensee HG, Fink PJ, Bevan MJ. Functional clonal deletion of class I-specific cytotoxic T lymphocytes by veto cells that express antigen. J Immunol 1984; 133(5):2390-2396.

17. Fink PJ, Shimonkevitz RP, Bevan MJ. Veto cells. Ann Rev Immunol 1988; 6:115-137.

18. Miller RG. The veto phenomenon and T-cell regulation. Immunol Today 1986; 7(4):112-114.

19. Rammensee HG. Veto function in vitro and in vivo. Int Rev Immunol 1989; 4(2):175-191.

20. Claesson MH, Ropke C. Antiself suppressive (veto) activity of responder cells in mixed lymphocyte cultures. Curr Top Microbiol Immunol 1986; 126:213-223.

21. Kiziroglu F, Miller R. In vivo functional clonal deletion of recipient CD4+ T helper precursor cells that can recognize class II MHC on injected donor lymphoid cells. J Immunol 1991; 146(4):1104-1112.

22. Kisielow P, Bluthmann H, Staerz UD, Steinmetz M, von Boehmer H. Tolerance in T cell receptor transgenic mice involves deletion of nonmature CD4+CD8+ thymocytes. Nature 1988; 333:742-746.

23. Hiruma K, Nakamura H, Henkart PA, Gress RE. Clonal deletion of postthymic T cells: veto cells kill precusor cytotoxic T lymphocytes. J Exp Med 1992; 175:863-868.

24. Roberts JL, Sharrow SO, Singer A. Clonal deletion and clonal anergy in the thymus induced by cellular elements with different radiation sensitivities. J Exp Med 1990; 171:935-940.

25. Brochu S, Roy DC, Perreault C. Tolerance to host minor histocompatibility antigens after allogeneic bone marrow transplantation. J Immunol 1992; 149(10):3135-3141.

26. van Twuyver E, Kast WM, Mooijaart RJD, Wilmink JM, Melief CJM, de Waal LP. Allograft tolerance induction in adult mice

associated with functional deletion of specific CTL precursors. Transplantation 1989; 48(5):844-847.

27. Azuma T, Sato S, Kitagawa S, et al. Tolerance induction of allo-class I H-2 antigen-reactive Lyt-2+ helper cells and prolonged survival of the corresponding class I H-2-disparate skin graft. J Immunol 1989; 143:1-8.

28. Kitagawa S, Sato S, Azuma T, Shimizu J, Hamaoka T. Heterogeneity of CD4+ T cells involved in anti-allo-class I H-2 immune responses. J Immunol 1991; 146:2513-2521.

29. Ryan JJ, Gress RE, Hathcock KS, Hodes RJ. Recognition and response to alloantigens in vivo. II. Priming with accessory cell-depleted donor allogeneic splenocytes: Induction of specific unresponsiveness to foreign major histocompatibility complex determinants. J Immunol 1984; 133(5):2343-2350.

30. Hori S, Sato S, Kitagawa S, et al. Tolerance induction of allo-class II H-2 antigen-reactive L3T4+ helper T cells and prolonged survival of the corresponding class II H-2-disparate skin graft. J Immunol 1989; 143(5):1447-1452.

31. Sato S,, Iwata H,, Kitagawa S,, et al. The lymphoid cell populations required for induction of tolerance of different subsets of alloantigen-reactive T cells. Transplantation 1991; 52:862-867.

32. Hori S, Kitagawa S, Iwata H, et al. Cell-cell interaction in graft rejection responses: Induction of anti-allo-class I H-2 tolerance is prevented by immune responses against allo-class II H-2 antigens coexpressed on tolerogen. J Exp Med 175:99-109.

33. Maeda T, Eto M, Nishimura Y, Nomoto K, Kong YY. Role of peripheral hemopoietic chimerism in achieving donor-specific tolerance in adult mice. J Immunol 1993; 150(3):753-762.

34. Thomas JM, Verbanac KM, Thomas FT. The veto mechanism

in transplant tolerance. Transplant Rev 1991; 5(4):209-229.

35. Thomas JM, Verbanac KM, Carver FM, et al. Veto cells in transplantation tolerance. Clin Transplantation 1993; (in press)

36. Thomas JM, Carver FM, Kasten-Jolly J, Haisch CE, Thomas FT. Transplantation tolerance in nonhuman primates: a case for veto-cells. Transplantation Science 1993; 3(1):66-68.

37. Miller RG, Muraoka S, Claesson MH, Reimann J, Benveniste P. The veto phenomenon in T-cell regulation. Ann NY Acad Sci 1988; 532:170-176.

38. Dorsch S, Roser B. Suppressor cells in transplantation tolerance: I. Analysis of the suppressor status of neonatally and adoptively tolerized rats. Transplantation 1982; 33(5):518-524.

39. Lance EM, Medawar PB. Survival of skin heterografts under treatment with antilymphocyte serum. Lancet 1968; 1(553):1174-1176.

40. Monaco AP, Wood ML, Russell PS. Studies on heterologous anti-lymphocyte serum in mice. III. Immunological tolerance and chimerism produced across the H-2 locus with adult thymectomy and anti-lymphocyte serum. Ann NY Acad Sci 1966; 129:190.

41. Hartner WC, DeFazio SR, Markees TG, Maki T, Monaco AP, Gozzo JJ. Specific tolerance to canine renal allografts following treatment with fractionated bone marrow and antilymphocyte serum. Transplant Proc 1987; XIX(1):476-477.

42. Gozzo JJ, Crowley M, Maki T. Functional characteristics of a ficoll separated mouse bone marrow cell population involved in skin allograft prolongation. J Immunol 1982; 129:1584.

43. Wood ML, Monaco AP. The effect of timing of skin grafts on subsequent survival in ALS-treated, marrow-infused mice. Transplantation 1977; 23:78.

44. Ildstad ST, Wren SM, Bluestone JA, Barbiero SA, Sachs DH. Characterization of mixed allogeneic chimeras. J Exp Med 1985; 162:231.

45. Sykes M, Sachs DH. Mixed allogeneic chimerism as an approach to transplantation tolerance. Immunol Today 1988; 9(1):23-27.

46. Slavin S, Reitz BA, Bieber CP, Kaplan HS, Strober S. Transplantation tolerance in adult rats using total lymphoid irradiation: permanent survival of skin, heart and marrow allografts. J Exp Med 1978; 147:700-707.

47. Myburgh JA, Smit JA, Hill RRH, Browde S. Transplantation tolerance in primates following total lymphoid irradiation and allogeneic bone marrow injection. II. Renal allografts. Transplantation 1980; 29:405-408.

48. Pierce GE, Watts LM. Do donor cells function as veto cells in the induction and maintenance of tolerance across an MHC disparity in mixed lymphoid radiation chimeras. Transplantation 1993; 55(4):882-887.

49. Cobbold SP, Martin G, Qin S, Waldmann H. Monoclonal antibodies to promote marrow engraftment and tissue graft tolerance. Nature 1986; 323:164.

50. Sharabi Y, Sachs DH. Mixed chimerism and permanent specific transplantation tolerance induced by a nonlethal preparative regimen. J Exp Med 1989; 169:493-502.

51. Thomas J, Alqaisi M, Cunningham P, et al. The development of a posttransplant TLI treatment strategy that promotes organ allograft acceptance without chronic immuno-

suppression. Transplantation 1992; 53:247-258.

52. Matzinger P, Guerder S. Does T-cell tolerance require a dedicated antigen-presenting cell? Nature 1989; 338:74-76.

53. Shimonkevitz RP, Bevan MJ. Split tolerance induced by the intrathymic adoptive transfer of thymocyte stem cells. J Exp Med 1988; 168:143-156.

54. Goss JA, Nakafusa Y, Flye MW. Donor-specific cardiac allograft tolerance without immunosuppression after intrathymic injection of donor allonantigen. Transplant Proc 1992; 24(6):2879-2880.

55. Goss JA, Nakafusa Y, Flye MW. Intrathymic injection of donor alloantigens induces donor-specific vascularized tolerance without immunosuppression. Ann Surg 1992; 216(4):409-416.

56. Ohzato H, Monaco AP. Induction of specific unresponsiveness (tolerance) to skin allografts by intrathymic donor-specific splenocyte injection in antilymphocyte serum-treated mice. Transplantation 1992; 54(6):1090-1095.

57. Thomas JM, Carver M, Scott J, Williams E, Thomas F. Effect of rabbit anti-human thymocyte globulin on lymphocyte subpopulations and functions following allotransplantation in the rhesus monkey. Transplantation 1979; 27(3):163-170.

58. Thomas FT, Carver FM, Foil MB, et al. Longer-term incompatible kidney survival in outbred higher primates without chronic immunosuppression. Ann Surg 1983; 198(3):370-375.

59. Thomas J, Carver F, Fahrenbruch G, Hall G, Deepe R, Thomas F. A prostaglandin-dependent immunoregulatory mechanism activated by in vivo administration of antithymocyte globulin (ATG). Surgery 1983; 94(3):384-389.

60. Kirklin J, Bourge R, White-Williams C, et al. Prophylactic therapy for rejection following cardiac transplantation - A comparison of RATG and OKT3. J Thorac Cardiovasc Surg 1990; 99(4):716-724.

61. Thomas FT, Griesedieck C, Thomas J, et al. Differential effects of horse ATG and rabbit ATG on T cell and T cell subset levels measured by monoclonal antibodies. Transplant Proc 1984; 16(6):1561-1563.

62. Rebellato LM, Gross U, Verbanac KM, Thomas JM. A comprehensive definition of the major antibody specificities in polyclonal rabbit antithymocyte globulin (RATG). Transplantation 1993; (in press).

63. Thomas JM, Carver FM, Haisch CE, Fahrenbruch G, Deepe RM, Thomas FT. Suppressor cells in rhesus monkeys treated with antithymocyte globulin. Transplantation 1982; 34(2):83-89.

64. Rebellato L, Gross U, Carver M, et al. Treatment of rhesus monkey allograft recipients with a combination of anti-T-cell antibodies. Transplant Proc 1993; 25(1):598-599.

65. Thomas JM, Carver FM, Kasten-Jolly J, et al. Further studies of veto reactivity in rhesus monkey bone marrow in relation to allograft tolerance and chimerism. Transplantation 1993; (in press)

66. Streilein JW, Socarras S, Powell TJ. Influence of I-E expression on induction of neonatal transplantation tolerance. Eur J Immunol 1991; 21:261-266.

67. Thomas J, Carver M, Rebellato L, Sash C, Cunningham P, Thomas F. Analysis of cytotoxic lymphocyte precursor frequency during kidney transplant rejection in rhesus monkeys. Transplant Proc 1988; 20(2):233-235.

314

68.   Verbanac KM, Carver M, Haisch CE, Thomas JM. Transforming growth factor-Beta (TGF-β) may function in the veto mechanism in transplant tolerance. Transplantation 1993; (in press)

69.   Kaplan D, Hambor J, Tykocinski M. An immunoregulatory function for the CD8 molecule. Proc Natl Acad Sci 1989; 86:8512-8515.

70.   Carver M, Thomas J, Saldanha C, Matthews C, Sash C. In vitro suppression of alloreactivity by rhesus monkey bone marrow cells. Transplant Proc 1989; 21(1):231-232.

71.   Thomas JM, Carver M, Cunningham P, Sash C, Park K, Thomas F. Promotion of incompatible allograft acceptance in rhesus monkeys given posttransplant antithymocyte globulin and donor bone marrow: II. Effects of adjuvant immunosuppressive drugs. Transplantation 1989; 47(2):209-215.

72.   Kosaka H, Sprent J. Tolerance of CD8 + T cells developing in parent--F1 chimeras prepared with sublethal irradiation: Step-wise induction of tolerance in the intrathymic and extrathymic environments. J Exp Med 1993; 177:367-378.

73.   Thomas J, Carver M, Cunningham P, Saldanha C, Thomas F. Mechanism of immunosuppression in long surviving (LS) monkey allograft recipients. Transplant Proc 1989; 21(1):388-390.

74.   Ljunggren HG, Karre K. In search of the "missing self": MHC molecules and NK cell recognition. Immunol Today 1990; 11:237-244.

75.   Bishop DK, Ferguson RM, Orosz CG. Differential distribution of antigen-specific helper T cells and cytotoxic T cells after antigenic stimulation. J Immunol 1990; 144:1153-1160.

76. Ascher NL, Hoffman R, Hanto D, Simmons R. Cellular basis of allograft rejection. Immunol Rev 1984; 77:217-232.

77. Carver M, Thomas J, Gonder P, Cunningham P, Park K, Thomas F. Unresponsiveness to kidney transplants in primates: Immunohistologic studies of long-surviving grafts. Transplant Proc 1987; 19(1):501-503.

78. Cassell D, Forman J. Two roles for CD4 cells in the control of the generation of cytotoxic T lymphocytes. J Immunol 1991; 146:3-10.

79. Uberti J, Martilotti F, Chou TH, Kaplan J. Human lymphokine activated killer (LAK) cells suppress generation of allospecific cytotoxic T cells: Implications for use of LAK cells to prevent graft-versus-host disease in allogeneic bone marrow transplantation. Blood 1992; 79(1):261-268.

80. Carver M, Thomas J. Natural killer cells in rhesus monkeys: Properties of effector cells which lyse Raji targets. Cell Immunol 1988; 117:56.

81. Gengozian N, Langley RE, Filler J, Good RA. Natural killer cells in the blood and bone marrow of the rhesus monkey. Cell Immunol 1986; 101:24.

82. Thiele DL, Lipsky PE. Mechanism of L-leucyl-L-leucine methyl ester-mediated killing of cytotoxic lymphocytes: Dependence on a lysosomal thiol protease, dipeptidyl peptidase I, that is enriched in these cells. Proc Natl Acad Sci 1990; 87:83-87.

83. Thiele DL, Lipsky PE. The action of leucyl-leucine methyl ester on cytotoxic lymphocytes requires uptake by a novel dipeptide-specific facilitated transport system and dipeptidyl peptidase I-mediated conversation to membranolytic products. J Exp Med 1990; 172:183-194.

84. Pecora AL, Bordignon C, Fumagalli L, et al. Characterization of the in vitro sensitivity of human lymphoid and hematopoietic progenitors to L-leucyl-L-leucine methyl ester. Transplantation 1991; 51:524-531.

85. Pierce G, Steers J. Thy1+ donor cells that promote allograft tolerance in sublethally irradiated MHC-disparate hosts. Transplantation 1991; 52:526-530.

86. Thomas R, Davis LS, Lipsky PE. Isolation and characterization of human peripheral blood dendritic cells. J Immunol 1993; 150(3):821-834.

87. Vremec D, Zorbas M, Scollay R, et al. The surface phenotype of dendritic cells purified from mouse thymus and spleen: Investigation of the CD8 expression by a subpopulation of dendritic cells. J Exp Med 1992; 176:47-58.

88. Inaba K, Steinman RM, Witmer-pack M, et al. Identification of proliferating dendritic cell precursors in mouse blood. J Exp Med 1992; 175:1157-1167.

89. Bowers WE, Berkowitz MR. Differentiation of dendritic cells in cultures of rat bone marrow cells. J Exp Med 1986; 163:872-883.

90. Agger R, Crowley MT, Witmer-Pack MD. The surface of dendritic cells in the mouse as studied with monoclonal antibodies. Immunol Rev 1990; 6(2-3):89-102.

91. Budjoso R, Hopkins J, Dutia BM, Young P, McConnell I. Characterization of sheep afferent lymph dendritic cells and their role in antigen processing. J Exp Med 1989; 170:1285-1302.

92. Gruschwitz MS, Hornstein OP. Expression of transforming growth type beta on human epidermal dendritic cells. J Invest Dermatol 1992; 99:114-116.

93. Ranges GE, Figari IS, Espevik T, Palladino MA. Inhibition of cytotoxic T cell development by transforming growth factor-beta and reversal by recombinant tumor necrosis factor-alpha. J Exp Med 1987; 166:991-998.

94. Mule JJ, Schwartz SL, Roberts AB, Sporn MB, Rosenberg SA. Transforming growth factor-beta inhibits the in vitro generation of lymphokine-activated killer cells and cytotoxic T cells. Cancer Immunol Immunother 1988; 26:95-100.

95. Smyth MJ, Strobl SL, Young HA, Ortaldo JR, Ochoa AC. Regulation of lymphokine-activated killer activity and pore-forming protein gene expression in human peripheral blood CD8+ T lymphocytes: Inhibition by transforming growth factor-beta. J Immunol 1991; 146(10):3289-3297.

96. Bursch W, Oberhammer F, Jirtle RL, et al. Transforming growth factor-β1 as a signal for induction of cell death by apoptosis. Br J Cancer 1993; 67(1):531-536.

97. Rotello RJ, Lieberman RC, Purchio AF, Gerschenson LE. Coordinated regulation of apoptosis and cell proliferation by transforming growth factor Beta 1 in cultured uterine epithelial cells. Proc Natl Acad Sci USA 1991; 88:3412-3415.

98. Lin JK, Chou CK. In vitro apoptosis in the human hepatoma cell line transforming growth factor beta. Can Res 1992; 52:385-388.

99. Pietenpol JA, Moran E, Yaciuk P, et al. TGF-β1 inhibition of c-myc transcription and growth in keratinocytes is abrogated by viral transforming proteins with pRB binding domains. Cell 1990; 61:735-738.

100. Laiho M, DeCaprio JA, Lulow JW, Livingston DM, Massague J. Growth inhibition by TGF-beta linked to suppression of retinoblastoma protein phosphorylation. Cell 1990; 62:175-185.

101. Howe PH, Draetta G, Leof EB. Transforming growth factor-beta inhibition of phosphorylation and histone H1 kinase activity is associated with G1/S-phase growth arrest. Mol Cell Biol 1991; 11(3):1185-1194.

102 Halloran PF, Schault J, Solez K, Srinivasa NS. The significance of the anti-class I response. Transplantation 1992; 53(3):550-555.

103 Wasowska B, Baldwin WM, Sanfilippo F. IgG alloantibody responses to donor specific blood transfusion in different rat strain combinations as a predictor of renal allograft survival. Transplantation 1992; 53(1):175-180.

104. Thomas JM, Carver FM, Cunningham PR, et al. Donor bone marrow infusion suppresses alloantibody response in RATG-treated recipients: A correlate of long survival. Transplant Proc 1993; 25(1):342-343.

105. Halloran PF, Schlaut J, Solez K, Srinivasa NS. The significance of the anti-class I response II. Clinical and pathologic features of renal transplants with anti-class I-like antibody. Transplantation 1992; 53(3):550-555.

106. Knechtle SJ, Wang J, Burlingham WJ, Beeskau M, Subramanian R, Sollinger HW. The influence of RS-61443 on antibody-mediated rejection. Transplantation 1992; 53(3):699-701.

107. Carpenter CB, d'Apice AFJ, Abbas A. The role of antibodies in the rejection and enhancement of organ allografts. Adv Immunol 1976; 22:1.

108. Tilney NL, Whitley WD, Diamond JR, Kupiec-Weglinski JW, Adams DH. Chronic rejection-an undefined conundrum. Transplantation 1991; 52(3):389-398.

109. Paul LC, Benediktsson H. Chronic transplant rejection: Magnitude of the problem and pathogenetic mechanisms. Transplant Rev 1993; 7(2):96-113.

110. Stetson CA. The role of humoral antibody in the homograft reaction. Adv Immunol 1963; 3:97-130.

111. Braun WE. Donor-specific antibodies. Clinical relevance of antibodies detected in lymphocyte crossmatches. Clin Lab Med 1991; 11:571-602.

112. Holan V. Modulation of allotransplantation tolerance induction by IL1 and IL2. J Immunogenet 1988; 15:331-337.

113. Suciu-Foca N, Reed E, D'Agati VD, et al. Soluble HLA antigens, anti-HLA antibodies, and antiidiotypic antibodies in the circulation of renal transplant recipients. Transplantation 1991; 51:593-601.

114. Thomas JM, Thomas FT, Kaplan AM, Lee HM. Antibody-dependent cellular cytotoxicity and chronic renal allograft rejection. Transplantation 1976; 22(2):94-100.

115. Olerup O, Zetterquist H. HLA-DR typing by PCR amplification with sequence-specific primers (PCR-SSP) in 2 hours: An alternative to serological DR typing in clinical practice including donor-recipient matching in cadaveric transplantation. Tissue Antigens 1992; 39:225-235.

116. Lagaaij E, Hennemann P, Ruigrok M, et al. Effect of one-HLA-Antigen-matched and completely HLA-DR-mismatched blood transfusions on survival of heart and kidney allografts. N Eng J Med 1989; 321(11):701-705.

117. de Waal LP, van Twuyver E. Blood transfusion and allograft survival: Is mixed chimerism the solution for tolerance induction in clinical transplantation? Crit Rev Immunol 1991; 10(5):417-425.

320

118. Benichou G, Takizawa PA, Olson CA, McMillan M, Sercarz EE. Donor major histocompatibility complex (MHC) peptides are presented by recipient MHC molecules during graft rejection. J Exp Med 1992; 175:305-308.

119. Dalchau R, Fangmann J, Fabre JW. Allorecognition of isolated, denatured chains of class I and class II major histocompatibility complex molecules. Evidence for an important role for indirect allorecognition in transplantation. Eur J Immunol 1992; 22:669-677.

120. Fangmann J, Dalchau R, Fabre JW. Rejection of skin allografts by indirect allorecognition of donor class I major histocompatibility complex peptides. J Exp Med 1992; 175:1521-1529.

121. Braun MY, McCormack A, Webb G, Batchelor JR. Mediation of acute but not chronic rejection of MHC-incompatible rat kidney grafts by alloreactive CD4 T cells activated by the direct pathway of sensitization. Transplantation 1993; 55(1):177-182.

122. Sykes M, Sheard MA, Sachs DH. Effects of T cell depletion in radiation bone marrow chimeras: II. Requirement for allogeneic T cells in the reconstituting bone marrow inoculum for subsequent resistance to breaking of tolerance. J Exp Med 1988; 168:661.

123. Sharabi Y, Abraham VS, Sykes M, Sachs DH. Mixed allogeneic chimeras prepared by a non-myeloablative regimen: Requirement for chimerism to maintain tolerance. Bone Marrow Transplantion 1992; 9:191-197.

124. Stephenson SP, Dorsch S, Roser B, Godden U, Herbert J. The identity of suppressor cells in neonatal tolerance. Transplant Proc 1983; 15:850.

125. Dorsch S, Roser B. Suppressor cells in transplantation. Transplantation 1982; 33(5):518-524.

126.   Mohler K, Strome P, Streilein J. Allo-I-J determinants participate in maintenance of neonatal H-2 tolerance. J Immunol 1987; 138(1):70-77.

127.   Maki T, Gottschalk R, Wood M, Monaco A. Specific unresponsiveness to skin allografts in anti-lymphocyte serum treated, marrow injected mice; participation of donor marrow derived suppressor T cells. J Immunol 1981; 127(4):1433-1438.

128.   Starzl TE, Demetris AJ, Murase N, Ildstad S, Ricordi C, Trucco M. Cell migration, chimerism, and graft acceptance. Lancet 1992; 339:1579-1581.

129.   Lubaroff DM, Silvers WK. Importance of chimerism in maintaining tolerance of skin allografts in mice. J Immunol 1973; 111(1):65-71.

130.   Streilein JW, Levy RB, Ruiz P, Matriano J, Socarras S. Multiple mechanisms induce and maintain neonatal transplantation tolerance. Transplant Science 1993; 3:11-16.

131.   Goodnight JE, Coleman DA, Steinmuller D. Serum-blocking factors versus specific cellular tolerance in long-term survival of rat heart allografts. Transplantation 1976; 22(4):391-397.

132.   Billingham RE, Brent L, Medawar PB. Actively allergized tolerance of foreign cells. Nature 1953; 172:603.

133.   Hutchinson IV. Suppressor T cells in allogeneic models. Transplant Rev 1986; 41(5):547-555.

134.   Hilgert I. The involvement of activated specific suppressor T cells in maintenance of transplantation tolerance. Immunol Rev 1979; 46:27-53.

135.   Qin S, Cobbold SP, Pope H, et al. "Infectious" transplantation tolerance. Science 1993; 259:974-977.

136. Okada S, Palathumpat V, Strober S. Identification of donor derived antigen specific suppressor cells in murine bone marrow chimeras prepared with total lymphoid irradiation. Transplantation 1983; 36(4):417-422.

137. Orita M, Iwahana H, Kanazawa H, Hayashi K, Sekiya T. Detection of polymorphisms of human DNA by gel electrophoresis as single-strand conformation polymorphisms. Proc Natl Acad Sci 1989; 86:2766-2770.

138. Lo YMD, Patel P, Mehal WZ, Fleming KA, Bell JI, Wainscoat JS. Analysis of complex genetic systems by ARMS-SSCP: Application to HLA genotyping. Nucleic Acids Research 1992; 20:1005-1009.

139. Guild BC, Finer MH, Housman DE, Mulligan RC. Development of retrovirus vectors useful for expressing genes in cultured murine embryonal cells and hematopoietic cells in vivo. J Virol 1988; 62(10):3795-3801.

140. Smith JP, Kasten-Jolly J, Thomas FT, Field LJ, Thomas JM. Assessment of donor bone marrow cell-derived chimerism in transplantation tolerance using transgeneic mice. Transplantation 1993; (in press)

141. Wood ML, Monaco AP. Suppressor cells in specific unresponsiveness to skin allografts in ALS-treated, marrow-injected mice. Transplantation 1980; 29(3):196-200.

142. Alqaisi M, Carver M, Cunningham P, Kasten-Jolly J, Thomas F, Thomas J. Effect of depleting CD3+ cells from DR- donor bone marrow to facilitate kidney graft tolerance in recipients given total lymphoid irradiation. Transplant Proc 1993; 25(1):344-345.

143. Strober S. Natural suppressor cells, neonatal tolerance and lymphoid irradiation: Exploring obscure relationships. Ann Rev Immunol 1984; 84(2):219.

144. Myburgh JA, Smit JA, Myers AM. Total lymphoid irradiation in renal transplantation. World J Surg 1986; 10:369-380.

145. Strober S. Total lymphoid irradiation: Basic and clinical studies in transplantation immunity. Prog Clin Biol Res 1986; 224:251.

146. Bieber CP, Jamieson S, Raney A, et al. Cardiac allograft* survival in rhesus primates treated with combined total lymphoid irradiation and rabbit antithymocyte globulin. Transplantation 1979; 28(4):347-350.

147. Rynasiewicz J, Sutherland DE, Kawahara K, Najarian JS. Total lymphoid irradiation: Critical timing and combination with cyclosporine A for immunosuppression in a rat heart allograft model. J Surg Res 1981; 30:365-371.

THE ROLE OF PASSENGER LEUKOCYTES IN REJECTION AND

"TOLERANCE" AFTER SOLID ORGAN TRANSPLANTATION: A POTENTIAL

EXPLANATION OF A PARADOX

Anthony J. Demetris[1], M.D.

Noriko Murase[2], M.D.

Abdul S. Rao[1,2], M.D., D. Phil.

Thomas E. Starzl[2], M.D., Ph.D.

From the Pittsburgh Transplant Institute, Departments of
Pathology[1] and Surgery[2], University of Pittsburgh Medical
Center, Pittsburgh, Pennsylvania, 15213.

Aided by Project Grant No. DK 29961 from the National
Institutes of Health, Bethesda, Maryland.

Address correspondence to: Thomas E. Starzl, M.D., Ph.D.,
3601 Fifth Avenue, 5C Falk Clinic, University of Pittsburgh,
Pittsburgh, Pennsylvania, 15213.

J. L. Touraine et al. (eds.), Rejection and Tolerance, 325–392.
© 1994 Kluwer Academic Publishers.

INTRODUCTION

The concept that passenger leukocytes are more "immunogenic" and thus initiate rejection, which is ultimately directed against the parenchyma and vessels of solid organ allografts, was first proposed by Snell (1) and later proved by Steinmuller (2). Steinman and Cohn (3-6) subsequently showed that a distinct type of passenger leukocyte, the dendritic cell, provides the most potent of the allogeneic stimuli. Besides dendritic cells, which reside in the interstitium of all allografts, every organ also carries with it a variable number of T and B lymphocytes, macrophages and myeloid cells. Therefore, each type of allograft presents a heterogenous stimulatory profile as well as the potential for graft-versus-host (GVH) reactions.

Based on the seemingly logical assumption that the highly immunogenic passenger leukocytes are deleterious to graft survival, attempts have been made to deplete donor hematolymphoid cells from organs prior to transplantation (7-10). While this approach can clearly yield improved short-term results, leukocyte-depleted allografts are still eventually rejected. Even epidermal allografts, which consist of pure keratinocyte cultures are rejected (11).

In a seeming paradox, donor hematolymphoid cells, particularly those from the bone marrow, are known to carry with them the ability to render the recipient's immune system specifically unresponsive to subsequent organ allografts (12-19). Owen (20) was the first to show that cattle fetuses whose individual placentas had placental cross-circulation (freemartins) subsequently developed "chimeric" hematolymphoid systems. The chimerism, which was a mixture of the ABO (and presumably other) phenotypes of the fetuses persisted, for a lifetime and was associated with subsequent cross-tolerance to tissue and whole organ (kidney) grafts (21).

The lead provided by Owen caused Burnet and Fenner (22) to predict the feasibility of iatrogenetically producing acquired tolerance by exposing fetuses to immunologically active adult tissues in utero, and this feat was accomplished in 1953 with spleen cells in mice by Billingham, Brent, and Medawar (12,23) in what was a decisive stimulus toward the ultimate development of clinical transplantation. Ensuing experimental models of radiation and monoclonal antibody-induced mixed hematolymphoid chimeras in adults are based on this principle. In general, these models attempt to recapitulate development of the neonatal immune system in a "twin-like" environment. First, the recipient's immune system is disabled with drugs or radiation, which is followed by an infusion of donor hematolymphoid cells. In this paradigm, uncommitted stem cells which have seeded the bone marrow, produce progeny that are educated in the recipient's thymus and immune system. Eventually, tolerance to a subsequent solid organ allograft is produced, but how this occurs is poorly understood.

Although Owen's original observations in freemartin cattle were of mixed chimerism, as opposed to the full chimerism of the Billingham-Brent-Medawar model, this crucial difference was seldom emphasized. The association of acquired tolerance with full chimerism, meaning complete replacement of the host hematolymphopoietic system with that of the donor, was so strong following the Billingham-Brent-Medawar reports that stable and permanent mixed chimerism as a means of tolerance induction was rarely mentioned again for almost 4 decades. In fact, hematolymphopoietic replacement was the dogma by which bone marrow transplantation per se was developed experimentally and ultimately used clinically (24,25). This approach was long envisioned to be the potential means by which tolerance could be induced for whole organ grafts (13).

Using the total bone marrow conditioning approach, permanent tolerance to a variety of organs has been produced across partial and full MHC, and even across species barriers (13-19). However, there were two major drawbacks which prevented clinical application. One was that the conditioning regimens necessary to ensure donor bone marrow engraftment were extreme, with an inherent short- and long-term morbidity. The second and more fundamental problem first described by Billingham and Brent (26) in mice was the development of graft versus host disease (GVHD). The risk from this complication in which the new immunologic apparatus destroyed the host was directly related to the degree of histoincompatibility between donor and recipient (27), restricting the marrow or other similar conditioning strategies to patients with perfect MHC-matched donors (24,25,28,29).

The entrenchment and durability of this therapeutic doctrine as a rational approach to tolerance induction for whole organs is really quite remarkable in view of the obvious fact that it was not fundamentally feasible. In the meanwhile, an important but long unexploited experimental observation by Liegeois et al (30,31) suggested as early as 1974 that complete extirpation and replacement of the recipient hematolymphopoetic system was not an absolute requirement for engraftment of donor bone marrow and the consequent induction of tolerance for other donor tissues and organs. These investigations were performed in Paris in an attempt to explain donor specific nonreactivity to skin grafts induced first by Monaco, Wood, and Russell (32) and then by Wood, Monaco, Gozzo, and Liegeois (33) with antilymphocyte serum (ALS) plus delayed intravenous bone marrow infusion one week later. Using karyotyping techniques, Liegeois et al (30,31) demonstrated progressively declining (always small) numbers of replicating donor bone marrow cells in the recipient's spleens as long as 134 days after the bone marrow-skin transplantations, a condition which they termed microchimerism. Although Liegeois et al (30,31) and Monaco (34) were intrigued by this finding, their assumption and that of others was that the decline in identifiable donor cells was premonitory to their extinction. This point of view that these chimeric cells were transient, prevented the recognition of the full significance of Liegeois's findings. In addition, these findings following bone marrow infusion were not suspected to pertain also to passenger leukocytes from whole organs.

In principle, Slavin and Strober et al (14-16) showed the same thing as Liegeois in 1977, but with the additional information that the mixed microchimerism could be persistent and stable for long periods. In rats treated with total lymphoid (not total body) irradiation (TLI) and donor bone marrow infusion, they produced mixed chimerism, emphasized the lack of GVHD in their animals, and showed that the donor and recipient were reciprocally tolerant --- analogous to Owens' freemartin cattle (20). Subsequently, Ildstad and Sachs (17) provided convincing confirmation by

cytoablating recipients and reconstituting them with mixed
donor and recipient marrow, with consequent mixed allogeneic
or xenogeneic chimerism. Slavin and Strober's experiments
led to clinical trials of kidney and liver transplantation
with donor bone marrow augmentation more than a decade ago
(35-42), but these were abandoned because of the conviction
that the bone marrow was an unnecessary adjuvant to the TLI,
and was potentially harmful (38-42).

Nearly a decade after the reports by Billingham, Brent,
and Medawar (12,23), a seemingly different therapeutic dogma
was developed with continuous chemical immunosuppression
that allowed increasingly successful whole organ
transplantation with graft acceptance by what were widely
construed as different immunologic mechanisms (44-51). This
misconception was dispelled in 1992 with the demonstration
that long-surviving human kidney, liver, and other whole
organ recipients had low level mixed allogeneic chimerism
(52-57) from dissemination and survival of passenger
leukocytes leaving the graft. The pattern and time course
of the cell migration and the movement into the graft of
recipient cells of the same lineages could be easily
identified after liver transplantation in experimental
animals (58,59). This was a mechanism that defied the logic
of the diametrically opposite strategy of trying to deplete
the passenger leukocytes described in the introduction of
this article.

Definition of a Paradox

Although donor hematolymphoid cells have been identified both as the most immunogenic (1-11) and the most tolerogenic cells (12-19) associated with solid organ allografts, there have been few attempts until recently to reconcile these apparently paradoxical roles. One reason apparently has been the assumption that the passenger leukocytes transferred with a solid organ were fundamentally different from those found in the bone marrow. In addition, many investigators have also assumed that the number of transferred donor hematolymphoid cells was insignificant and the cells were rapidly destroyed. The recent studies in humans and experimental animals have shown that both of these assumptions were invalid (52-59). In fact, we have proposed that persistence of rare passenger leukocytes in recipient tissues is conducive to, and the explanation of, graft acceptance. Properly addressing this opposite effect paradox may yield a different perspective of transplantation biology.

The following is not intended as a review of the area of passenger leukocytes in transplantation biology. Rather this manuscript should be considered as a hypothesis to explain how donor hematolymphoid cells transferred with the graft could assist in graft acceptance. A brief description

of the their role in provoking rejection and tolerization is
also presented. This aspect is particularly important to
development of the hypothesis.

Passenger Leukocytes Under Temporary Immunosuppression
or in Untreated Organ Allograft Recipients

The Liver --- The early events leading to the chimeric
state after liver transplantation have been studied in rats
(58) and mice (59), including the pathways of passenger
leukocyte dissemination. Within minutes or hours, some of
these cells leave the liver and home to the spleen, lymph
nodes, thymus, and bone marrow where they are destroyed by
rejection in most animals models except those using mice as
subjects. However, under temporary immunosuppression in
rats (2 weeks daily FK 506), these mononuclear cells pause
for about 2 weeks in the lymphoid organs, but then break out
and move secondarily to all recipient tissues (58). Rat
liver recipients treated in this way (for example, Lewis
[LEW] to Brown Norway [BN]) survive indefinitely without
further treatment and retain their graft and systemic
chimerism.

Interestingly, permanent survival of the engrafted
livers occurs without any immunosuppression in some rat
strain combinations of which BN to LEW has been most

completely studied (60), and it occurs without treatment in virtually all mouse strain combinations no matter how severe the histoincompatibility (59). The heavy endowment of the liver with potentially migratory white cells is thought to be the basis for the previously inexplicable phenomenon of "hepatic tolerogenicity".

In fact, we believe that the foregoing migration and repopulation is the central mechanism of acceptance of all whole organ grafts (52-59). Although this is a generic process, there are quantitative differences between organs in the density of the potentially migratory dendritic cells, macrophages, and lymphoid collections. The heavy endowment of the liver with the foregoing leukocyte lineages (including Kupffer cells) is a particularly striking feature that invites further speculation about the role of these cells in the well known tolerogenicity of this organ.

The immunologic advantage of the liver relative to other organs includes a greater ease of inducing the acceptance of hepatic allografts (described above) or xenografts after a limited course of immunosuppression (47,49,61,62) or in swine (63-65) and some rat strain combinations (60,66) with no treatment at all. In addition, the transplanted liver graft is relatively resistant to the preformed antigraft antibodies that cause hyperacute rejection of the kidney and heart (67-70). Another quality

is its unusual ability to induce a state of unresponsiveness
to other tissues and organs transplanted concomitantly or
subsequently from the donor or donor strain (66,68,71) and
even shield these organs from the hyperacute rejection
caused by preformed allospecific (70) or xenospecific (72)
antidonor antibodies. In all of these circumstances, the
liver appears to quickly transform the recipient environment
to one more favorable for all donor tissues including
itself. All of these qualities of the liver are evident in
practically every mouse strain combination, no matter what
the degree of histoincompatibility (59).

Other Organs --- The foregoing observations have been
attributed to "hepatic tolerogenicity", incorrectly we
believe, because the term implies that the hepatocytes are
responsible. We have proposed that the crucial variable
distinguishing the tolerogenicity of one organ graft from
another under effective immunosuppression (or in some animal
models without treatment) is its leukocyte, not its
parenchymal component (56-59). This is a reversal of the
immunogenic role described classically for the "passenger"
white cells (1-10,73-76). Thus, because of its dense
constituency of these migratory leukocytes, the liver is
high on the favorable tolerogenic list with the lung and
intestine following and the kidney and heart bringing up the
rear. Experimental studies showing less striking
tolerogenicity of the lymphoreticular-rich spleen (77-79),

intestine (80), and lung (81,82) are compatible with this generalization.

Sites of Alloactivation and Tolerization
with Particular Reference to Leukocyte-Poor Organs

By the end of 1992, it was concluded that all whole organs underwent the same process of potential tolerance induction as the liver, although the dynamics were not so easy to study except with the leukocyte-rich intestine (80,83-85). However, the same kind of traffic in the context of alloactivation and rejection rather than tolerization, had been well worked out earlier with the so-called lymphoid-poor organs including the kidney. Studies in untreated animals have shown that the alloreaction starts in 2 general sites, peripherally in the graft and centrally in the recipient lymphoid tissues.

Central Alloactivation --- In a very complete study in 1981 of untreated rat kidney recipients, Hayry and Nemlander and their associates (86) demonstrated extensive leukocyte migration to the spleen and elsewhere. If Hayry had given one or two doses of cyclosporine in his kidney transplantation experiments (which were with an "easy" strain combination) and had followed his animals further, he almost certainly would have uncovered the events of cell migration and long term repopulation that awaited another dozen years for exposure with the liver (58). Larsen et al (87) found that donor dendritic cells from heterotopic cardiac allografts were released into the circulation, where they eventually homed into the T-cell areas of the recipient spleen. In the spleen, the donor cells initiate proliferation of recipient cells, and vice versa (86-90). This reaction might be thought of as an in vivo mixed lymphocyte response (MLR) and epitomizes central allosensitization with potential tolerization.

Intragraft Alloactivation --- Allosensitization (and tolerization) presumably also occurs within the graft. Forbes et al (89) showed that clustering of recipient lymphocytes occurs around donor dendritic cells in the interstitium of cardiac grafts, within a few days after transplantation. The recipient lymphoid cells were undergoing blastogenesis and proliferation in these clusters. We have described analogous events in rejecting rat livers (88).

In human recipients of kidney grafts (91,92) under cyclosporine-prednisone immunosuppression, Hayry and Willebrand noted what appeared to be a bidirectional MLR in needle aspiration biopsies. When studied with the Staphylococcus aureus assay and alloantibodies to non-shared donor and recipient allelic specificities, most of the collected blast cells in some cases were derived from the donor or else the response was split, "resembling a bidirectional mixed lymphocyte reaction in vitro" (91).

In these models, the difference from the experiments with liver transplantation appear to be quantitative. With the smaller number of passenger leukocytes, there is a greater tendency to allosensitization and less to tolerogenicity. Nevertheless, Corry (93) and Russell et al (94) showed that tolerance without drug induction could be induced by heart and kidney transplantation between weakly MHC incompatible strains of mouse recipients.

The Parking Experiments --- Earlier evidence that the disseminated passenger leukocytes play a crucial role in allograft rejection came from elegant studies by Lechler and Batchelor (75,76), who demonstrated that rat allogeneic kidneys were indefinitely accepted if they were first "parked" in the immunosuppressed recipient and subsequently re-transplanted secondarily into naive animals syngeneic to the recipient strain (75,76). However, these kidneys were acutely rejected if the animals receiving the re-transplants were intravenously injected with donor strain dendritic cells (76). This was the first direct evidence that the immunogenecity of a passenger cell depleted allograft and could be restored by addition of donor strain dendritic cells. Similar observations were also made by Benson et al, (95) who showed that deoxyguanosine treated fetal thymus

allografts were rejected if transplanted into animals primed
with donor-strain dendritic cells.

Unfortunately, results with the experimentally useful
parking model have been extrapolated overly freely to
discussions and criticisms of the cell migration and
microchimerism concepts. In the parking experiment, neither
the host immunocytes (including those that home to the
parked organ) nor the donor leukocytes seeded ubiquitously
in the recipient remain the same. The changes have been
shown dramatically in rat liver transplant experiments in
which the "passenger leukocyte" load brought in with the
liver was augmented by donor bone marrow simultaneously or
at an earlier time. Staged delivery of the donor leukocytes
caused fulminant GVHD. Aside from clarifying limitations in
interpretation of parking experiments, these studies have
significant clinical implications in planning the staged use
of bone marrow for the augmentation of passenger leukocytes
(58).

The Fate of Passenger Leukocytes in Treated Recipients

Immunosuppressive drugs such as FK 506 do not grossly
alter the migration of donor hematolymphoid cells out of an
allograft (58,96,97). However, almost all
immunosuppressants markedly reduce the infiltration of
recipient cells into the graft. They also protect the graft

from injury and prolong the survival of donor passenger leukocytes, both within the graft and peripherally in the recipient tissues (58,96,97). Additionally, neither FK 506 nor cyclosporine abolish the immune response in recipient's lymphoid tissues provoked by the passenger leukocytes (58,98,99). They merely diminish it, and possibly alter the response in a qualitative fashion (58,98,99).

Over time, the peripheralized donor cells can be identified in the recipient's skin, visceral organs and lymphoid tissues, including the bone marrow and thymus (58,97). This ubiquitous distribution argues against passive spread via draining lymphatics. Moreover, homing of the donor cells to the same anatomic locations as their phenotypically identical counterparts argues for the existence of preprogrammed migratory routes, which are independent of allogeneic barriers (99-102). Thus, immunosuppressive drugs regardless of their molecular site of action, appear to have a permissive and regulatory, rather than a purely inhibitory effect on the interactions between donor and recipient hematolymphoid cells (56,58).

Even under the protection of continuous immunosuppression, the number of donor cells that have emigrated out of transplanted organs gradually decreases with time (58,59). One likely explanation for this finding is that the majority of the transferred donor cells have a mature phenotype, and therefore are eventually eliminated by the recipient's immune system. Or if they are terminally differentiated and are incapable of further division, they simply die out. Finally, it is possible that a few donor progenitor cells "engraft" and produce a very small number of peripheralized donor cells, which can persist for many years in the tissues of stable organ allograft recipients.

To designate this condition, we have used the term "micro-chimerism" that was originally coined by Liegeois et al (30,31) and popularized by Monaco (34). If, however, "microchimerism" is of importance in tolerance, any hypothesis explaining the mechanisms must account for an effect of the donor cells, which far exceeds their number (52-59).

Macro- versus Microchimerism

Because these 2 terms have been used in different ways, it is important for this discussion to define our meaning. It is generally accepted that stable hematolymphoid macrochimerism is synonymous with allogeneic tolerance. Radiation models, such as those described by Ildstad and Sachs (17) and the human fetal-liver recipients described by Touraine (103), have defined mixed hematopoietic macrochimerism using flow cytometric studies. This technology can confidently discriminate between allogeneic populations when one component is as small as 1.0%. Although, individual contributions to the total pool reciprocally may vary between 10 and 90 percent, hematopoietic cell lineages from both donor and recipient can usually be detected.

In vitro immunologic testing in the mouse models of macrochimerism reveals a donor specific proliferative defect and lack of donor-directed cytolytic activity, while the same responses to third party lymphocytes remain intact (17). This in vitro state of nonreactivity may not be absolute in higher species. For example, the human macrochimeras reported by Touraine and Roncarolo et al (103) show host reactive cells in vitro. Yet, such patients have no obvious GVHD and the donor cells appear to be under a regulatory influence, perhaps mediated by cytokines or other cells.

In a different context, Thomas et al have used the word microchimerism to describe nodules of donor leukocytes found on the capsule of renal allografts in subhuman primates rendered donor specific tolerant by adjuvant bone marrow infusion and ALG plus total lymphoid irradiation (104).

"Microchimerism" as reported by us in humans (52-57) and in animals (58,59) refers to the diffuse rather than localized presence in recipient tissues of donor cells at

levels below the detection threshold of flow cytometry, thus
requiring alternative methods of identification (52-59).
Donor cell labeling using immunocytochemistry with anti-MHC
monoclonal antibodies or in situ hybridization for
mismatched sex chromosomes can detect donor cells present in
recipient tissues in concentrations between 1:1000 and
1:5000. Polymerase chain reaction studies for mismatched
HLA-DR alleles or the Y chromosome is even more sensitive.
As few as one cell in 40,000 can be identified.

Because of the paucity of cells present in
microchimerics, it is difficult to define multiple lineages
in a single stable patient. However, multilineage chimerism
has been shown in several humans (105-107) after liver
transplantation. In rat and mouse studies (58,59),
different lineages are found as long as 300 days after
transplantation.

In vitro immunologic testing of "microchimeras" may
show donor specific hyporeactivity, but intact MLR and CML
responses may also be seen (49,59,104,108,109). This is not
surprising, since Strelein et al (110) has shown before in
neonatal chimeras, that in vitro immunologic testing may not
always reflect, or predict, in vivo tolerance. No matter
what the outcome of in vitro assays, recipients often
tolerate allografts in vivo in the same way as the

macrochimeric recipients cited above
(49,59,104,108,109,111).

The Commonality of Treatment Regimens
to Induce Chimerism and Tolerance in Adults

Regimens used to induce allogeneic tolerance in the
adult animal (or in humans) have in common two factors,
donor allo-antigen, which is a specific requirement, and
non-specific immunosuppression for variable periods (13-19).
With the possible exception of the liver (59), donor bone
marrow has been the best source of "tolerogenic
alloantigen". The best choice of immunosuppression remains
controversial, but virtually all potent modalities achieve
the same end result in spite of their widely variable
mechanisms. For example, cytotoxic drugs that inhibit DNA
synthesis, cyclosporine, FK 506, monoclonal antibodies,
radiation, cytokine therapy, or nothing at all except donor
tissue have all been used to induce tolerance with variable
success (13-19,52-59).

A very important concept that emerges in the
development of all of these regimens is that too much
immunosuppression can block the induction of tolerance
(112), implying that it is an active process. Wood et al
(112) and Liegeois et al (30,31) have particularly
emphasized this point as well as the dynamic nature of

tolerance. It is also known that the dose and timing of alloantigen presentation influences the final outcome of tolerance induction (13-19,30,31,52-59). These considerations are not different from those required to induce tolerance to self or other non-allogeneic antigens (106,113,114).

Because of the passenger leukocyte migration and repopulation that now are known to be a generic phenomena after the engraftment of all whole organs, every such clinical operation has the theoretic potential for initiating tolerance induction. However, this does not happen reliably, and despite the co-existence of both alloantigen and immunosuppression, drug-free graft acceptance is an uncommon clinical outcome. Nevertheless, the ability to eventually withdraw immunosuppressive drugs without initiating graft rejection has often been documented in clinical reports, particularly after liver transplantation (57,115), and can be routinely accomplished in numerous experimental transplantation models (58,59). Drug withdrawal is least often achieved without complications in kidney and heart allograft recipients (57).

One obvious difference between these organs is the number of passenger leukocytes, which is higher in the bone marrow and liver than in heart or kidney. However, in the ensuing paragraphs, we will first globally and then specifically attempt to describe how the presence of donor leukocytes, even in small numbers, can promote allograft acceptance. Our hypothesis is based on a network viewpoint of the immune system (116-123).

Global Hypothesis

Transplantation of a solid organ without the need for continual immunosuppression requires in some respect, redefinition of the recipient's immunologic self (116). Co-transplantation of a fragment of the donor's immune system (i.e., passenger leukocytes of solid organ grafts, or bone marrow augmentation), whose normal function is to define the donor's immunologic self, would appear to be most capable of achieving this task (116-117). In fact, the desire to induce hematolymphoid chimerism for promoting allograft acceptance is knowingly or unknowingly, based on this idea and in essence, is an attempt to merge two different immune systems.

This merger however is resisted by mature cells in both immune networks, which mediate classical alloimmune reactions and NK cells, which can prevent allogeneic progenitor cell engraftment (124,125). Any maneuver that results in the combination of less immunogenic and more plastic donor and recipient hematolymphoid progenitor cell populations lessens the resistance. Therefore, most investigators have used depletion of mature cells from the donor inoculum and ablation of donor reactivity in the recipient by cytoreductive or radiation therapy (13-19). It is now realized that transplant surgeons have been unknowingly protecting the passenger leukocyte (donor immune system) by various forms of immunosuppression while it carried out immunologic redefinition of the recipient (52-57).

The concept of MHC restriction however, appears to limit the interactions that could occur between allogeneic lymphoid cells to antagonistic ones. But, if these engagements are viewed as receptor-ligand interactions of varying "fits" or affinities, the possibility of cooperative interactions occurring between allogeneic cells is not unreasonable (116-123). In fact, effective collaboration between allogeneic APC's and lymphocytes within a single chimeric immune network has been shown before in a chimeric human (103). "Cross-talk" between the allogeneic cells of both populations comprising a fully integrated chimeric immune system is the ultimate goal.

The key component for establishing and maintaining tolerance in a chimeric allogeneic network would be donor cells or antigen if immunologic self definition is maintained by self assertion as Coutinho suggests (116). This requirement for the presence of the tolerated antigen

is not different from that of classical explanations of
allogeneic tolerance (114,126-128). The major difference
between these two views turns on whether tolerance is an
active or passive process. Under either circumstance, the
donor cells provide the necessary signals to imprint
specificity and inhibit the development of effector
responses (112,114,126).

From this viewpoint, it becomes very difficult to
dispute that hematopoietic chimerism is essential for
successful organ engraftment, whether this is at a macro or
micro level. The direct relation of acquired tolerance (and
GVHD) with chimerism discovered by Billingham, Brent and
Medawar (12,23) was formally verified by Russell (129) who
reversed both tolerance and --- runt disease (GVHD) with the
elimination of the chimerism with antidonor leukocyte
antibodies. The only debate is the quantity of donor
leukocytes required. This may be a moot point if the
iterative and metadynamic properties of an immune network
are considered (116-123). The mobile donor hematolymphoid
cells released from the graft during the first week or so
after transplantation provoke an initial burst of
alloreactivity in the recipient's lymphoid tissue. Under
the protection of immunosuppression they also begin to
participate alongside recipient cells in preprogrammed
migratory routes (e.g. through the thymus and lymphoid
tissues) (58,97). Exposure of immature recipient cells to

donor dendritic and other leukocyte populations during
thymic or early post-thymic maturation gradually erodes the
basis for alloreactivity and the singular identity of the
recipient's "immunologic self".

The education or re-education process is made easier if
the merging populations consist of relatively immature and
more malleable uncommitted progenitor cells, like those seen
in neonates. Such cells have more ready access to
"immunologic privileged" sites such as the thymus and spleen
and serve as a renewable source of cells. However,
regardless of their age, mixing of allogeneic hematolymphoid
populations would eventually exert selection pressures on
various receptor specificities, such that evolution of the
chimeric mixture would occur. Genetic restriction of
receptor configurations may ultimately determine whether a
dynamic equilibrium is ever reached (116-123).

MECHANISTIC HYPOTHESIS

A network-based viewpoint categorizes immune responses
as receptor-ligand interactions, occurring between the
receptors on various participating cellular populations
(116-123). For example, CD4+ T cells are originally
selected in the thymus on the basis of their affinity for
self-MHC class II antigens, that are expressed on the
surface of antigen presenting cells(APC) (130,131). Cells

with an extremely high or low affinity or "fit" for self MHC class II are negatively selected and therefore not represented in the peripheral T cell pool. Cells with receptors of intermediate affinity are positively selected on the basis of limited "autoreactivity (anti-self class II)", and released from the thymus to participate in immune responses.

In the periphery, alterations of self-MHC class II on an APC, induced by binding of an exogenous peptide, changes the affinity of these cells for receptors on CD4+ T cells, which in turn results in T cell activation (132-134). The activated CD4+ T cells then develop idiotypes that are antigenic to a subgroup of anti-idiotypic regulatory T cells. The regulatory cells are thought to recognize the class II MHC/T-cell receptor complex present on the activated CD4+ T cells (anti-anti-self) (Figure 1) and thereby prevent uncontrolled autoreactivity. The anti-anti self MHC class II/receptor on the regulatory T-cells resemble the self-MHC class II antigens present on the original stimulatory APC's, and because of this have been called "MHC-image" (MHCi) cells (119,120). Such cells have been identified during and after exposure to toxins, nominal antigens and graft- versus-host and allogeneic reactions (135-142). We would suggest however, that antibodies also could provide an MHCi, and function with the regulatory MHCi cells in a "suppressor-like" fashion, showing high network

Figure 1. Diagrammatic presentation of the theory of "Network Focusing".

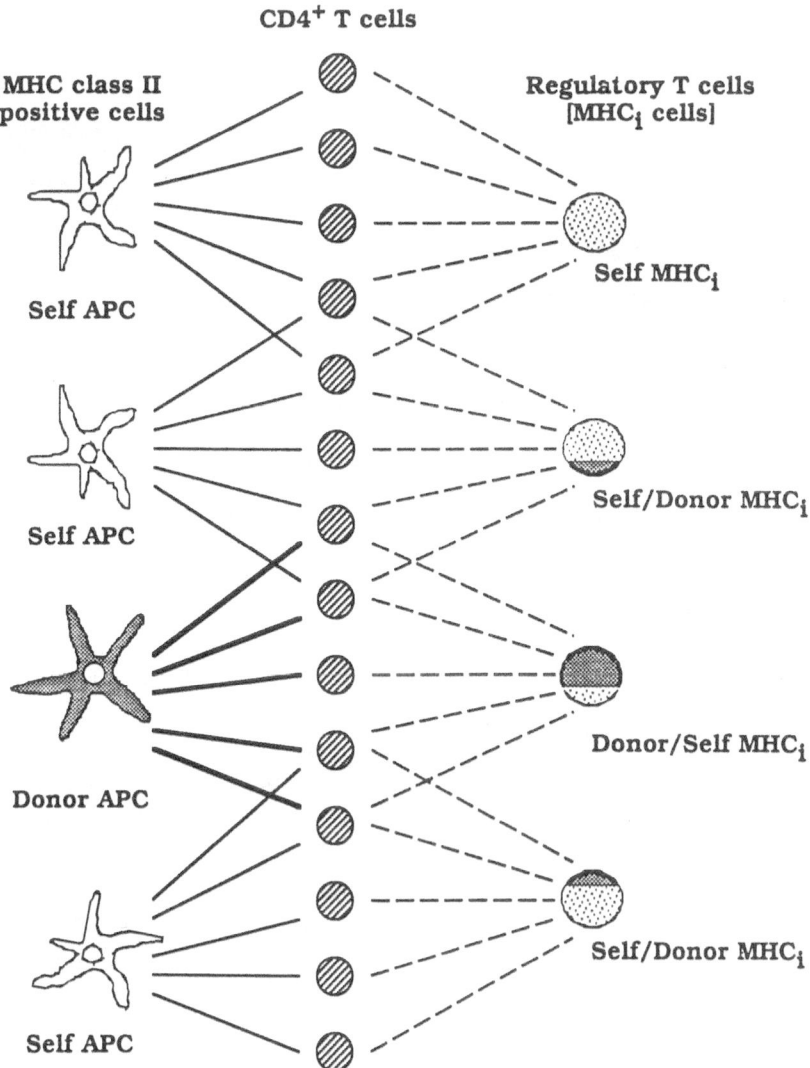

connectivity (i.e few cells would regulate many others)
(116-123). The entire concept is illustrated in Figure 1
has been referred to as "network focusing" (119,120).

We propose that an alloreaction is not fundamentally
different from other immune responses. It is subject to
similar regulatory controls. In fact, the essence of our
hypothesis is that *the alloreaction itself gives birth to
the tolerogenic cells by imprinting on the recipient's
immune network an internal image of the donor*. Furthermore,
allogeneic tolerance is maintained by specific autoimmune
reactions, which are fueled by the presence of donor
hematolymphoid cells(Figure 2). Over time the continued
participation of donor cells in the recipient's immune
network gradually erodes the previously strong barriers that
prevent effective cooperation between allogeneic networks
(58,143). The following paragraphs describe how this could
occur.

Spontaneously alloreactive T cells comprise about 1% of
the total peripheral T cell pool, and have been shown to
crossreact with self-APC bearing a nominal antigen (132-
134). Because of this crossreactivity, an immune network
would likely be unable to reliably distinguish between an
alloreaction and response to other antigens (132-134).
However in an alloresponse, the MHCi cells are selectively
stimulated on the basis of receptor complementarity to

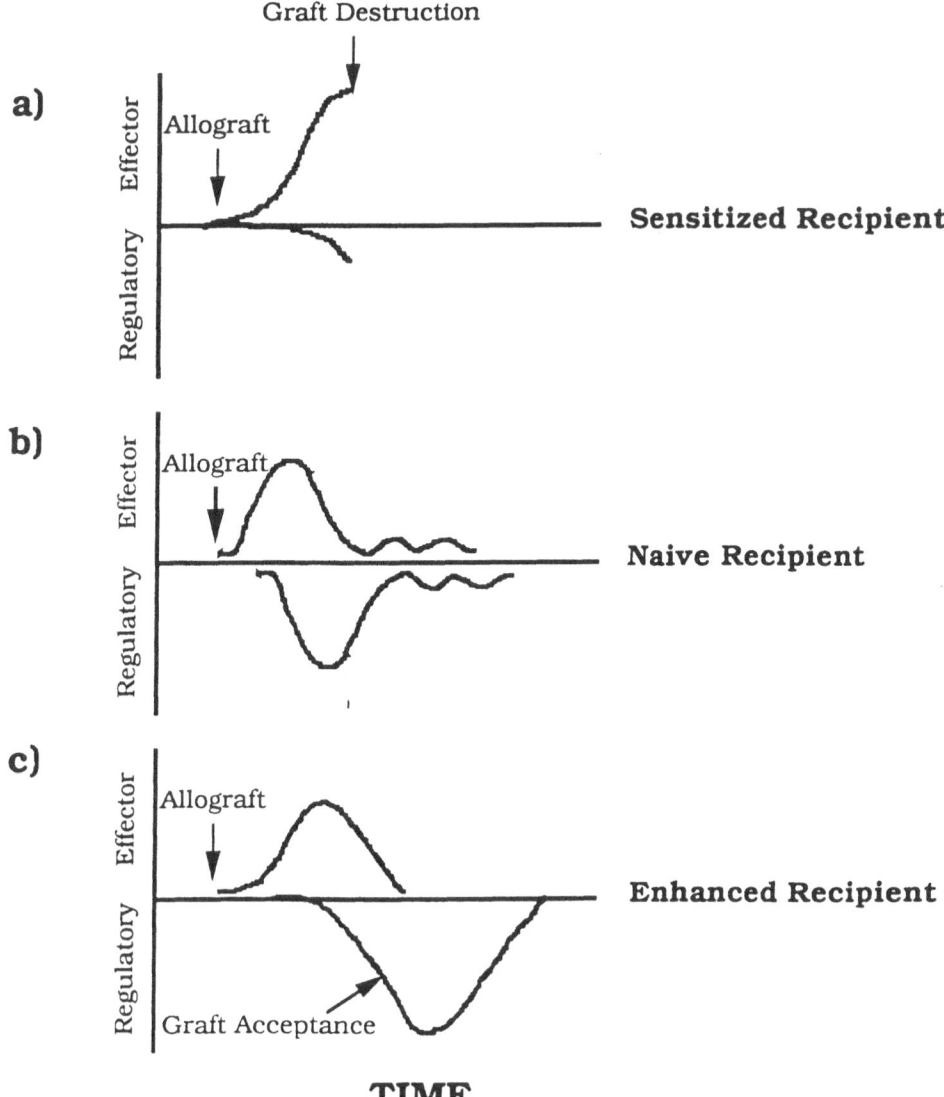

Figure 2. Schematic representation of an alloresponse of a sensitized (a); naive (b); and enhanced (c) recipients. Time post-transplant is represented on the X-axis. The positive displacement on the Y-axis symbolizes the strength of the effector phase [i.e. rejection reaction]. The negative quadrant on the Y-axis represents the regulatory responses, which at present are poorly understood.

alloreactive CD4+ T cells (anti, anti-donor MHC). Suciu-Foca et al (136,137) have provided direct evidence that such cells do indeed exist. They have shown that alloactivated T cells develop idiotypic-like determinants, which elicit an autologous mixed lymphocyte response. This active response was shown to exhibit both specificity and memory in the primed lymphocyte test, which failed to exhibit secondary reactivity to autologous blasts primed against a different allospecificity (136,137). Thus, the early brisk alloreaction provoked by the initial influx of donor cells into recipient lymphoid tissues, would begin to create an internal image of the donor in the recipient's immune system (58,98,99).

The initial alloreaction also generates effector mechanisms, which have the potential to damage both the graft and mobile cells. If however, the graft and the migratory cells survive the effector response, the regulatory reaction described above, which is 180 degrees out of phase with the effector response (Figure 2), will eventually self-limit the rejection. Continual restimulation of the alloreaction, as would be seen with the survival of microchimeric hematolymphoid cells, would in turn also recruit the regulatory cells carrying the donor-MHCi. Thus, alloreactive and auto-alloreactive MHCi regulatory reactions would be in a constant flux, resulting in a dynamic and at times unstable equilibrium (116).

Meanwhile, the continued trafficking and participation of donor hematolymphoid cells in the recipient's immune system eventually would result in further erosion of the basis for alloreactivity (58,143).

The explanation of donor specificity of allogeneic tolerance is obvious from our hypothesis. It is also clear how too much immunosuppression could prevent tolerance induction. Specificity is conferred by the presence of donor cells, or antigen maintaining the donor MHCi. Overly aggressive immunosuppression would not only inhibit the regulatory reactions, but also prevent donor cell division, which is particularly important during the formative stages of tolerance induction. Elegant studies by Russell et al (144,145) illustrate these points.

They attempted to provoke destruction of an accepted kidney allograft in a "tolerant" recipient by infusion of syngeneic lymphoid cells, which had already been sensitized to the donor. Although they succeeded in causing graft rejection, it was only transient. The graft recovered and the recipient returned to a tolerant state (144,145). Complete immunologic graft destruction required treatment with donor leukocytes (antigen), combined with cyclophosphamide pretreatment and/or continual BCG immunostimulation after delivery of the donor cells. These manipulations would either prevent or overwhelm respectively the regulatory responses.

Actively enhanced recipients, when subsequently challenged with an allograft, initially experience rejection that spontaneously resolves (146). This includes marked upregulation of donor MHC antigens (146), which has led several authors to conclude that the pretransplant blood transfusions are powerfully immunosuppressive. The active components in transfusions are known to be class II-bearing donor hematolymphoid cells (147-151). It is proposed that this form of pre-transplant conditioning (active enhancement) bolsters the regulatory reactions, outlined above and represent a "vaccination" or an indirect stimulation of donor MHCi cells. When the enhanced subject is subsequently challenged with an allograft, rejection is internally controlled before it is able to destroy the graft (Figure 2).

Wotherspoon et al (152) have provided more direct evidence that the alloreactive cell are capable of tolerance induction. They showed that cells capable of transferring allogeneic tolerance (or resistance to GVHD) also bear receptors for the tolerated alloantigen. Strelein et al (153) have summarized a similar experience in neonatal chimeras by showing the importance of "tolerogen-specific T cells" in the maintenance of tolerance. Qin et al (154) provided evidence that tolerance could be transferred with T cells across as many as four generation, a phenomenon he called "infectious" tolerance. We believe that idiotypic determinants on T-cells provide a rational explanation for the above observations, and are similar to the reasoning behind using effector cell vaccination for preventing autoimmune allergic encephalitis (155).

The association and importance of "autoimmune reactions" in the establishment and maintenance of allogeneic tolerance has been particularly well studied in neonatal chimeric mice (153,156-161). Briefly, chimeric donor B and possibly other cells are thought to constantly stimulate recipient CD4+ cells, that show a TH2-type profile. These tolerogen-specific, TH2-type alloreactive CD4+ cells are unable to coordinate an effective rejection reaction, and in fact, inhibit the response through the secretion of IL-4 and possibly other TH2-type cytokines (153,159,160). The elevated IL-4 also results in upregulation of class II MHC on the chimeric donor B-cells, B-cell hyperactivity and secretion of autoantibodies directed at DNA, smooth muscle cells and basement membrane constituents (153,156-161).

Autoimmune reactions triggered by heavy metal injections or transient cyclosporine therapy share many features of the autoimmunity observed in the chronic GVHD

models (162-166) described above. The BN rat is
particularly sensitive to both of these syndromes, which
appear to be dependent on autoreactive anti-Ia CD4+ T cells
(162-165). Zhang et al (166) have shown that these autoreactive T cells are capable of prolonging heart allograft
survival, and we have recently shown that BN recipients of
LEW liver allografts also retain hematolymphoid chimerism
for more than 300 days after liver transplantation, even
without continual immunosuppressive therapy (58). More
interestingly, BN recipients of LEW intestinal or liver
allografts experience a lethal graft versus host disease,
even when the percentage of donor cells is <5% of the total
lymphoid cell population (167). We currently are testing
the hypothesis that although LEW donor cells are fewer in
number, they receive assistance from "autoimmune" reactions
precipitated by the alloreaction in the recipient's immune
network.

The above hypothesis is similar to the hypotheses of
van Rood et al (151) and Dorsch and Roser (168,169),
although, there are key differences as well. Both of the
groups just mentioned, stress the need for hematolymphoid
chimerism and anti-idiotypic-like reactions. However, they
also stress the necessity of MHC restriction and view the
relationship between the two immune systems as one of
antagonism. In contrast, we stress the possibility of
effective collaboration across MHC barriers with "auto-

reactivity" ultimately being responsible for graft
acceptance. Furthermore, we feel that the "autoimmune"-type
reactions described in the preceding pages are likely part
of the repertoire of a normally functioning immune network
(116-123).

It should be mentioned that Shearer et al (170) and
Hoffman et al (171) have used the concept of network
focusing to explain the pan-immunologic deficit of the
Acquired Immune Deficiency Syndrome (AIDS). They suggested
that the combination of allogeneic lymphoid cells and HIV
trigger chronic GVH and autoimmune reactions, which are
internally directed against the CD4+ components of the
immune network. The end result is overactivity of the MHCi
system, which produces an immune defect that is far greater
than would be expected if the virus alone were causing the
disease.

From the preceding discussion, it would appear that
specific allogeneic tolerance is something easily and
reproducibly achieved. Such is not the case in clinical
organ transplantation and therefore immunosuppressive
protocols tend to be designed to completely abolish all
alloreactivity. Our hypothesis would suggest that such an
approach is not conducive to tolerance induction and
eventual drug withdrawal. We now know that there are many

more considerations to the induction of tolerance besides the elimination of rejection.

In fact, without alloactivation, there will be no tolerance. Effective immunosuppressants appear to function at least in part by permitting regulatory responses to occur, while protecting both the peripheralized donor hematolymphoid cells and graft from injury (52-58,98,99). All the while, donor cells are assimilated into the recipient's immune network. In addition, FK 506 and cyclosporine change thymic physiology, by increasing the emigration into peripheral tissue of immature thymocytes (172,173), and increasing the recruitment into the thymus of immature medullary dendritic cells (174).

The type of allograft may also play an important role in the induction of transplantation tolerance. For example, the liver contains a large number of natural killer cells, which can assist in donor hematolymphoid cell engraftment (175). The liver also is known to be intimately involved with regulation of hematopoietic stem cell activity in the bone marrow (176,177). All of the considerations in the preceding two paragraphs could potentially influence the merging of two immune systems.

At present however, we do not know how to measure or control potentially beneficial regulatory responses. More importantly, we also do not know which factors dictate whether an alloantigen exposure will result in sensitization or tolerance. These two seemingly opposite reactions are obviously quite closely related. Nevertheless, empiric observations have shown that increasing the donor's immune system representation is advantageous for tolerance induction. Therefore, non-cytotoxic regimens are needed to enhance the survival or permit engraftment of donor hematolymphoid cells to accomplish immunologic redefinition of the recipient. Regardless of the specific approach, increasing attention to the network properties of immune systems will likely be required.

REFERENCES

1. Snell GD. The homograft reaction. Ann Rev Microbiol 11:439-458, 1957.

2. Steinmuller D. Immunization with skin isografts taken from tolerant mice. Science 158:127-129, 1967.

3. Steinman RM, Cohn ZA. Identification of a novel cell type in peripheral lymphoid organs of mice. I. Morphology, quantitation, tissue distribution. J Exp Med 137:1142-1162, 1973.

4. Steinman RM, Cohn ZA. Identification of a novel cell type in peripheral lymphoid organs of mice. II. Functional properties in vitro. J Exp Med 139:380-397, 1974.

5. Steinman RM, Lustig DS, Cohn ZA. Identification of a novel cell in peripheral lymphoid organs in mice. III. Functional properties in vivo. J Exp Med 139:1431-1445, 1974.

6. Steinman RM. The dendritic cell system and its role in immunogenicity. Ann Rev Immunology 9:271-296, 1991.

7.   Talmage DW, Dart G, Radovich J, Lafferty KJ.   Activation of transplant immunity; effect of donor leukocytes in thyroid allograft rejection.   Science 191:385-387, 1976.

8.   Lafferty KJ, Bootes A, Dart G, Talmage DW.   Effect of organ culture in the survival of thyroid allografts in mice. Transplantation 22:138-149, 1976.

9.   Faustman D, Hauptfeld V, Lacy P, Davie J.   Prolongation of murine islet allograft survival by pretreatment of islets with antibody directed to Ia determinants.   Proc Natl Acad Sci USA 78:5156-5159, 1981.

10.   Austyn JM, Steinman RM.   The passenger leukocyte - a fresh look.   Transpl Rev 2:139-176, 1988.

11.   Fabre JW.   Epidermal allografts.   Immunology Letters 29:161-166, 1991.

12.   Billingham RE, Brent L, Medawar PB.   Actively acquired tolerance of foreign cells.   Nature 172:603-606, 1953.

13.   Main JM, Prehn RT.   Successful skin homografts after the administration of high dosage X radiation and homologous bone marrow.   J Natl Cancer Inst 15:1023-1029, 1955.

364

14.   Slavin S, Strober S, Fuks Z, Kaplan HS. Induction of specific tissue transplantation tolerance using fractionated total lymphoid irradiation in adult mice.   Long-term survival of allogeneic bone marrow and skin grafts.   J Exp Med 146:34-48, 1977.

15.   Slavin S, Reitz B, Bieber CP, Kaplan HS, Strober S. Transplantation   tolerance in adult rats using total lymphoid irradiation: permanent survival of skin, heart and marrow allografts.   J Exp Med 147:700-707, 1978.

16.   Slavin S, Fuks Z, Weiss L, Morecki S. Mechanisms of tolerance in chimeric mice prepared with total lymphoid irradiation.   ICN-UCLA Symp. Mol Cell Biol 17:383, 1980.

17.   Ildstad ST, Sachs DH.   Reconstitution with syngeneic plus allogeneic or xenogeneic bone marrow leads to specific acceptance of allografts or xenografts.   Nature 307:168-170, 1984.

18.   Myburgh JA, Smit JA, Stark JH, Browde S.   Total lymphoid irradiation in kidney and liver transplantation in the baboon: prolonged graft survival and alteration in T cell subsets with low cumulative dose regimens.   J Immunol 132:1019-1025, 1984.

19. Mayumi H, Himeno K, Tanaka K, Tokuda N, Fan J, Nomoto K. Drug induced tolerance to allografts in mice. XII. The relationships between tolerance, chimerism and graft-versus-host disease. Transplantation 44:286-290, 1987.

20. Owen RD: Immunogenetic consequences of vascular anastomoses between bovine twins. Science 102:400-401, 1945.

21. Anderson D, Billingham RE, Lampkin GH, Medawar PB: The use of skin grafting to distinguish between monozygotic and dizygotic twins in cattle. Heredity 5:379-397, 1952.

22. Burnet FM, Fenner F: The Production of Antibodies. 2nd ed Melbourne, Macmillan 1949. pp: 1-142

23. Billingham R, Brent L, Medawar P: Quantitative studies on tissue transplantation immunity. III. Actively acquired tolerance. Philos Trans R Soc Lond (Biol) 239:357-412, 1956.

24. Gatti RA, Meuwissen HJ, Allen HD, Hong R, Good RA: Immunological reconstitution of sex-linked lymphopenic immunological deficiency. Lancet 2:1366-1369, 1968.

25. Thomas ED: Allogeneic marrow grafting - A story of man and dog. In Terasaki PI and Cecka JM, eds. Clinical Transplants, 1991 UCLA Press pp: 381-390.

26. Billingham R, Brent L: Quantitative studies on transplantation immunity. IV. Induction of tolerance in newborn mice and studies on the phenomenon of runt disease. Philos Trans R Soc Lond (Biol) 242:439-477, 1956.

27. Billingham RE. Reactions of grafts against their hosts. Transplantation immunity works both way-hosts destroy grafts and grafts may harm hosts. Science 130:947-953, 1959.

28. Good RA: Immunologic reconstitution: The achievement and its meaning. Hospital Practice 1969, 4:41-47.

29. Rapaport FT, Bachvaroff RJ, Mollen N, Hirasawa H, Asano T, Ferrebee JW: Induction of unresponsiveness to major transplantable organs in adult mammals. Ann Surg 1979, 190:461-473.

30. Liegeois A, Charreire J, Brennan LB: Allograft enhancement induced by bone marrow cells. Surg Forum 25:297-300, 1974.

31. Liegeois A, Escourrou J, Ouvre E, Charreire J: Microchimerism: A stable state of low-ratio proliferation of allogeneic bone marrow. Transplant Proc 9:273-276, 1977.

32. Monaco AE, Wood ML, Russell PS: Studies of heterologous anti-lymphocyte serum in mice. III. immunologic tolerance and chimerism produced across the H-2 locus with adult thymectomy and anti-lymphocyte serum. Annals of the New York Academy of Sciences. 129:190-209, 1966.

33. Wood ML, Monaco AP, Gozzo JJ, Liegeois A: Use of homozygous allogeneic bone marrow for induction of tolerance with antilymphocyte serum: Dose and timing. Transplant Proc 3:676-683, 1971.

34. Monaco AP, Wood ML, Maki T, Gozzo JJ: Post transplantation donor-specific bone marrow transfusion in polyclonal antilymphocyte serum-treated recipients: The optimal cellular antigen for induction of unresponsiveness to organ allografts. Transplant Proc 20:1207-1212, 1988.

35. Myburgh JA, Smit JA, Hill RRH, Browde S: Transplantation tolerance in primates following total lymphoid irradiation and allogeneic bone marrow injection. Transplantation 29:405-408, 1980.

36. Myburgh JA, Smit JA, Browde S, Hill RRH: Transplantation tolerance in primates following total lymphoid irradiation and allogeneic bone marrow injection. I. Orthotopic liver allografts. Transplantation 29:401-404, 1980.

37. Saper V, Chow D, Engleman ED, Hoppe RT, Levin B, Collins G, Strober S: Clinical and immunological studies of cadaveric renal transplant recipients given total-lymphoid irradiation and maintained on low-dose prednisone. Transplantation 45:540-546, 1988.

38. Najarian JS, Ferguson RM, Sutherland DER, Slavin S, T
Kim, Kersey T, Simmons RL: Fractionated total lymphoid
irradiation as preparative immunosuppression in high-risk
renal transplantation. Ann Surg 196:442-452, 1982.

39. Waer M, Vanrenterghem Y, Roels L, Ang KK, Bouillon R,
Lerut T, Gruwez J, van der Schueren E, Vandeputte M,
Michielsen P: Immunological and clinical observations in
diabetic kidney graft recipients pretreated with total-
lymphoid irradiation. Transplantation 43:371-379, 1987.

40. Cortesini R, Molajoni ER, Berloco P, Bachetoni A, Cinti
P, Trovati A, Sallusto F, Pretagostini, Iapelli M, Caricato
M, Rossi M, Alfani D: Long-term follow-up of kidney grafts
in high-risk patients under TLI and CsA therapy. Transplant
Proc 21:1790-1792, 1989.

41. Myburgh AJ, Smit AJ, Meyers MA, Botha JR, Browde S,
Thomson PD: Total lymphoid irradiation in renal
transplantation. World J Surg 10:369-380, 1986.

42. Myburgh JA, Meyers AM, Thomson PD, Botha JR, Margolius
L, Lakier R, Smit JA, Stark JH, Gray C: Total lymphoid
irradiation-current status. Transplant Proc 21:826-828,
1989.

43. Medawar PB: Transplantation of tissues and organs: introduction. Br Med Bull 21:97-99, 1965.

44. Weber RA, Cannon JA, Longmire WP: Observations on the regrafting of successful homografts in chickens. Ann Surg 139:473-477, 1954.

45. Murray JE, Sheil AGR, Moseley R, Knight R, McGavic Dickinson J, Dammin GJ: Analysis of mechanism of immunosuppressive drugs in renal homotransplantation. Ann Surg 160:449-473, 1964.

46 Starzl TE: Host-Graft Adaptation. In: Experience in Renal Transplantation WB Saunders Company, Philadelphia PA 1964. pp: 164-170.

47. Starzl TE: Efforts to Mitigate or Prevent Rejection. In: Experience in Hepatic Transplantation WB Saunders Company, Philadelphia PA 1969. pp: 203-206, 216-220, 226-233.

48. Levey RH: Immunological tolerance and enhancement: A common mechanism. Transplant Proc 3:41:48, 1971.

49. Murase N, Kim DG, Todo S, Cramer DV, Fung JJ, Starzl TE: FK 506 suppression of heart and liver allograft

rejection II: The induction of graft acceptance in rat. Transplantation 50:739-744, 1990.

50. Streilen JW: Neonatal tolerance of H-2 alloantigens. Procuring graft acceptance the "old-fashioned" way. Transplantation 52:1-10, 1991.

51. Eto M, Mayumi H, Nishimura, Maeda T, Yoshikai T, Nomoto K: Similarity and difference in the mechanisms of neonatally induced tolerance and cyclophosphamide-induced tolerance in mice J Immunol 147:2439-2446, 1991.

52 Starzl TE, Demetris AJ, Murase N, Ildstad S, Ricordi C, Trucco M: Cell migration, chimerism, and graft acceptance. Lancet 339:1579-1582, 1992.

53. Starzl TE, Demetris AJ, Trucco M, Ramos H, Zeevi A, Rudert WA, Kocoua M, Ricordi C, Ildstad S, Murase N: Systemic chimerism in human female recipients of male livers. Lancet 340:876-877, 1992.

54. Starzl TE, Demetris AJ, Trucco M, Ricordi S, Ildstad S, Terasaki P, Murase N, Kendall RS, Kocoua M, Rudert WA, Zeevi A, Van Thiel D: Chimerism after liver transplantation for type IV glycogen storage disease and Type I Gaucher's disease. New Engl J Med 328:745-749, 1993.

55. Starzl TE, Demetris AJ, Trucco M, Zeevi A, Ramos H, Terasaki P, Rudert WA, Kocova M, Ricordi C, Ildstad S, Murase N: Chimerism and donor specific nonreactivity 27 to 29 years after kidney allotransplantation. Transplantation 55:1272-1277, 1993.

56. Starzl TE, Demetris AJ, Murase N, Thomson AW, Trucco M, Ricordi C: Cell chimerism permitted by immunosuppressive drugs is the basis of organ transplant acceptance and tolerance. Immunol Today 14(No.6):326-332, 1993.

57. Starzl TE, Demetris AJ, Trucco M, Murase N, Ricordi C, Ildstad S, Ramos H, Todo S, Tzakis A, Fung JJ, Nalesnik M, Rudert WA, Kocova M: Cell migration and chimerism after whole organ transplantation: The basis of graft acceptance. Hepatology 17(6):1127-1152, 1993.

58. Demetris AJ, Murase N, Fujisaki S, Fung JJ, Rao AS, Starzl TE: Hematolymphoid cell trafficking, chimerism, and tolerance after liver, bone marrow, and heart transplantation: Rejection, GVHD and the merging of immune systems. J Exp Med

59. Qian S, Demetris AJ, Fu F, Li Y, Sun H, Lan G, Thai N, Dahman U, Murase N, Fung JJ, Starzl TE: Murine liver allograft transplantation: tolerance and donor cell chimerism. Hepatology

60. Murase N, Demetris AJ, Kim DG, Todo S, Fung JJ, Starzl TE: Rejection of the multivisceral allografts in rats: A sequential analysis with comparison to isolated orthotopic small bowel and liver grafts. Surgery 108:880-889, 1990.

61. Starzl TE, Marchioro TL, Porter KA, Taylor PD, Faris TD, Herrmann TJ, Hlad CJ, Waddell WR: Factors determining short- and long-term survival after orthotopic liver homotransplantation in the dog. Surgery 58:131-155, 1965.

62. Valdivia LA, Fung JJ, Demetris AJ, Starzl TE: Differential survival of hamster-to-rat liver and cardiac xenografts under FK 506 immunosuppression. Transplant Proc 1991; 23:3269-3271.

63. Garnier H, Clot J, Bertrand M, Camplez P, Kumlim A, Gorim JKP, LeGoaziou F, Levy R, Cordier G: Liver transplantation in the pig: surgical approach. Cr Acad Sci, Paris 260:5621-5623, 1965.

64. Peacock JH, Terblanche J: Orthotopic homotransplantation of the liver in the pig. In: Read AE (ed.): The Liver, London, Butterworth & Co., Ltd., 1967, pp:333-336.

65. Calne RY, White HJO, Yoffa DE, Maginn RR, Binns RM, Samuel JR, Molina VP: Observations of orthotopic liver transplantation in the pig. Br Med J 2:478-480, 1967.

66. Zimmerman FA, Butcher GW, Davies HS, Brons G, Kamada N, Turel O: Techniques for orthotopic liver transplantation in the rat and some studies of the immunologic responses to fully allogeneic liver grafts. Transplant Proc 11:571-577, 1979.

67. Starzl TE, Ishikawa M, Putnam CW, Porter KA, Picache R, Husberg BS, Halgrimson CG, Schroter G: Progress in and deterrents to orthotopic liver transplantation, with special reference to survival, resistance to hyperacute rejection, and biliary duct reconstruction. Transplant Proc 6:129-139, 1974.

68. Kamada N, Davies HFFS, Roser B: Reversal of transplantation immunity by liver grafting. Nature 292:840-842, 1981.

69. Houssin D, Gugenheim J, Bellon B, Brunard M, Gigou M, Charra M, Crougneau S, Bismuth H: Absence of hyperacute rejection of liver allografts in hypersensitized rats. Transplant Proc 17:293-295, 1985.

70. Fung J, Makowka L, Tzakis A, Klintmalm G, Duquesnoy R, Gordon R, Todo S, Griffin M, Starzl TE: Combined liver-kidney transplantation: Analysis of patients with preformed lymphocytotoxic antibodies. Transplant Proc 1988; 20 (Suppl. 1):88-91.

71. Calne RY, Sells RA, Pena JR, Davis DR, Millard PR, Herbertson BM, Binns RM, Davies DAL: Induction of immunological tolerance by porcine liver allografts. Nature 233:472-474, 1969.

72. Valdivia L, Demetris AJ, Fung JJ, Celli S, Murase N, Starzl TE: Successful hamster to rat liver xenotransplantation under FK 506 immunosuppression induces unresponsiveness to hamster heart and skin. Transplantation 55:659-661, 1993.

73. Hart DNJ, McKenzie JL: Interstitial dendritic cells. Int Rev Immunol 6:128-149, 1990.

74. Hart DNJ, Winearls CG, Fabre JW: Graft adaptation: studies on possible mechanisms in long-term surviving rat renal allografts. Transplantation 30:73-80, 1980.

75. Batchelor JR, Welsh KI, Maynard A, Burgos H: Failure of long surviving, passively enhanced allografts to provoke T-dependent alloimmunity: I. Retransplantation of (AS X

AUG)F1 kidneys into secondary AS recipients. J Exp Med
150:455-464, 1979.

76.   Lechler RI, Batchelor JR: Restoration of immunogenicity
to passenger cell-depleted kidney allografts by the addition
of donor-strain dendritic cells. J Exp Med 155:31-41,
1982.

77.   Marchioro TL, Rowlands DT Jr, Rifkind D, Waddell WR,
Starzl TE, Fudenberg H: Splenic homotransplantation. Ann
NY Acad Sci 120:626-651, 1964.

78.   Wakely E, Oberholser JH, Corry RJ: Elimination of
acute gvhd and prolongation of rat pancreas allograft
survival with DST, cyclosporine, and spleen transplantation.
Transplantation 49:241-245, 1990.

79.   Bitter-Suermann H, Save-Soderbergh JS: The course of
pancreas allografts in rats conditioned by spleen
allografts. Transplantation 26:28-34, 1978.

80.   Murase N, Demetris AJ, Matsuzaki T, Yagihasi A, Todo S,
Fung J, Starzl TE: Long survival in rats after
multivisceral versus isolated small bowel
allotransplantation under FK 506. Surgery 110:87-98,
1991.

81. Prop J, Kuijpers K, Petersen AH, Bartels HL, Nieuwenhuis P, Wildevuur CRH: Why are lung allografts more vigorously rejected than hearts? Heart Transplantation 4:433-436, 1985.

82. Westra AL, Prop J, Kuijpers KC, Wildevuur CRH: A paradox in heart and lung rejection. Transplantation 49:826-828, 1990.

83. Iwaki Y, Starzl TE, Yagihashi A, Taniwaki S, Abu-Elmagd K, Tzakis A, Fung J, Todo S: Replacement of donor lymphoid tissue in human small bowel transplants under FK 506 immunosuppression. Lancet 337:818-819, 1991.

84. Murase N, Demetris AJ, Woo J, Furuya T, Nalesnik M, Tanabe M, Todo S, Starzl TE: Lymphocyte traffic and graft-versus-host disease after fully allogeneic small bowel transplantation. Transplant Proc 23:3246-3247, 1991.

85. Murase N, Demetris A, Woo J, Tanabe M, Furuya T, Todo S, Starzl TE: Graft versus host disease (GVHD) after BN to LEW compared to LEW to BN rat intestinal transplantation under FK 506. Transplantation 55:1-7, 1993.

86. Nemlander A, Soots A, Willebrand EV, Husberg B, Hayry P: Redistribution of renal allograft responding leukocytes during rejection. II. Kinetics and specificity. J Exp Med 156:1087-1100, 1982.

87. Larsen CP, Morris PJ, Austyn JM: Migration of dendritic leukocytes from cardiac allografts into host

spleens. A novel route for initiation of rejection. J Exp Med 171:307-314, 1990.

88. Demetris AJ, Qian S, Sun H, Fung JJ, Yagihashi A, Murase N, Iwaki Y, Gambrell B, Starzl TE: Early events in liver allograft rejection. Am J Pathol 138:609-618, 1991.

89. Forbes RD, Parfrey NA, Gomersail M, Darden AG, Guttmann RD: Dendritic cell-lymphoid aggregation and major histocompatibility antigen expression during rat cardiac allograft rejection. J Exp Med 164:1239-1258, 1986.

90. van Schlifgaarde R, Hermans P, Terpstra JL, van Breda Vriesman PJC: Role of mobile passenger lymphocytes in the rejection of renal and cardiac allografts in the rat. Transplantation 29:209, 1989.

91. Hayry and Willebrand. <u>Transplantation and Clinical Immunology</u>. Volume 15, Immunosuppression. 15th International Course, Lyon, (eds., Touraine, Thaegen, Betuel, Brochier, Dubernard, Revillard, & Triau). Excerpta Medica, Amsterdam, 1983.

92. von Willebrand E, Taskinen E, Ahonen J, Hayry P: Recent modifications in the fine needle asipration biopsy of human renal allografts. Transplant Proc 15:1195-1197, 1983.

93. Corry RJ, Winn HJ, Russell PS: Primary vascularized allografts of hearts in mice: The role of H-2D, H-2K and non-H-2 antigens in rejection. Transplantation 16:343-350, 1973.

94. Russell PS, Chase CM, Colvin RB, Plate JMD: Kidney tranpslants in mice. An analysis of the immune status of mice bearing long-term G-2 incompatible transplants. J Exp Med 147:1449-1468, 1978.

95. Benson MT, Buckley G, Jenkinson EJ, Owen JJ. Survival of deoxyguanosine treated fetal thymus allografts is prevented by priming with dendritic cells. Immunology 60(4):593-596, 1987.

96. Demetris AJ, Murase N, Starzl TE. Donor dendritic cells in grafts and host lymphoid and non-lymphoid tissues after liver and heart allotransplantation under short term immunosuppression. Lancet 339:1610, 1992.

97. Srlwatanawongsa V, Davies HffS, Brons IGM, Aspinall R, Thiru S, Jamieson NV, Calne SRY. Continued presence of donor leukocytes in recipients of liver grafts. Transplant Proc 25:371-372, 1993.

98.   Kroczek RA, Black CDV, Barbet J, Shevach EM.
Mechanisms of action of cyclosporine A in vivo.   J Immunol.
139:3597-3603, 1987.

99.   Clerici M, Shearer GM.   Differential sensitivity of
human T helper cell pathways by in vitro exposure to
cyclosporine A.   J Immunol 144:2480-2485, 1990.

100.   Austyn JM, Kupiec-Weglinski JW, Hankins DF, Morris PJ.
Migration patterns of dendritic cells in the mouse: Homing
to T-cell dependent areas of spleen, and binding with
marginal zone.   J Exp Med 167:646-651, 1988.

101.   Nieuwenhuis P, DeVries-Bos L, Opstelten D, Deenen GJ,
Stet RJM, Rozing J, 1983.   Lymphocyte migration across major
histocompatibility barriers in splenectomized rats.   Immunol
Rev. 73:53-70, 1983.

102.   Austyn JM, Larsen CP.   Migration patterns of dendritic
leukocytes.   Transplantation 49:1-7, 1990.

103.   Roncarlo MG, Touraine JL, Banchereau J.   Cooperation
between major histcompatibility complex mismatched
mononuclear cells from a human chimera in the production of
antigen-specific antibody.   J. Clin. Invest. 77:673-680,
1986.

104. Thomas J, Carver M, Cunningham P, Park K, Gonder J. Promotion of incompatible allograft acceptance in rhesus monkeys given posttransplant antithymocyte globulin and donor bone marrow. I. In vivo parameters and immunohistologic evidence suggesting microchimerism. Transplantation 43:332-338, 1987.

105. Roberts JP, Ascher NL, Lake J, Capper J, Purohit S, Garovoy M, Lynch R, et al. Graft versus host disease after liver transplantation in humans. A report of four cases. Hepatology 14:274-281, 1991.

106. Collins RH, Anastasi J, Terstappen LWWM, Nikaein A, Feng J, Fay JW, Klintmalm G, Stone MJ: Brief Report: Donor-derived long-term multilineage hematopoiesis in a liver-transplant recipient. New Engl J Med 328:762-765, 1993.

107. Comenzo ROL, Malachowski ME, Rohrer RJ, Freeman RB, Rabson A, Berkman EM. Anomalous ABO phenotype in a child after an ABO-incompatible liver transplantation. N. Engl. J. Med. 326:867-889, 1992.

108. Monaco AP and Wood ML. Studies on heterologous antilymphocyte serum in mice. VII. Optimal cellular antigen for induction of immunologic tolerance with ALS. Transplant Proc 2:489-496, 1970.

109.   Monaco AP, Wood ML, Maki T, Gozzo JJ.   Post transplantation donor-specific bone marrow transfusion in polyclonal antilymphocyte serum-treated recipients.   The optimal cellular antigen for induction of unresponsiveness to organ allografts.   Transplant Proc. 20:1207-1212, 1988.

110.   Strelein JW, Strome P, Wood PJ.   Failure of in vitro assays to predict accurately the existence of neonatally induced H-2 tolerance.   Transplantation 48:630- 1989.

111.   Mayumi H, Himeno K, Tokuda N, Fan JL, Nomoto K.   Drug induced tolerance to allografts in mice.   X Augmentation of split tolerance in murine combinations disparate at both H-2 and Non-H-2 antigens by the use of spleen cells from donors preimmunized with recipient antigens.   Immunobiol. 174:274-291, 1987.

112.   Wood KJ.   Alternative approaches for the induction of transplantation tolerance.   Immunology Letters 29:133-138, 1991.

113.   Miller JFAP.   Post-thymic tolerance to self antigens. Journal of Autoimmunity 5:27-35, 1992.

114. Ramsdell F, Fowlkes BJ. Maintenance of in vivo tolerance by persistence of antigen. Science 257:1130-1134, 1992.

115. Reyes J, Zeevi A, Ramos HC, Tzakis A, Todo S, Demetris AJ, Nour B, Nalesnik M, Trucco M, Abu-Elmagd K, Fung JJ, Starzl TE: The frequent achievement of a drug free state after orthotopic liver transplantation. Transplant Proc (In Press).

116. Coutinho A. Beyond clonal selection and network. Immuno Rev. 110:63-87, 1989.

117. Perelson AS. Immune Network Theory. Immunol Rev. 110:5-36, 1989.

118. Hoffmann GW, Kion TA, Forsyth RB, Soga KG, Cooper-Willis A. In: Theoretical immunology, ed. Perelson AS. (Addison-Wesley. Redwood City, CA, pp. 291-319, 1988.

119. Hoffmann GW. In: Regulation of immune response dynamics, eds. DeLisi, C. & Hiernaux, J. (CRC, Boca Raton, FL). pp. 137-162, 1982.

120. Hoffmann GW. In The Semiotics of cellular communication in the immune system, eds. Sercarz, E.E.,

Celada. F., Mitchiso, .AA. & Tada, T. (Springer, New York), pp. 257-271, 1988.

121. Cohen IR. The cognitive paradigm and the immunological homunculus. Immunology Today 13:490-494, 1992.

122. Perelson AS, Weisbuch G. Modeling immune reactivity in secondary lymphoid organs. Bulletin of Mathematical Biology. 54:649-672, 1992.

123. De Boerts RJ, Segel LA, Perelson AS. Pattern formation in one- and two-dimensional shape-space models of the immune system. J Theor. Biol 155:295-333, 1992.

124. Rolstad B, Benestad HB. Spontaneous alloreactivity of natural killer (NK) and lymphokine-activated killer (LAK) cells from athymic rats against normal haemic cells. NK cells stimulate syngeneic but inhibit allogeneic haemopoiesis. Immunol 74:86-93, 1991.

125. Vaage JT, Dissen E, Ager A, Fossum S, Rolstad B. Allospecific recognition of hemic cells in vitro by natural killer cells from athymic rats; evidence that allodeterminants coded for by single major histocompatibility complex haplotypes are recognized. Eur J Immunol 21:2167-2175, 1991.

384

126. Miller JFAP, Morahan G. Peripheral T Cell Tolerance.
Ann Rev Immunol 10:31-69, 1992.

127. Nossal GJV. Immunologic tolerance: Collaboration
between antigen and lymphokines. Science 245:147-153, 1989.

128. Matzinger P, Guerder S. Does T cell tolerance require
a dedicated antigen presenting cell? Nature 338:74-76,
1989.

129. Russell PS: Modification of runt disease in mice by
various means. In: Transplantation: Ciba Foundation
Symposium (Wolstenholme CEW, Cameron MP, London J,
Churchill A, eds), Little Brown and Co., Boston, MA 1962
pp: 350-383

130. Kappler JW, Roehm M, Marrack P. T cell tolerance by
clonal elimination in the thymus. Cell 49:273-280, 1987.

131. Zinkernagel RM, Hengartner H. T cell receptor Vβ use
predicts reactivity and tolerance to Mlsa-encoded antigens.
Nature 332:40-45, 1988.

132. Finberg, R, Burkakoff SJ, Cantor H, Benacerraf B.
Biological significance of alloreactivity: T cells
stimulated by Sendai virus-coated syngeneic cells

specifically lyse allogeneic targets cells. Proc Natl Acad Sci USA 75:(10) 5145-5149, 1978.

133. Gaston JSH, Waer, M. Virus-specific MHC-restricted T lymphocytes may initiate allograft rejection. Immunol Today 6: 237-???, 1985.

134. Benacerraf, B. Significance and biological function of Class II MHC molecules. Am J Pathol 120:334-343, 1985.

135. Belligrau D, Wilson DB. Immunological studies of T-cell receptors. J Exp Med 103-114.

136. Suciu-Foca N, Rohowsky C, Kung P, King DW. Idiotype-like determinants on human T lymphocytes alloactivated in mixed lympocyte culture. J Exp Med 156:283-288, 1982.

137. Suciu-Foca N, Rohowsky C, Kung P, Lewison A, Nicholson J, Reemstsma K, King DW. MHC-specific idiotypes on alloactivated human T cells: In vivo and in vitro studies. Transplant Proc XV:784-789, 1983.

138. Kimura H, Pickard A, Wilson DB. Analysis of T cell populations that induce and mediate specific resistance to graft-versus-host disease in rats. J Exp Med 160:652-658, 1984.

139. Saito K, Tamura A, Narimatsu H, Tadakuma T, Nagashima M. Cloned auto-Ia-reactive T cells elicit lichen planus-like lesion in the skin of syngeneic mice. Journal of Immunology 137:2485-2495, 1986.

140. Sainis K, Datta SK. CD4+ T cell lines with selective patterns of autoreactivity as well as CD4- CD8- T helper cell lines augment the production of idiotypes shared by pathogenic anti-DNA autoantibodies in the NZB X SWR model of lupus nephritis. Journal of Immunology 140:2215-2224, 1988.

141. Pelletier L, Pasquier R, Rossert J, Vial MC, Mandet C, Druet P. Autoreactive T cells in mercury-induced autoimmunity. Journal of Immunology 140:750-754, 1988.

142. Cornacchia E, Golbus J, Maybaum J, Strahler J, Hanash S, Richardson B. Hydralazine and procainamide inhibit T cell DNA methylation and induce autoreactivity. Journal of Immunology 140:2197-2200, 1988.

143. Palathumpat V, Sobis H, Vandeputte M, Michielsen P, Waer M. Induction of mixed lymphocyte reaction nonresponsiveness after chimeric thymus transplantation. Transplant Int 3:217-221, 1990.

144. Russell PS, Chase CM, Colvin RB, Plate JMD. Kidney transplants in mice. An analysis of the immune status of

mice bearing long-term, H-2 incompatible transplants. J Exp Med 147(5):1449-1468, 1978.

145. Russell PS, Chase CM, Colvin RB, Plate JMD. Induced immune destruction of long-surviving, H-2 incompatible kidney transplants in mice. J Exp Med 147(5):1469-1486, 1978.

146. Armstrong HE, Botton EM, McMillan I, Spencer SC, Bradley JA. Prolonged survival of actively enhanced rat renal allografts despite accelerated cellular infiltration and rapid induction of both class I and class II MHC antigens. J. Exp. Med. 164:891-907, 1987.

147. Opelz G, Mickey MR, Terasaki PI: Blood transfusions and unresponsiveness to HL-A. Transplantation 16:649-656, 1973.

148. Fabre JW, Morris PJ: Dose response studies in passive enhancement of rat renal allografts. Transplantation 15:397-403, 1973.

149. Bradley JA. The blood transfusion effect: experimental aspects. Immunol Lett 29:127-132, 1991.

150. de Waal LP, van Twuyver E. Blood transfusion and allograft survival: Is mixed chimerism the solution for

388

tolerance induction in clinical transplantation?   Immunol
10:417-425,1991.

151.   van Rood JJ, Claas FHJ.   The influence of allogeneic
cells on the human T and B cell repertoire.   Science
248:1388-1393, 1990.

152.   Wotherspoon JS, Dorsch SE.   Graft-versus-host
resistance induced by tolerant cell populations.
Transplantation 47:528-532, 1989.

153.   Strelein JW, Levy RB, Ruiz P, Matriano J, Socarras S.
Multiple mechanism induce and maintain neonatal
transplantation tolerance.   Transplant Sci. 3:11-16, 1993.

154.   Qin S, Cobbold SP, Pope H, Elliott J, Kioussis D,
Davies J, Waldmann H.   "Infectious" transplantation
tolerance.   Science 259:974-977, 1993.

155.   Herber-Katz E, Acha-Orbea H: The V-region disease
hypothesis: evidence from autoimmune encephalomyelitis.
Immunology Today 10:164-169, 1989.

156.   Goldman M, Feng HM, Engers H, Hochman A, Louis J,
Lambert PH.   Autoimmunity and immune complex disease after
neonatal induction of transplantation tolerance in mice.
Journal of Immunology 131:251-258, 1983.

157. Merino J, Schurmans S, Luzuy S, Izui S, Vassalli P, Lambert PH. Autoimmune syndrome after induction of neonatal tolerance to alloantigens: effects of in vivo treatment with anti-T cell subset monoclonal antibodies. 139:1426-1431, 1988.

158. Goldman M, Abramowicz D, Lambert P, Vandervorst P, Bruyns C, Toussaint C. Hyperactivity of donor B cells after neonatal induction of lymphoid chimersim in mice. Clin Exp Immunol 72:79-83, 1988.

159. Schurmans S, Heusser CH, Qin HY, Merino J, Brighous G, Lambert PH. In vivo effects of anti-IL-4 monoclonal antibody on neonatal induction of tolerance and or an associated autoimmune syndrome. Journal of Immunology 145:2465-2473, 1990.

160. Abramowicz D, Vandervorst P, Bruyns C, Doutrelepont JM, Vandenabeele P, Goldman M. Persistence of anti-donor allohelper T cells after neonatal induction of allotolerance in mice. Eur J Immunol 20:1647-1653, 1990.

161. Guery JC, Tournade V, Pelletier L, Druet O, Druet P. Rat anti-glomerular basement membrane antibodies in toxin-induced autoimmunity and in chronic graft vs host reaction share recurrent idiotypes. Eur J Immunol 20:101-105, 1990.

162. Tournade H, Pelletier L, Pasquier R, Vial MC, Mandet C, Druet P. Graft-versus-host reactions in the rat mimic toxin-induced autoimmunity. Clin Exp Immunol 81:334-338, 1990.

163. Pelletier L, Pasquier R, Guetttier C, Cecile Vial M, Mandet C, Nochy D, Basin H, Druet P. HgC12 induces T and B cells to proliferate and differentiate in BN rats. Clin Exp Immunol 71:336-342, 1988.

164. Aten J, Veninga A, De Heer E, Rozing J, Nieuwenhuis P, Hoedemaeker PJ, Weening JJ. Susceptibility to the induction of either autoimmunity or immunosuppression by mercuric chloride is related to the major histocompatibility complex class II haplotype. Eur J Immunol 21:611-616, 1991.

165. Goldman M, Druet P, Gleichmann E. TH2 cells in systemic autoimmunity: insights from allogeneic diseases and chemically-induced autoimmunity. Immunology Today 12:223-227, 1991.

166. Zhang H, Hortitz L, Fischer AC, Laulis M, Colombani PM, Hess AD. Adoptive transfer of cyclosporine-induced MHC class II autoreactive cells prolongs heart allograft survival. Transplant Sci 3:17-19, 1993.

167. Tanabe M, Murase N, Demetris AJ, Hoffman RA, Nakamura K, Fujisaki S, Galvao FHF, Todo S, Fung J, Starzl TE: The influence of donor and recipient strains in isolated small bowel transplantation in rats. Gastroenterology (In Press).

168. Dorsch S, Roser B. Suppressor cells in transplantation tolerance. Transplantation 33:518-524, 1982.

169. Dorsch S, Roser B. Suppressor cells in transplantatio tolerance II. Transplantation 33:525-529, 1982.

170. Shearer GM. Allogeneic leukocytes as a possible factor in induction of AIDS in homosexual men. N Engl J Med 308:223-224, 1983.

171. Hoffmann GW, Kion TA, Grant MD. An idiotypic network model of AIDS immunopathogenesis. Proc Natl Acad Sci 88:3060-3064, 1991.

172. Hosseinzadeh H, Goldschneider I. Demonstration of large-scale migration of cortical thymocytes to peripheral lymphoid tissues in cyclosporine A-treated rats. J Exp Med (in press).

173. Hosseinzadeh H, Goldschnedier I. Recent thymic emigrants in the rat express a unique antigenic phenotype

and undergo post-thymic maturation in peripheral lymphoid tissues. J Immunol 150:1670-1679, 1993.

174. de Waal EJ, Rademakers LH, Schuurman HJ, van Lovesen H. Interdigitating cells in the rat thymus during cyclosporin A treatment: ultrastructural observations. Thymus 20:163-170.

175. Lafreniere R, Borkenhagen K, Bryant LD, Anton AR, Chung A, Poon MC. Analysis of liver lymphoid cell subsets pre- and post-in vivo administration of human recombinant interleukin 2 in a C57BL/6 murine system. Cancer Research 50:1658-1666, 1990.

176. Sakamoto T, Saizawa T, Mabuchi A, Norose Y, Shoji T, Yokomuro K. The liver as a potential hematolymphoid organ examined from modifications occurring in the systemic and intrahepatic hematolymphoid system during liver regeneration after partial hepatectomy. Regional Immunology 4:1-11, 1992.

177. Sakamoto T, Maabuchi A, Kuriya SI, Sudo T, Aida T, Asano G, Shoji T, Yokomuro K. Production of granulocyte-macrophage colony-stimulating factor by adult murine parenchymal liver cells (hepatocytes). Regional Immunology 3:260-267,1990.

POSTERS

PART : A

TOLERANCE AND HISTOCOMPATIBILITY

INTRATHYMIC ALLOGENIC ISLET-CELL TRANSPLANTATION IN RATS FAILS TO INDUCE DONOR-SPECIFIC UNRESPONSIVENESS FOR WHOLE PANCREAS TRANSPLANTATION.

OSCAR CHAPA, MOHAMED FAKIR, JEAN-MICHEL RACE, MARC LEGRELLE, NEGIB ELIAN, CAROLINE BENSIMON, JEAN-JACQUES ALTMAN .
Laboratoire de recherche sur la transplantation d'îlots et de pancréas, Hôpital Laënnec et INSERM Unité 341, Hôpital Hôtel-Dieu, Paris, France.

Introduction: The role of the thymus in the induction of self tolerance is well established and makes it a unique transplant site. Rat islet-cell allografts transplanted into the thymus of recipients treated with a single injection of anti-lymphocyte serum, survived indefinitely and induced donor-specific unresponsiveness. The prolonged stay of allogenic islets in the thymus induces unresponsiveness to islets transplanted extrathymically from the same donor[1].

The aim of this study was to determine whether Lewis rat islet-cell transplanted in the thymus of MHC-incompatible Wistar-Furth rat, could induce donor-specific unresponsiveness to total pancreas transplantation without immunosuppression.

Material and Method : Six Wistar-Furth rats, 8 to 10 weeks old, in which diabetes was induced 2 weeks earlier with intravenous streptozotocine, were transplanted with isolated islets according to Gotoh method, from Lewis rats. A total of 750 freshly prepared islets were introduced into the thymus by direct injection into each lobe together with an intraperitoneal administration of 1ml of antilymphocyte serum. Total pancreas from Lewis rats were transplanted into those Wistar-Furth rats 2 months after thymic Lewis islet grafting. For control group, six Wistar-Furth rats were transplanted with total pancreas from same strain donor or from Lewis donor but without prior thymic injection.

Results: All rats in the study survived total pancreas transplantation and showed immediate metabolic normalisation. No satisfactory diabetes control was achieved following islet grafting alone. Only transient, short-term and incomplete normalisation of glycemia was observed. Thymus histology consistently revealed islet allogenic survival for several weeks. Pancreas allogenic grafts following tolerance induction were rejected after the same period, 10 days, as grafts without tolerance induction by intrathymic islet injection. Only in the isogenic control group, the grafted pancreas survived indefinitely.

Discussion: Our study fails to demonstrate that transplantation of islet-cells into the thymus induces donor-specific unresponsiveness for total pancreatic transplantation. Even when a transient metabolic response was obtained for a few days, normalisation of glycemia was not observed. Remuzzi et al.[2] showed that isolated glomeruli from Brown-Norway rat kidneys inoculated into the thymus of MHC—incompatible Lewis rats, subsequent to a two-day immunosuppression, allowed indefinite survival of a kidney graft from the same donor. In their work, it is conceivable that antigen pre-treatment with immunusuppressants could have induce unresponsiveness to donor antigen. Intravenous antigen (with whole blood, bone-marrow cells, splenocyte or extracted histocompatibility antigens) pre-treatment, independantly of any thymic manipulation, when combined with immunosuppressive agents, induces peripheral tolerance and unresponsiveness to donor antigen[3].

In our study, despite survival of islets in the thymus as confirmed by partial normalisation of glycemia and by histology, intra-thymic islet graft did not induce immunological tolerance of a heterotopic transplanted pancreas which harbours more complex and numerous antigens. The role of factors on graft survival such as hyperglycaemia prior and following the intrathymic islet cell inoculation and acute immunosuppression accompanying islet cell grafting, have to be evaluated.

1. AM. Posselt, CF. Barker, JF. Tomaszewski JF. Markmann, MA. Choti, A. Naji
   Induction of donor-specific unresponsiveness by intrathymic islet transplantation
   Science, 249,1293-1295, 1990.
2. M. Remuzzi, M. Rossini, O. Imberti, N. Perico : Kidney graft survival in rats without immuno-suppressants after intrathymic glomerular transplantation.
   Lancet 337, 30, 750-752, 1991.
3. DJ. Propper, J. Woo, AW. Thomson, GRD. Catto, AM. MacLeod,
   FK-506: its influence on anti-class I MHC alloantibody responses to blood transfusion.
   Transplantation, 50, 267-271, 1990.

Integration of human fetal xenografts in the adult rat brain: delayed vascularization and replacement of graft microglia by host microglia.

Christian Geny, Souad Naimi-Sadaoui, Abd el Madjid Belkabi,*Roland Jeny, £Sharon L. Juliano and Marc Peschanski, INSERM CJF 91-02, UFR de Médecine, 94010 Créteil cedex , France;*Hôpital Esquirol, Saint-Maurice, France £USUHS, Bethesda USA.

Transplantation of neural tissue from human fetuses is presently used as a therapeutics in patients with Parkinson's disease. Human neurons xenografted in the brain of adult immunosuppressed rats mature anatomically and functionally. This model can therefore be used to mimic the situation one expects to obtain in patients. Microglial cells are the principal antigen presenting cells of the brain. They play an important role in the rejection of xenografts. They act as immunostimulatory cells of T helper cells and enhance the killer activity of host T cells. Our study is devoted to the immunohistochemical analysis of the vascularization and the microglial cells of the host and the graft in a xenograft paradigm allowing clear distinction of the origin of the cells.

Spinal and brainstem neural tissue obtained from routine suction abortion was transplanted as a cell suspension into the thalamus of adult rat previously lesioned. Rats were sacrificed 3 to 12 weeks after transplantation. Histochemical and immunohistochemical techniques revealed neurons, endothelial cells, microglial cells and metabolic activity (cytochrome oxidase, glucose consumption with ^{14}C-2DG).

Human xenografts do not contain any blood vessel up to 1 month after transplantation, even though neural tissue in the foetus was clearly vascularized. Over the following two months, rare capillaries - develop in the peripheral and central portions of the transplant. At three months, the amount of blood vessels in the graft is lower than in the host rat brain This delayed vascularization is accompanied by an almost total lack of metabolic activity. One month after transplantation, the human microglial cells present in the graft have phenotypic features of ameboid microglia. The rat microglial cells have started to invade the graft. At three months, the number of human microglial cells is dramatically lower than that of rat microglial cells within the graft. There is neither signs of rejection nor T lymphocytes infiltration.

Our results indicate that human neural tissue remains in a quite abnormal state for several months after transplantation, as far as vascularization and metabolic activity are concerned, even though transplanted neurons survive and develop. The mechanisms underlying the restriction of vascularization are not known With regards to therapeutic transplantation, it will be of utmost importance to determine whether this situation benefits neural development.

Human microglial cells do not increase in number after transplantation and even are apparently progressively eliminated. Our data clearly demonstrate that presence of a large number of host microglial cells in the graft is not necessarily associated with rejection. This work suggests that the host microglia replaces the graft microglia leading to a chimera of xenogenic neuronal tissue with host microglia.

Supported by A.N.R.S. and Sandoz Labs.

SPLIT TOLERANCE IN CHIMERIC GVH MICE

C. BARON, V. BIERRE, G. ROSTOKER, B. WEIL, P. LANG *

The iv inoculation of parental spleen cells into adult F1 hybrid mice results in a GVH reaction. In the strain combination B10.D2->(B10.BRxB10.D2)F1 this reaction is associated with thymic injury and cellular immune deficiency. This study was performed to further elucidate the immune status of these mice 60 days after GVH induction .

Phenotypic studies of spleen cells performed by fac's analysis showed that these mice were repopulated with parental cells resulting in a high degree of chimerism (85%). In vitro functional studies showed that these mice were unresponsive against F1 cells in MLR but exhibit normal reactivity in MLR and CTL assays against third party allogeneic targets. NK activity was decreased. In vivo functional studies showed that chimeric cells did not induce GVH and using mixing experiments we did not detect any suppressor activity. The immune status of the chimeric state was further studied after lethal irradiation and bone marrow (BM) reconstitution .

Surprisingly F1 BM cells were unable to reconstitute these mice whereas D2 parental BM cells were fully effective, indicating a split tolerance. ^{125}IUdr assay confirmed that F1 clls were indeed rejected. Grafting a neonatal F1 thymus prevented the rejection of semiallogeneic cells but did not reconstitute T cells functions. In contrast after parental thymus grafting CTL activity was restored

In conclusion: the chimeric state induced by GVH reaction is associated with a split tolerance which can be circumvented by parental thymus grafting.

* Unité INSERM U 139 Service de Néphrologie Hôpital Henri Mondor CRETEIL .

Tolerance to host antigens in H-2-incompatible chimeric mice is maintained by non-deletional mechanisms and is dependent on the persistence of the tolerogen.

Abdelouahab AITOUCHE and Jean-Louis TOURAINE (Lyon).

Mechanisms of induction of transplantation tolerance are believed to be a complex of different processes acting differently but contributing together to maintain a state of non-responsiveness *in vivo* towards self antigens and other tolerogens. In chimeric mice, mechanisms underlying donor-to-host and host-to-donor tolerance may differ according to the way tolerance is achieved and regarding thymus function. We constructed [BALB/c→CBA, i.e.; H2d→H2k] allochimeras using lethally irradiated adult CBA (H2-k) mice reconstituted with BALB/c (H2-d) 14 day-fetal liver cells and thus became permanently tolerant to BALB/c skin allografts. Hæmatopoietic chimerism which ensues is entirely of the donor BALB/c origin. Newly supplied naive but not allo-sensitized host-type hæmatopoietic cells containing alloreactive T cell clones failed to break down the established tolerance in [BALB/c→CBA] chimeras pretreated or not with anti-mouse lymphocyte serum (ALS). At first sight this may suggest an active suppression of non-expanded alloreactive clones via suppressor cells or tolerance "infectious" cells. We then assessed whether the chronic presence of the CBA host tolerogens is essential for the maintenance of the established tolerance. We transferred [BALB/c→CBA] chimeric cells tolerant to the CBA host, without *in vitro* treatment, into lethally irradiated BALB/c mice (a murine environment free of the CBA antigens), then challenged the mice four weeks later with CBA test skin grafts. The BALB/c mice, reconstituted with bone marrow and spleen cells from [BALB/c→CBA] chimeras, rejected CBA allografts acutely in 10.0±1.4 days (n=8) while normal BALB/c controls rejected in 10.7±0.8 days (n=6). Our results show that [BALB/c→CBA] chimeric cells tolerant to their CBA host, once parked for one month in an environment free of the H-2k tolerogens fully recover their reactivity against CBA skin allografts (host-type antigens). This clearly shows that T cell clones reacting with the host CBA antigens were not deleted in the [BALB/c→CBA] chimeras. Clonal anergy therefore is responsible for the tolerance to CBA host antigens and CBA antigens appear to be required for the maintenance of this anergic state. The accelerated rejection of CBA skin allografts (second-set like response in 5/8 mice which rejected the graft in 9 days), as compared to control mice may suggest that expansion of BALB/c anti-CBA clones occurred during tolerance induction but that such clones were anergized before the expression of their anti-host effector phase.

Alive human HLA chimeras.

Gebuhrer L., Lambert J., Labonne M.P., Mollet I., Souillet G.*, Philippe N*.,,Touraine J.L°.,
Roncarolo M.G.°°., Betuel H.
Pediatrics Department. LYON.*; St ETIENNE **, Transplantation Unit. Hôpital E.
Herriot°., DNAX Institute, PALO ALTO, USA°°., Histocompatibility Laboratory. C.T.S.1-3
rue du Vercors. 69007. LYON. France.

Infants presenting a Severe Combined Immuno Deficiency (SCID), without HLA identical
sib can be successfully treated in utero and/or after birth by transplantation of foetal liver
and thymus cells originating from multiple donors. Identification of HLA antigens (ag.) of
the donor by serology and by DNA typing (PCR/ASO) allows the follow-up of graft take
at different periods. We present 6 cases of SCID who had normal expression of HLA ag.,
now 3 to 17 years old, alive, in whom coexist self HLA ag. and those of the donors. Two
situations were observed :
1°/ **Persistence of a weak T cell population of HLA Class I from the donors (1 case).**
a) Brus (born (b) 18.3.87) 6 grafts after birth from 4 to 12 months (m).

2°/ **Clear chimerism of HLA Class I, Class II ag. for T cells (5 cases).**
In all cases, HLA ag. of the donor(s) are present at the surface of T cells only, which also
bear HLA Class II genes. The recipient retains self HLA Class I, Class II ag.on B cells. The
proportion of T cells bearing HLA Class I from the donor is variable.

(i) *Coexistence of 20% HLA Class. I of the donor(s). 1 case*
b) Com (b. 16.2.77) 5 grafts after birth from 6 to 26 m.

(ii) *Progressive predominance of HLA Class I of the donor(s) 1 case.*
c) Hor (b.7.8.89) 1 graft in utero, 8 after birth. Appearance at day 20 of HLA Class I ag.
from the donor on peripheral T cells, representing at 3 years 80% of the T cell population.

(iii) *Exclusive presence of HLA Class of the donor. 2 cases.*
d) Samp. (b.2.10.76) 2 grafts after birth at 1 and 4 m. Presently the four Class I ag. from the
2 donors are detectable on peripheral T cells (80% and 20% respectively). The two DRB1
genes of the 2 donors and of the recipient are identified. He has thus 6 different DRB1
alleles.

e) Val. (b.30.5.86) 7 grafts after birth from 12 to 18 months. At 24 m. , exclusive presence of
Class I ag. from the donor on T cells, HLA Class I genes are also detected. The B
lymphocytes carry self ag. and genes of Class I and Class II.

These observations demonstrate that in spite of total disparity between T cells of the
donor and B cells of the recipient, a state of tolerance develops without
immunosuppression. Furthermore immunological defence against common pathogens
exists, since these children lead a normal life.

INFLUENCE OF POSTTRANSPLANTATION BLOOD TRANSFUSION ON KIDNEY ALLOGRAFT SURVIVAL : A SINGLE CENTER DOUBLE-BLIND PROSPECTIVE RANDOMIZED STUDY COMPARING CRYOPRESERVED (CRBC) AND FRESH RED BLOOD CELL CONCENTRATES (FRBC)

P. LANG, P. BIERLING, C. BUISSON, G. FRUCHAUD, M. BUSSON, C. BARON,
D. BELGHITI, T. SEROR, D. DAHMANE, F. BEAUJAN, A. BENMAADI, D. CHOPIN,
C. ABBOU; B. BOURGEON, G. ROSTOKER, P. REMY, B. WEIL.

It has been reported that posttransplantation infusion of donor specific bone-marrow improved human cadaveric kidney allograft survival. Considering the beneficial effect of pre-transplantation blood transfusion and the logistic difficulties of specific bone-marrow collection, we investigated whether random FRBC could also mediate a tolerogenic effect. In order to exclude any bias in the management of the patients, we performed a double blind prospective randomized study comparing CRBC (deleucocyted) with FRBC (non deleucocyted) in 100 consecutive non immunized cadaveric renal transplant recipients. All these patients had received at least 3 random FRBC before transplantation. Posttransplantation protocol consisted in transfusion of 3 RBC on day 8, 14, and 21. In case of additional blood requirement, the RBC were chosen according to the initial randomization. Patients with either technical failures (n=8) before day 8, or who had received additional transfusions not corresponding to the randomization (n=2) were excluded from the study. Both groups were well-matched for age, sex, ischemic times, number of HLA compatibilities and for the therapeutic regimen which included anti-lymphocyte globulin for the first two weeks.

RESULTS	CRYOPRESERVED RBC n = 43	FRESH RBC n = 47	
1 year patient survival	93 %	100%	NS
1 year graft survival	84 %	96 %	$p < 0.05$
No of rejection / patient	0.85	0.78	NS
% of patients with rejection	60	55	NS
1 year serum creatinine (µmol/l)	154.6 ± 55	146.2 ± 41	NS
% of patients with PRA	15	25	NS
% of CMV infection	56	49	NS

No case of HBS, HCV or HIV infection was noted.

Conclusion : Posttransplant FRBC may improve kidney allograft survival, however the non negligible risk of sensitization must be taken into account whenever blood transfusions are required in kidney transplant patients.

Service de Néphrologie – C.D.T.S.
Hôpital Henri Mondor – 94. CRETEIL

UNUSUAL CD8+ T CELLS LYMPHOCYTOSIS IN STABLE TRANSPLANT RECIPIENTS

J.J. LLOVERAS, J. TKACZUK, D. DURAND, L. ROSTAING, N. MAILLARD, M.H. CHABANNIER, M. ABBAL, E. OHAYON, J.M. SUC, A. MODESTO-SEGONDS
Toulouse - France

We report an unusual feature of CD8+ T Cells increase in peripheral blood occurred in 4 transplant recipients, without malignancy, active viral infection, or rejection.

Since 1988, the different peripheral blood lymphocyte subsets are systematically studied in the transplant recipients during the post-operative period if an infectious (viral or bacterial) or a rejection episode is suspected, then yearly. Three color flow-cytometric analysis was used to determine proportions of CD2+, CD3+, CD4+, CD8+ T cells, and among these later, the cells expressing the phenotypes CD45 RA, CD45 RO and/or HLA DR. Absolute counts of these cells are calculated thereafter. Four patients exhibited a sharp lymphocytosis, persistent at least five years after transplantation, with uneventful evolution.

	Pt 1	Pt 2	Pt 3	Pt 4
Sex/Age	M/28	M/37	F/48	M/37
Transplant/Year	Kidney/87	Kidney/87	Kidney /85	Liver/87
Treatment	CsA-Aza-MP	CsA-Aza-MP	CsA-MP	CsA-MP
Time of lymphocytosis	2 months	11 months	2 months	2 months
Course post-transplantation	- CMV not treated - Chronic hepatitis (HBV, HCV)	- CMV not treated	-	- CMV disease (lung, liver), treated - Recurrence at one year - Chronic HCV hepatitis
Immunofixation	Ig ↑	Monoclonal	Normal	Ig ↑
Other events	Splenectomy	-	Splenectomy	Splenectomy
CD2+	4665 ± 755	4150 ± 1087	2987 ± 459	4035 ± 361
CD3+	4562 ± 737	4040 ± 1030	2561 ± 246	3918 ± 315
CD4+	1456 ± 296	1118 ± 264	1021 ± 70	1608 ± 195
CD8+	3061 ± 485	1974 ± 401	1531 ± 175	2423 ± 101
% CD8 (CD45 RA+)	49 ± 7	92 ± 2	63 ± 0	73 ± 1
% CD8 (CD45 RO+)	79 ± 7	23 ± 3	56 ± 5	30 ± 15
% CD8 (DR+)	36 ± 7	33 ± 1	30 ± 4	12 ± 3
CD 19+	329 ± 159	42 ± 11	248 ± 5	325 ± 104

Values are mean ± SD of the different counts obtained at least five years after the transplantation.

Three patients (1,2,3) underwent regular myelograms and osteomedullar biopsies disclosing a tumoral proliferation. Of note, a splenectomy was performed in three cases before (pts 1,3) or during (pt 4) the transplantation. In all the cases, the CD4+ T Cells were slightly increased, while the total CD8+ T Cells count was much more larger than the observed value in a control group of 7 patients ; these kidney transplant recipients (mean age = 43 ± 9 ; 4 M ; 3 F), did not exhibit rejection episode, clinical CMV infection or hepatitis during their course and had a normal renal function (112 ± 12 µmol/l) 4 to 5 years after the transplantation, when peripheral blood lymphocyte subsets were studied : CD4+ : 678 +/- 258/mm3 ; CD8+ : 360 +/- 210/mm3 ; CD19+ : 97 +/- 33/mm3.

The CD8+ T Cells, or "suppressive-cytotoxic" T Cells may share the CD45 determinant under two different isoforms : RA ("naïve cells") or RO ("memory primed cells"). This late form has been predominantly found in kidney transplants during acute rejection or in subendothelial space of heart transplant arteries during coronary artery disease. This led to the hypothesis of a cytotoxic activity supported by these cells. However in two patients (1,3) most of the CD8+ T Cells were RO+ and in each case, the absolute count of this subset was increased, without adverse event.

In conclusion, we report 4 cases of a steady peripheral blood CD8+ T Cells lymphocytosis in transplant recipients with stable graft function, without infection or malignancy. Its significance is not clear but could suggest, under particular conditions, the presence of the isoform CD45 RO+, among CD8+ cells, CD45 RO+ without cytotoxic activity.

INFLUENCE OF HLA MATCHING ON THE OUTCOME OF KIDNEY TRANSPLANTS: SIX YEARS EXPERIENCE OF RENAL TRANSPLANTATION; DATA OF 107 CASES

Immunology : R. Bardi , KH. Ayed.
Nephrology : T. Ben Abdallah , A. El Matri , H. Ben Maïz ,
Urology : M. Chebil , M. El Ouakdi , M. Ayed
Charle Nicolles Hospital ; Tunis - Tunisia .

The beneficial effect of optimal HLA matching on the outcome of renal transplantation is still mater in debate . Different results have been reported . For many centers the best 5 years graft and patient survival was obtained in recipients who received a graft without HLA A , B and DR missmatches and who were treated with cyclosporin .The importance of HLA matching observed in large multicenter studies , apparently does not apply to individual units , but HLA matching appears very important for highly sensitized patients .

The aim of our study is to calculate patient and graft survival according to the number of missmatches on the HLA A , B and DR locus .

Renal transplant therapy was introduced in Tunisia At Charle Nicolles Hospital In June 1986 . 107 kidney transplantations have been performed between June 1986 and December 1992 . Only those kidneys with a follow up of at least three years have been taken into account for analysis of HLA typing in this study . Among 107 patients 75 were men and 32 were women . All patients were first transplants (only 2 second transplants) . An overall of 26 % had cytotoxic antibodies (Pretransplant Panel Antibodies) : 10% had antibodies > 30% and 16% had PRA < 30% of reactivity with T cells . The basis of immunosuppressions was a standard triple drug therapy . HLA typing was performed using a classical microlymphocytotoxicity technique . Our minimal immunologic recquirement were pairs HLA haplo-identical or HLA identical (for living related donor) and negative cross matches with current and historical sera . All patients received non specific blood transfusion .

Comparing the results of 0 , 1 and 2 mismatchs in HLA A locus there is no statistical significant difference on graft survival . The same was true for HLA B locus . Only in the HLA DR locus there is a statistical difference between zero and one missmatch . Patients with 0 missmatch in DR locus had best graft survival and less graft rejection than the other groups.

RELEVANCE OF FLOW CYTOMETRY CROSS MATCH
TO RENAL TRANSPLANTATION

V. FOURNIER, B. HORY, E. LEGRAND, C. BRESSON-VAUTRIN,
D. SALARD, E. RACADOT, Y. SAINT-HILLIER
Service de Néphrologie Transplantation renale
CHU 2, place Saint Jacques 25000 BESANCON FRANCE

A positive flow cytometry cross match (FCCM) has been reported to correlate with inferior graft outcome and a greater incidence of rejection episode. We studied 172 recipients of renal allografts to determine the impact of a positive FCCM on immediate and one year outcome.

METHODS

All patients were tested with an immunomagnetic cross match (IM CM) : lymphocytotoxicity assay on antibody coated microspheres (T and B cross match)(DYNEABEADS DYNAL AS NORWAY) . Detection of IgM (DTT) and auto-cross match were performed in case of positive IMCM.

172 recipients were transplanted on the basis of a negative IM T cell cross-match. FCCM was performed using a dual color flow cytometric binding assay. A positive FCCM was determined by a fluorescence increase of 20 %. Antibodies detected were IgG reacting with T or B cells.

RESULTS

151 patients were negative using IMCM and FCCM (gr I), 14 had positive B cell IMCM and 2 of them had also T cell positive FCCM (gr II), 7 others patients had only positive FCCM, 4 with T cells and 3 with B cells (gr III).

1) <u>Graft survival</u> : At one year, patient survival of group I and group II was not different (96 % gr I, 86 % gr II) but patients of group III had a worse prognosis(71 % gr III) (p < 0.001). At one year, graft survival of the 3 groups was not different (90 % gr I, 83 % gr II and 70 % gr III)(NS). However the percentage of patients without rejection was 55 % in gr I, 43 % in gr II and 14 % in gr III (p < 0.02).
2) <u>Kidney function</u> : At 3 months, mean creatininemia of gr II was significantly higher than creatinemia of gr I (205 ± 154 versus 151 ± 68) (p < 0.05). Creatinemia of gr I and gr III were not different (151± 68 versus 197 ± 62) but 2 of the 7 recipients of this group lost their graft during the first month.

CONCLUSION

We confirm that low complement fixing antibodies giving a negative reaction in the cytotoxic assay are associated with immunological complication. Detection of non complement fixing HLA reactive IgG antibodies using FCCM could lead to a reduced frequency of early acute rejection and inversible graft losses.

PART : B

FOLLOW-UP OF TRANSPLANT PATIENTS

AND IMMUNOLOGICAL MONITORING

Two patterns of cytokines secretion by graft infiltrating T cells (GIC) in human renal allograft rejection

C LAMBERT, P MERVILLE*, C POUTEIL-NOBLE#, JL TOURAINE#, F BERTHOUX, J BANCHEREAU*

dpt Nephrology, CHU St Etienne, #dpt Transplantation CHU E Herriot, Lyon, *Lab Immunology research Schering Plough, Dardilly, France

In a previous study, we have shown, by ELISPOT method, that GIC (mainly composed of granulomatous CD14 + and T cells CD3+) secrete high amounts of γIFN and Il10. Using the same approch, we analyzed the ability of FACS-sorted CD3+CD4+ and CD3+CD4- cells to secrete these cytokines and their regulation by Il4, Il10 and γIFN.

CD3+ CD4+ cells represented from 4 to 22% and CD3+CD4- from 12 to 65% of GIC. Following stimulation by solid phase anti-CD3, two patterns of cytokines secretion could be identified among 4 rejected kidneys tested. In two kidneys, (group I), we observed a high frequency of Il-10 secreting cells in both CD4+ (mean 1.4%) and CD4- (mean 0.8%) while the other two kidneys, (group II), had less Il-10 secreting cells (CD4+: 0.16%, CD4-: 0.17%). Interestingly, the frequency of γIFN producing cells in group I (CD4+: 1.3%, CD4-: 0.8%) was lower than that in group II (CD4+: 4.6%, CD4-: 7,1%).

Il4 strongly decreased the frequency of γIFN secreting CD4+ in group II (from 4.6 to 0.25%) but not in group I (from 1.3% to 1.5%). In contrast, Il4 weakly affected the frequency of γIFN secreting cells of the CD3+CD4- compartment. `

This observation illustrates a balance between γIFN and Il10 with distinct pathways of regulation within Graft infiltrating T cells subpopulations.

Natural soluble TNF antagonists in End Stage Renal Failure (ESRF) and early events in renal transplantation (RTP)

Lambert C, Jurine J, Vindimian M, Berthoux P, Berthoux F.
Nephrology, Dialysis and Transplantation,
CHRU 42055 St ETIENNE, Cedex2, FRANCE

TNF is clearly involved in rejection. It induces the release of soluble part of its receptors (sTNFr p75 and p55) which can antagonize its effects. We analyzed the kinetics of both sTNFrs in renal recovery after RTP.

Methods: sTNFr and sIl2r were measured by ELISA and TNF by RIA. Serial analysis (3 times a week) were performed 53 RTP patients.

Results:

Both cytokines receptors were high in ESRF:

- sTNFr p75: **52,9** ± 28 ng/ml, N: 5.5 ± 2.0,
- sTNFr p55: **57,3** $\pm 35,6$ng/ml, N: 2.8 ± 0.5)
- TNF 23 ± 14 ng/ml, N<15 and
- sIL2r 159 ± 100 nmol/ml, N:70 ± 45.

Following RTP, all values decreased progressively (p<0,0001) reaching normal ranges by one month. sTNFr55 (MW below glomerular sieving coefficient) decreased more rapidly. sTNFr p55 (which molecular weight is below the glomerular sieving point) decreased more rapidly. Both sTNFrs levels were correlated together (p<0,0007, r2 = 0,92) but never with the TNF levels.

Just before transplantation, sTNFr levels were not correlated to Serum Creatinin but the relation appeared when the graft started to function: p55 from day 8, p<0.01, r2 = 0,71), p75 from day 15. Then p55 were also correlated to sIL2r (p<0,004, r2=0,77). Levels did not raised significantly in cellular acute rejection. Anti-lymphocyte serum treatment induced sTNFr rise(p<0,001) as well as TNF and sIl2r.

Conclusion: sTNFr were very high in renal failure. Levels decreased progressively with renal function recovery. Because of the high accumulation in due to renal failure, no significant changes could be observed in early rejections events. No protective effect on rejection risk or gravity could be demonstrated.

HILDA/LIF secretion during infections in kidney transplant recipients

D.Morel, J.L. Taupin, E.Leguen, L.Potaux, N.Gualde, J.F.Moreau

Hôpital Pellegrin and URA CNRS 1456 33076 BORDEAUX FRANCE

The cytokine HILDA/LIF exerts a wide array of biological activities, some of them intricated with inflammatory phenomenons.It is secreted by activated monocytes, as well as T lymphocytes. It binds specifically with high affinity receptors on monocytes and macrophages surface. Besides, HILDA/LIF triggers the synthesis and release of acute phase proteins by hepatocytes HILDA/LIF urinary excretion is already known to increase during kidney tranplant rejection, blood levels remaining most of the time under the detection limits of a bio-assay.

Using the more sensible technique ELISA, we monitored HILDA/LIF urinary and blood levels in 23 kidney and 1 kidney and pancreas transplant recipients weekly then monthly during the first year post transplant. This sandwich ELISA combined two monoclonal antibodies recognizing two different epitopes on the soluble molecule, obtained in our laboratory. The threshold of detection is then arround 80 pg/ml.

In kidney transplants recipients without concomitant pathology, HILDA/LIF was usualy below 80 pg/ml in blood, urinary excretion being less than 300 ng/24h.

We report here on the correlation between the cytokine levels and isolated infectious episodes. The results are summarized as follows:

EVENTS	PATIENTS total number	PATIENTS + increased LIF in urines ng/24 h	PATIENTS + increased LIF in blood pg/ml	PATIENTS + no increase of LIF (blood or urin)
Urinary tract infections	n=8	n= 6 m=2498 (300-11115)	n=3 m=629 (322-980)	n=1
bronchitis	n=9	n=6 m=820 (178-1250)	n=4 m=287 (155-484)	n=1
CMV	n=6	n=6 m=2904 (500-6269)	n=3 m=219 (140-264)	n=0
orchi epidydimitis	n=2	n=1 2000	n=2 350-1000	n=0
wound suppuration	n=2	n=2 1423-2993	n=1 340	n=0
viral gastro enteritis	n=1	n=1 2522	n=1 426	n=0
esophageal candidiasis	n=3	n=2 368-600	n=0	n=1

HILDA/LIFurinary and blood levels decreased with the healing of the infection. Taken together, these data indicate a strong correlation between the development of infectious deseases and HILDA/LIF secretion. It therefore emphazises the involvment of these cytokine in clinical inflammation, even in immunocompromised patients.

Cellular immune responses in cyclosporine-treated patients followed repeatedly more than three years after heart transplantation.

S. VITSE*, F. PINATEL*, F. POITEVIN-LATER*, P. BOISSONNAT**, G. DUREAU**, J. NINET**, F. TOURAINE**.

* Laboratoire d'Immunologie - Hôpital Neurologique - ** Hôpital Cardiologique - BP 69394 Lyon Cedex 03.

Objective

The study was aimed at evaluating the level of immunosuppression in heart transplant patients, in view of treatment monitoring and complication prevention.

Materials and methods

100 heart transplant patients with various immunosuppressive therapies, grafted for more than 3 years, were investigated.
Three times, over six months, a blood sample was taken in order to evaluate both the plasmatic cyclosporinemia (PC) and the in vitro immunological state (lymphocyte count (LC), CD4+ and CD8+ lymphocyte absolute number, proliferative respons to mitogens : concanavalin A (ConA), phytohemagglutinin (PHA)).

Results

In eight of the 100 patients, a perfectly constant treatment was given throughout the study. The results in these 8 patients are shown in the table where it can be seen that the analyzed immunological parameters did not vary in correlation with cyclosporine levels, within the usual therapeutic levels.

Patients	PC µg/l	LC /mm3	CD4+ /mm3	CD8+ /mm3	ConA + PHA (dpm)
N° 1	138/121/90*	970/960/720	170/220/170	580/480/370	184400/182190/327470
N° 2	195/145/50	930/980/600	560/570/280	260/260/200	792792/846550/373040
N° 3	178/160/176	470/600/540	280/290/280	100/160/110	582832/205940/305650
N° 4	40/54/50	760/910/790	430/400/350	220/280/280	444720/440320/225540
N° 5	136/155/461	2860/2240/1850	1060/560/610	1490/1160/830	239650/221000/221550
N° 6	144/155/157	1520/1570/2040	670/660/980	630/680/880	315730/176050/541050
N° 7	173/166/196	1450/1300/1660	610/560/680	580/520/750	259420/367450/127570
N° 8	102/293/259	1710/1750/2310	380/510/440	870/680/1250	368490/573620/452520

*The 3 values correspond to the three assays carried out during the 6 month period.
Patients 1 to 4 : Azathioprine100 mg/day and Methylprednisolone 10 mg/day.
Patients 5 to 8 : Azathioprine 0 mg/day and Methylprednisolone 5 mg/day.

Conclusion

Variations of mitogenic responses or lymphocyte subsets depend on other factors more influent than cyclosporine dosage in heart transplant patients after more than three years. These results lead us to evaluate more precisely correlation between immune state and clinical complications.

Are CD4+ and CD8+ lymphocyte numbers or mitogen lymphocyte responses correlated to cyclosporine levels in heart transplant patients?

F. POITEVIN-LATER*, F. PINATEL*, C. MALCUS*, S. VITSE*, P. BOISSONNAT**, G. DUREAU**, J. NINET**, F. TOURAINE*.

* Laboratoire d'Immunologie - Hôpital Neurologique - ** Hôpital Cardiologique - BP 69394 Lyon Cedex 03.

Objective

This study was intended to determine whether transplant patients with different cyclosporinemia levels, in the long - term, had different immunological parameters in peripheral blood.

Materials and methods

100 heart transplant patients with various immunosuppressive therapies, grafted for more than 3 years, were investigated. They had immunological tests 3 times in a period of 6 months.
15 of these 100 patients were selected on the basis of low methylprednisolone therapy (5 mg/day) and absence of azathioprine. Cyclosporine was given to all patients, at different dosages. Plasmatic cyclosporinemia (PC), CD4+, CD8+ lymphocyte numbers (LC), proliferative responses to mitogens (ConA, PHA, PWM) were determined on peripheral blood. Two groups of patients, selected on the PC level were compared : 7 patients with PC < 170 µg/l, 8 patients with PC > 200 µg/l. The statistical non parametric Mann Whitney test was used for the comparison.

Results

No statistically significant difference was found between the two groups concerning the peripheral blood lymphocyte count, CD4+, CD8+ absolute number and responses to mitogens. The results are shown in the table :

	PC < 170 µg/l			PC > 200 µg/l	
	m	σ		m	σ
PC µg/l	133	39	p < 0,01	295	91
LC/mm^3	1066	243	NS	1462	730
CD4+/mm^3	382	153	NS	480	255
CD8+/mm^3	411	142	NS	595	409
ConA dpm	120317	43884	NS	130244	94680
PHA dpm	196675	87222	NS	135757	78394
PWM dpm	38781	12031	NS	37970	25314

Conclusion

In the therapeutic conditions of our heart transplant patients, relatively higher levels of cyclosporinemia certainly did not result in more profound lymphopenia, imbalance of T-cell subsets or decreased lymphoproliferative responses. Because of lack of correlation between these various parameters and since no single test is indicative of the immune status of the patient, immunological monitoring must rely on several tests.

FOLLOW-UP OF ALVEOLAR MACROPHAGE CYTOKINE PRODUCTION IN LUNG TRANSPLANT RECIPIENTS.

A. Magnan, M. Reynaud, L. Garbe, B. Meric, L. Viard, M. Badier, P. Thomas, B. Kreitman, R. Giudicelli, M. Noirclerc, A. Arnaud, P. Fuentes, J-L Mege.

Service de Pneumologie, CHU Nord, Marseille.
Laboratoire d'Immunologie, CHU Ste Marguerite, Marseille, France.
Groupe de Transplantations Pulmonaires, Marseille, France.

Alveolar Macrophages (AM) are believed to be involved in complications of lung transplantation such as acute rejection (AR), Cytomegalovirus Pneumonia (CMVP), and Obliterative Bronchiolitis (OB). IL-6, a pro-inflammatory cytokine, is increased in broncho-alveolar lavages (BAL) during CMVP and AR. To show that this over-secretion is the reflect of AM activation, and to study the evolution of this secretion after treatment, IL-6 and TNF-α were assayed in 147 supernatants of 24 hours-cultured AM (10^6 cells / ml of medium), obtained by BAL from 29 lung transplant recipients. IL-6 and TNF-α secretion was analysed in a radio-immunometric assay. Four groups were considered: AR (n=21), CMVP (n=12), BO (n=15), and controls (n=70). In 15 and 7 cases respectively, AM IL-6 and TNF-α production was assayed 15 and 30 days after the onset of AR. In 7 cases, this secretion was analysed 30 days after CMVP occured. Results are expressed as mean$\pm$ SEM (pg/ml).

AM TNF-α and IL-6 amounts were strongly correlated (y= 1,38 x +501,62, R2= 0,84, p<0,0001). AM TNF-α and IL-6 secretion was increased during acute rejection (3709$\pm$1409 , and 5482$\pm$2058, respectively,) versus controls (777$\pm$280, and 1055$\pm$311, respectively, p<0,005), and returned to control values within 15 days. This statistical difference was still observed during CMVP (5000$\pm$2773, and 12280$\pm$3939 respectively). AM Il-6 and TNF-α levels 30 days later were not different from controls . There was no statistical difference between levels of AM cytokine secreted by patients displaying BO and controls.

The strong correlation between IL-6 and TNF-α values suggest that the method used in this work, independent of BAL cell concentration and dilution, and specific for AM, is suitable for monitoring AM activation.

We undoubtebly show that AM are at least in part responsible for the increase of cytokine amounts in BAL during AR and CMVP. Furthermore, we show that treatment reverses this AM activation. Although there is no over-activation of AM during OB, mediators expressed during AR and CMVP favorise fibrotic processes and then may be involved in OB pathogenesis. Thus, these results plead for active treatment of lung graft complications.

LUNG TRANSPLANTATION FOR MAJOR EMPHYSEMA : 14 CASES

J.P. GAMONDES, M. BERTOCCHI, F. THEVENET, P. BRUN, O. BASTIEN, T. WIESENDANGER, T. GREENLAND, P. ADELEINE, M. CHUZEL, J.F. MORNEX , J. BRUNE.

HOPITAL LOUIS PRADEL - BP LYON MONTCHAT - 69394 LYON CEDEX 03 - FRANCE

Between March 89 and March 93 we performed 43 lung transplants of which 14 were for major emphysema (9 single lung : group I, and 5 double : group II). Patients were 11 men and 3 women with a mean age of 49 ± 7 yrs and were similarly distributed between the 2 groups. All patients were symptomatic at NYHA class III or IV, and 4 had abnormal @1 Anti-Trypsin. Right ventricular failure had occured at least once in 6 patients, and 9 had alveolar ventilatory insufficency necessitating oxygenotherapy. Mean right ventricular ejection fraction was 36 %. Operations were performed with cardio-pulmonary bypass in 5 cases (3 single lung and 2 double lung). Early death occured in 2 single transplanted patients (14 %) and 3 late deaths (2 single lung, 1 double lung) have occured (21 %) within a mean follow up time of 18 months, although bronchial stenosis and dyskinesia are present in one single lung and two double lung recipients : 5 COOK stents were used and two patients recieve a substitutive treatment with @1 Anti-Tryspin. The 9 survivors are presently well with a good quality of life. Functional and haemodynamic results of the survivors are presented. Significantly better results after double lung tranplants were obtained for FEV1/VC and cardiac output at excercise.

TABLE : LUNG FUNCTION AND PULMONARY HAEMODYNAMICS IN 9 LONG TERM TRANSPLANT RECIPIENTS

	Pre-op	Post-op		p Value
	n = 14	Group I	Group II	between Gr I and Gr II
		n = 5	n = 4	
FEV1/CV (%)	27±7	49±9	76±17	0.012*
DLCO/VA (% predicted)	37±17	91±12	103±15	0.56
PaO2 rest (kPa)	7±1.5	8.5±1.3	105±0.5	0.13
PaO2 excercise (kPa)	7.4±1.3	10±2	11±2	0.68
Cardiac ouptut rest (l.m-1)	4.3±1	4.3±2	6.7±1.5	0.14
Cardiac ouptut excercise (l.m-1)	6.2±1.7	7.8±1.8	10.8±0.1	0.04*
MPAP rest (mmHg)	28±16	21±8	22±3	0.82
MPAP excercise (mmHg)	44±9	41±16	43±16	0.89

* significant at 5 % confidence

FEV1/VC : Tiffeneau coefficient ; DLCO : diffusing capacity of carbon monoxide ; PaO2 : arterial oxygen tension
MPAP : mean pulmonary artery pressure.

RETROSPECTIVE STUDY OF TRANSBRONCHIAL LUNG BIOPSIES IN HEART LUNG AND LUNG TRANSPLANTATIONS.

N. Roux, Mornex JF, Loire R, Tabib A, Bertocchi M, Brune J. Hôpital Louis Pradel, Lyon, France.

Thirty nine lung transplant recipients (27 men, 12 women, mean age 38.3 years) were monitored by transbronchial lung biopsy. They included 15 heart lung, 18 simple lung and 6 double lung transplantation performed between 12/88 and 1/93. Indications for transplantation included : pulmonary vascular disease (11), emphysema (11), cystic fibrosis (5), histiocytosis X (3), pulmonary fibrosis (5) and others (4). The mean follow up was 21.11 month. Transbronchial lung biopsies were performed during a fiberoptic bronchoscopy either on a routine basis (every 2 month during the first year) or whenever dyspnea, fever, opacities on chest X ray, hypoxemia, decreased FEV1 occured. One thousand and ten specimen biopsies were retrospectivelly reassessed using the standard "working formulation". A total number of 428 biopsies were performed (i.e a mean of 10 biopsies/patient), of those 391 contained enough lung material to be used for diagnosis. The mean number of specimens was 2.5/biopsy. Among these 391 biopsies, 111 showed perivascular infiltrates consistent with the diagnosis of acute rejection : grade I in 97, grade II in 13, and grade III in 1. Additional features were observed. CMV pneumonitis was diagnosed in 10 instances based on typical cytopathic effect, furthermore a viral cytopathic effect occured repeatedly in 4 patients. Intra alveolar and intra bronchiolar buds (with a typical aspect of bronchiolitis obliterans organizing pneumonia) were observed in 19 patients. They occured either early during the first month in 6 instances or later in 14. Pure obliterative bronchiolitis was observed in 5 patients with a mean post transplant time of 4.6 month. Finally, acute bronchitis with lymphocyte and neutrophil infiltrate occured repeatedly in 10 patients, often at the same time as perivascular infiltrates.

In conclusion, transbronchial lung biopsy enables to make the diagnosis of acute rejection on the basis of perivascular infiltrate, it can disclose viral pneumonitis. Obliterative bronchiolitis (the major long term complication of lung transplantation) can not be appreciated by the method.

Long term evolution of erythropoietin after successfull renal transplantation

A. Hadj-Aïssa, P. Morel, C. Pouteil-Noble, J.L. Touraine, and N. Pozet, Lyon, France.

Earlier studies have shown that successful renal transplantation leads to normalization of erythropoietin (EPO) concentration and anemia. A first peak of EPO appears within the first three days after transplantation. This peak seems to be independent of graft function. A second peak occurs one month later and is associated with graft recovery and resolution of anemia. The EPO production by the grafted kidneys tends to decline again once anemia ameliorates, indicating an intact regulation of erythropoiesis. These studies were performed up to three months following transplantation, and the respective longterm evolution of EPO levels and graft function has not been clearly defined. Morever graft function is usually assessed by serum creatinine which is known not to be the most accurate index of renal function.

Patients and method. We measured plasma EPO levels (Enzyme Immuno-Assay), GFR (inulin clearance) and hematocrit (Ht) at month 1, 3, 6, and 12 after successful renal transplantation. Thirty four patients with stable graft function between the 1st and the 12th month after renal transplantation were enrolled. All patients were cadaveric kidney graft recipients and received conventional immunosuppressive treatment with ciclosporin, azathioprine and prednisolone.

Results. GFR remained unaltered during the 12 months observation period according to the criteria of selection (55 ± 3, 60 ± 3, 61 ± 3 and 57 ± 3 ml/min/1.73 m2 at month 1, 3, 6, and 12 after transplantation). However EPO decreased between the 1st and the 3rd month, and remained stable thereafter above normal values (3.7-15.1 mU/ml). Ht shows an opposite evolution, but reached normal values from the 3rd month. There was no correlation between EPO and GFR or Ht.

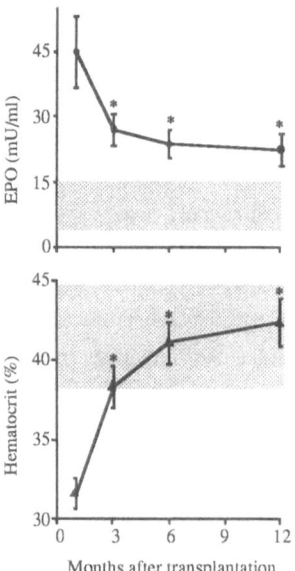

Conclusion. These data show that, unlike other published results, the improvement of the erythropoietic response to EPO, which occurs between the 1st and the 3rd month after successfull renal transplantation, does not depend on a further recovery of renal function. Moreover, while GFR remained stable during one year after transplantation, EPO concentrations plateaued from the 3rd month without reaching normal values. This later result suggests that, in contrast to patients with chronic renal failure and similarly decreased GFR, grafted kidneys are able to produce EPO and that a higher level of EPO is needed to achieve normal erythropoiesis.

Renal function in patients with hemoglobinopathy before and after bone-marrow allograft.

A. Hadj-Aïssa [1], C. Wright [2], P. Cochat [2], G. Souillet [3], L. David [2], N. Philippe [3], N. Pozet [1]

[1] Exploration Fonctionnelle Rénale, [2] Néphrologie Pédiatrique and [3] Hématologie Pédiatrique
Lyon, France.

Seventeen children and young adults (10 femals), aged 1.8 to 21.4 yrs (11.8 ± 5.4), with sickle cell anemia (SC, n=10) or homozygous thalassemia (Th, n=7) underwent measurement of GFR (inulin clearance), renal plasma flow (RPF : PAH clearance), creatinine clearance and urinary osmolality (UOsm, after overnight fasting). Results were as follows (mean ± SEM)

	SC	Th	p
GFR (ml/min/1.73m^2)	163 ± 8	157 ± 14	ns
RPF (ml/min/1.73m^2)	953 ± 78	874 ± 77	ns
Ccr (ml/min/1.73m^2)	158 ± 11	145 ± 7	ns
UOsm (mOsm/kg)	439 ± 9	722 ± 84	< 0.05

Renal function evaluation was performed in 6 of these patients before and 1 year after bone-marrow allograft (BMG)

	Before BMG	After BMG	p
GFR(ml/min/1.73m^2)	149 ± 22	116 ± 28	< 0.05
RPF (ml/min/1.73m^2)	792 ± 128	620 ± 175	< 0.05
Filtration Fraction	0.19 ± 0,04	0.19 ± 0,03	ns
Ccr (ml/min/1.73m^2)	143 ± 16	110 ± 24	< 0.05
Pcr (µmol/l)	36 ± 8	49 ± 13	< 0.05

Conclusion : i) Patients with hemoglobinopathy showed an increase in renal hemodynamics probably due to the increase in cardiac output secondary to the anemia. ii) There was a defect in urinary concentration capacity in patients with SC. This could be in relation with renal medullary tissue alterations. ii) Renal function returned to normal level after BMG which corrects anemia, but associated treatments, in particular ciclosporine, may also account for these modifications.

NON PRIMARY FUNCTION OF RENAL GRAFT : RELAPSE OF HEMOLYTIC - UREMIC SYNDROME OR ACUTE REJECTION ?

CAVALIER - ARRIEU A., FISCHBACH M., URLACHER A., DESPREZ PH., TONGIO A.M., WOLFF PH., GEISERT J.
Unité de Néphrologie Dialyse Transplantation pour enfants.
HOPITAUX UNIVERSITAIRES DE STRASBOURG.

F.B. ten-year-old is admitted in the departement with acute abdominal pain, without diarrhoea but with subicterus. No cutaneous, articular or visceral lesions are noted. The blood pressure is 170/100 mmHg. Several convulsions occur. Laboratory data reveal intra-vascular extra-corpuscular acute regenerative hemolytic anemia (schizocytes+++), with thrombocytopenia (86000/mm3) and oligo-anuric acute renal failure (gross hematuria and proteinuria). No verotoxin secreting bacteria are found in stool. No inflammatory state is noted, no anti-neutrophil cytoplasm antibodies, anti-DNA antibodies nor disorder of complement system are found in blood. Renal biopsy shows arteriolar predominant microangiopathy . Hemolytic-uremic syndrome is diagnosed. Peritoneal dialysis is started, relayed later by hemodialysis.
A first renal transplantation is undergone in june 1990. Donor and recipient share one HLA antigen at each A,B,DR and DQ locus. The cross-Match is negative. Because of a reversible cardiac arrest (hyperkaliemia) during the operation, the removal of the bad vascularized graft is necessary after less than 30mn. Later, IgM anti HLA-class I (A3+B40) and IgG anti HLA-class II antibodies (DQ1) are detected, reacting specifically against the non shared antigens.
A second renal transplantation is undergone in august 1992; donor and recipient are identical for their HLA-class II antigens. A positive IgM B cross-match does not contra-indicate the transplantation. The graft is well-tolerated (no fever, no pain, no purpura) but immediately non functional (anuria). Laboratory data do not reveal hemolytic anemia, nor thrombopenia, nor schizocytosis. Histological study of second graft shows inflammatory infiltration and significant arteriolar obstruction caused by acute necrotizing aeteriolitis, compatible with thrombotic microangiopathy or vascular rejection. Ten days after surgery, the patient develops an anti-HLA broad hyperimmunisation due to IgM antibodies which persists until transplantectomy.
After that, only IgM antibodies of primo-immunisation against the first graft are found steadily, without any marks of immunisation against the second graft. Retrospective studies of class II HLA antigen of recipient and donors, by using molecular biology technique, may explain the immunologic course of our patient.
Acute rejection, simulating relapse of hemolytic-uremic syndrome, is to be evoked because of inflammatory infiltration, polyclonal activation of lymphocytes during second transplantation, and lack of clinical or biological signs of hemolytic-uremic syndrome.

Is the incidence of kidney rejection episodes higher in combined kidney/pancreas (CKP) than in single kidney (SK) transplant patients ?

D. Cantarovich, M. Hourmant, J. Dantal, M. Giral, J. Paineau, G. Karam and J.P. Soulillou.
Service de Néphrologie et Immunologie Clinique, Nantes University Hospital, 44035 Nantes, France.

To determine whether the incidence of rejection episodes is different following CKP or SK transplantation, we retrospectively analysed 67 consecutive CKP and 100 consecutive SK transplant patients. The CKP group consisted of 35 men and 32 women, aged 20 to 61 years (mean 39), which had been insulin-dependent for 5 to 35 years (mean 24). 32% of patients were not on dialysis at the time of transplantation. The non-diabetic SK group consisted of 64 men and 36 women, aged 13 to 65 years (mean 41.5). 12% of patients were not on dialysis at the time of transplantation. In both groups, induction immunosuppression consisted of azathioprine (Aza; 2 mg/kg/day), prednisolone (Pred; 0.5 mg/kg/day in the CKP group, and 1 mg/kg/day in the SK group), antithymocyte globulin or an anti-IL2-R monoclonal antibody, and cyclosporine (CsA; introduced on postoperative day 3 (1 to 10) in the CKP group and systematically on postoperative day 10 in the SK group). Maintenance immunosuppression consisted of CsA and Aza in the CKP group and CsA monotherapy in the SK group.

During the first 3 postoperative months, the incidence of rejection was 33% in the CKP group and 28.5% in the SK group (p= NS). After the third month, the incidence of rejection was 8% in the CKP group and 5% in the SK group (p= NS). Although the first-line treatment of the rejection episode differed between both groups (OKT3 in the CKP group and methylprednisolone pulses in the SK group), the number of patients requiring "rescue" treatment was similar in both groups (3 in the CKP group and 3 in the SK group). One year mean serum creatinine level was lower but not significantly different in the CKP group (137 versus 166 μmol/L). The one year kidney actuarial survival rates were similar in both groups: 90.5% in the CKP group and 85% in the SK group (p= NS). The one year actuarial patient survival rates were 95.2% in the CKP group and 96% in the SK group (p= NS). Although analyses were done retrospectively and immunosuppression was not identical, this data suggests that diabetic recipients of CKP transplants experienced a similar incidence of kidney rejection episodes as compared to non-diabetic recipients of SK transplant. Whether CKP transplant patients do require heavier immunosuppression than SK transplant patients remains to be determined with randomised trials.

Circadian blood pressure (BP) profile in kidney graft patients (KGP)

J HACINI, J BOULAHROUZ, A ZIANE, C LAMBERT, F BERTHOUX
Nephrology, Dialysis and Transplantation dpt, CHU 42055 St ETIENNE Cedex 2

The aim of that study was to analyze the circadian BP profile, the efficiency of anti-hypertensive treatment and to compare ambulatory blood pressure monitoring to conventionnaly (>160/90) arm-cuff diagnosed hypertension (HT).

Method: Ambulatory BP monitoring was performed in 34 KGP, aged from 45 ±14 years old. A Nippon Collin (380G) type Holter monitor was used. Charge is the frequency of values >150/90 on daytime and >130/80 on night in each patients.

Results:

conventionnal:	controlled BP (n = 23)	Hypertension (n=24)
ambulatory monitoring		
daytime		
mean systolic BP	152±15*	132±12
systolic charge	.52±.33*	.13±.23
mean diastolic BP	94 ±7	76± 10
diastolic charge	.47±.3	.17±.18
nocturnal		
mean systolic BP	150±19*	127±10
systolic charge	.83±.27*	.41±.3
mean diastolic BP	87 ±15*	77± 9
diastolic charge	.66 ±.3	.27±.28

*$p<.01$

Conclusions:

Circadian cycles were reversed in 40% of hypertensive and in 28% of controlled BP in Kidney graft patients. Nocturnal systolic charge was prevalent. Nocturnal hypertension appeared in 28% of patients considered with normalized BP by conventional method.

PART : C

IMMUNOSUPPRESSIVE THERAPY

INFLUENCE OF CYCLOFOSFAMIDE ON MORPHOLOGICAL AND IMMUNOHISTOCHEMICAL FEATURES OF REJECTION IN THE HAMSTER-TO-RAT HETEROTOPIC HEART XENOTRANSPLANTATION (HHX)

M. Catena[1], S. Gatti[1], S. Celli[1], G. Ferla[1], N. Maggiano[2], G. Lattanzio[3] and P. Musiani[3]

[1]Dept. of Sciences and Biol. Technologies. - Univ. of Milan, Italy,
[2]Dept. of Pathology - Catholic University, Rome, Italy,
[3]Dept. of Pathology - University of Chieti, Italy.

Hamster to rat xenotransplantation has been always considered as a concordant transplant according to Calne's definition.

In our previus study we could demonstrate that rejection between these two "closely ralated" species is triggered by preformed natural antibodies against hamster endothelial cells, both in sensitized and non sensitized animals.

The aim of this study was to investigate the features of rejection in animals treated with Cyclophosphamide (CyP), analyzing the sequential ultrastructural and immunohistochemical changes occuring in myocardial and splenic tissue after an HHX between Hamster (donor) and rat (reciepient).

Animals were divided into 2 differently treated groups. **Group A:** 15 Lewis rats that recieved 15 Golden Syrian hamster hearts. Five recipients were sacrificed on the 3rd - 4th post operative day, which is the time of rejection in this model; the other ten were divided into five groups of 2 and sacrificed 12, 24, 36, 48 and 60 hours after HHX, respectively. **Group B:** 11 animals which were treated 5 days before and 1 day after transplantation with 50 mg/Kg i.p. of CyP; five of these were sacrificed at the time of rejection, the other six were divided into three groups and sacrificed 48, 72, 96 hours after HHX. Transplanted heart and native spleen from all recipients at the time of their sacrifice were obtained; sera of all animals for immunohistochemical testing were obtained. In group A, at time of rejection, it was possible to observe sequential antibody deposition on graft endothelium followed by vascular trombosis and hemorrhagic necrosis. At time of rejection the spleen showed a marked stimulation of white pulp marginal zones. In group B rejection occured on 4th - 5th post operative day (except one on 8th day); histologic and ultrastructural study on graft tissue revealed the presence of fibrosis starting from subpericardial and subendocardial areas in presence of activated fibroblasts: there was no evidence of lymphocitic and/or PMN infiltration (as also demonstrated immunohistochemically using monoclonal antibodies against mononuclear cell subpopulations). The spleen within 72-96 hours seemed to be completely depleted from immunoblasts and plasmacells. Also native spleen samples from animals treated but not transplanted, showed depletion of white pulp marginal zones 3 days after the second CyP administration. Immunoistochemical studies showed the presence of xenoantibodies in the sera of all animals, treated and untreated; their pathogenetic role in this HHX model is discussed.

LONG TERM RESULTS OF CYCLOSPORINE MONOTHERAPY AFTER HEART
TRANSPLANTATION IN PEDIATRIC AND ADULT PATIENTS

M. M. Koerner, H. Posival, G. Tenderich, E. zu Knypphausen, M.
C. Wilhelms, P. Stahlhut, A. El Banayosi, H. Koertke, H. Meyer,
R. Koerfer

Heart Center North Rhine Westphalia, University Hospital of
Bochum, Bad Oeynhausen, FR Germany

Since 4 years the long term immunosuppressive therapy (IST) of
choice after heart transplantation (HTx) is the double drug
therapy with Cyclosporine A (Cy) and Azathioprine (AZ) at our
center.

There is no monoclonal or polyclonal antibody prophylaxis.

About 65% of 464 patients (pts) after HTx received this IST. To
avoid side effects it is of benefit to reduce also this IST onto
a mimimal level. The records of 40 pts (32 men/8 women) aged 2
to 73 years (mean=44 years) were studied, who of them received
only Cy IST as monotherapy over a minimum of a 6 months period
up to 34 months after HTx. Target level of Cy in the specific
monoclonal RIA was 150 µg/l in adults and 200 µg/l in children.

During the follow up period there were no death. There were only
3 rejection episodes with the need of a cortison pulse. 2
episodes of these occurred after viral infection episodes, one
after a bacterial pneumonia.

Cy monotherapy is a safe and effective IST after HTx in a
special subgroup of pediatric and adult patients.

Effect of Plasmapheresis on kinetic of cyclosporin A.

DIAB N., LAMBERT C., MAACHI K. BERTHOUX F.

Nephrology, Dialysis and Transplantation, CHRU 42055 St ETIENNE, Cedex2, France

In transplantation, it is crucial to maintain blood cyclosporin A (CyA) levels in therapeutical ranges (TR) specially during rejection crisis. Plasma Exchanges (PE) are used in severe acute rejection. The purpose of that study was to determine the effect of PE on CyA kinetic.

Methods: 9 patients with stable CyA doses were analyzed: mean age 45 ± 13.2, 2 females, 7 males, mean body weight 62.3 ± 8.5 kg. No interfering drugs were introduced during that period. Liver functions were normal. 3 liters of plasma were replaced with human albumine and Ringer lactate solution on equal volume, by cytapheresis technique. CyA from total blood was measured by TDX method (Abott ltd: Therapeutical range from 267 to 612 µg/l)

Results: We observed a decrease of CyA trough levels from the day after the first session ($p<0,05$). The nadir appeared after the second exchange ($p<0,006$) and was below the TR in 44% of the patients. Previous levels were reached back by the fourth day after the last PE.

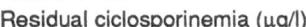
Residual ciclosporinemia (µg/l)

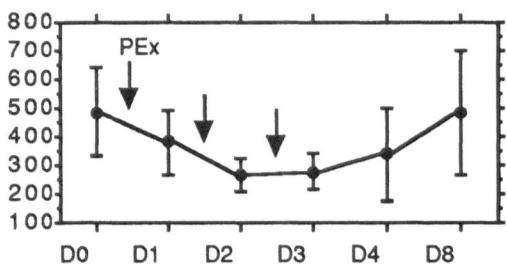

Blood hemoglobin did not change significantly and serum total protein slightly decreased.

Conclusion: CyA kinetic significantly decreased following plasma exchanges, often below therapeutical threshold and may impaire the cure of rejection crisis. The effect may be due to the clearance of lipo-proteins which carry one third of the blood content of the drug. Doses or timing of PE should be adapted.

In vitro effects of cyclosporine, FK506, 6-mercaptopurine and prednisolone on lymphokine-activated killer cells.

E. Alamartine, O. Sabido, F. Berthoux. Laboratoire de Néphrologie et Centre de Cytométrie en Flux, Faculté de Médecine, Saint-Etienne, FRANCE.

In transplant recipients, immunosuppressive regimens are deleterious on natural killer and lymphokine-acetivated killer cells, but the effects of each agent are not identical. We tested the influence of cyclosporine, FK506, 6-mercaptopurine and prednisolone in an *in vitro* IL-2 activation of LAK cells.

PBMC were obtained from healthy volunteers, and were incubated 2 days with either cyclosporine, FK506, 6-mercaptopurine or prednisolone, whose concentrations ranged from 0 to 10 µg/ml, in order to screen infra-therapeutic, therapeutic, and supra-therapeutic doses. Thereafter, 100 IU of IL-2 were added for a further 3-day culture. We performed 11 assays for each drug. Before and after the culture, we analysed 1-) the cell subsets by direct IF staining with anti CD3/CD16/CD56 antibodies, 2-) the LAK activity by the lysis of Daudi cells, 3-) the cell proliferation with a 24-Hr incorporation of thymidine.

The LAK cytotoxicity was correlated with the number of CD3⁻ CD16⁺ CD56⁺ cells, and increased with the incorporation of thymidine. The number of CD3⁻ CD16⁺ CD56⁺ cells, but not the number of CD3⁺ CD16⁻ CD56⁻ cells, was correlated with the incorporation of thymidine. Cyclosporine and FK506 did not impair the LAK cytotoxicity nor the number of LAK cells, whereas both prednisolone and 6-mercaptopurine decreased the LAK cytotoxicity, the number of CD3⁻ CD16⁺ CD56⁺ cells, and the thymidine incorporation.

We conclude that *in vitro*, the LAK activity is impaired by prednisolone and 6-mercaptopurine, but neither by cyclosporine nor FK506; and that the deficiency of the LAK cytotoxicity seems to be related to the decreased number of IL-2-activated NK cells.

CYCLOSPORIN A PROTECTS MURINE AND HUMAN B CELL LINES AGAINST CALCIUM-INDUCED APOPTOSIS.

N. Bonnefoy-Berard, M.T. Dearden-Badet, L. Genestier, M. Flacher and J.P. Revillard. Laboratory of immunology, INSERM U80 UCBL, Hôpital E. Herriot, 69437 Lyon cedex 03 France.

Apoptosis or programmed cell death (PCD) is a process of selective cell deletion characterized by activation of calcium-dependent endonucleases. PCD occurs during T as well as B cell ontogeny, leading to a normal selection process during cellular differentiation (1). The immunosuppressive agent cyclosporin A (CsA) has already been reported to inhibit TCR-mediated apoptosis in T cell hybridomas and thymocytes. Recently, an "unbalanced" signalling between the two arms of the classical phosphatidyl inositol pathway in favour of intracellular Ca^{2+} ion level has been suggested as a possible inducer of apoptosis in numerous cell lines.

Inhibition of Ca^{2+}-dependent activation pathways by CsA appears to require the formation of intracellular CsA-cyclophilin complexes which inhibit the activity of calcineurin, a Ca^{2+}- and calmodulin-dependent serine/threonine phosphatase. We report here that CsA inhibits apoptosis induced by calcium ionophore or receptor cross-linking in several human and murine B cell lines.

Group I Burkitt's lymphoma (BL) cell lines and other B cell lymphomas are susceptible to apoptosis induced by ionomycin or anti-mIg (2). In these conditions, CsA protects against cell death in a dose-dependent manner with a maximal activity at 50-100 ng/ml, without modifying Ca^{2+} elevation induced by ionomycin. CsA potentiates the protective effect of IFNα and TNFα on ionomycin-induced cell death. Conversely, CsA has no protective effect on Ca^{2+}-independent apoptosis induced by antilymphocyte (ALG) or antithymocyte globulins (ATG) in Apo-1 positive lines (3). In addition CsA up-regulates *bcl-2* gene expression and Bcl-2 protein synthesis, an effect which may contribute to the resistance to Ca^{2+}-induced apoptosis but does not affect Apo-1 mediated apoptosis.

The murine cell line WEHI-231 represents a model of immature B cells in which either ligation of surface IgM or ionomycin induces apoptosis by a mechanism leading to increased intracellular Ca^{2+} without protein kinase C (PKC) activation (4). CsA inhibits such cell death with a maximal activity at 50 ng/ml. A similar protective effect was achieved by PKC-activating phorbol esters and lipopolysaccharide.

This novel property of CsA on B cell lines is likely to involve the blockade of calcineurin phosphatase activity.

1- J.J. Cohen 1991, *Adv.immunol.* 50 : 55-85. 2- K.A. Knox *et al.* 1992, *Int. J. Cancer* 52 : 959-966. 3- N. Bonnefoy-Berard *et al.*1992, *Blood* 79 : 2164-2670. 4- P. Sarthou *et al.* 1989, *Eur. J. Immunol.* 19 : 1247-1252.

6 THIOGUANIDINE INTRA ERYTHROCYTE LEVEL IN TRANSPLANTED CHILDREN UNDERGOING AZATHIOPRINE TREATMENT

F.BOUISSOU, S.BILLY, B.MARTINEZ, C.GAY, M.REMESY, G.HOUIN, Ph BARTHE
Unité de Néphrologie Pédiatrique, Laboratoire de Pharmacocinétique -CHU PURPAN - TOULOUSE

Azathioprine (AZA), a widely used immunosuppressive drug in transplantation, has a variable pharmacokinetics both in adults and children ; its main plasmatic metabolite 6 Mercaptopurine (6MP) has been well studied, with a short plasmatic half-life and a very changeable bioavailability. In kidney transplanted children we have previously found a positive correlation between the 6MP area under curve at 3 hours (AUC 3) and the clinical immunosuppressive effect , with a lower incidence of acute rejection episodes during the first two years of transplantation when the AUC 3 was higher than 40 ng/ml/h .

However it is well known that both immunosuppressive and side effects depend of its intra cellular metabolites, mainly **6 Thioguanidine** which has a longer half-life of several days.

We report our experience with the monitoring of intra erythrocyte 6 Thioguanidine (E6TGN) in 43 children with a kidney transplant (mean age :12 years , 2 to 18 years ; time from transplantation : 2 to 10 years ; triple sequential therapy : ATG, Cyclosporine - Steroid - AZA ; the AZA dose was adapted to the 6 MP - AUC 3).
E6TGN level (64 determinations) was assessed by HPLC and UV detection at 342 n.meters. The results were expressed in picomol / 8.10^6 red blood cells. The correlations have been made with the clinical status (viral infections, rejection episodes), renal function, AZA dose, 6 MP kinetics and hematological parameters. A sequential evaluation of 6 TGN has been done in 15 children.

The mean level of E6TGN was 168 ± 15 pmol for 8.10^8 RBC (range 0-522) ; it did not increase with the time, and was remarkably stable in the sequential study, without any cumulative effect. But in two children an increasing dosage was followed by an increase of E6TGN.We did not find any correlation with age, renal function, AZA dose plasma , 6 MP kinetics, or hematological parameters.

Furthermore we demonstrated a **bimodal distribution** of E6TGN among the children : one group with a high level (10 children : 377 ± 298 range 251-522) and an other with a "normal" level (33 children 119 ± 6 range 0-215 ; $p = < 0.001$). These two groups were not different for age, renal function, time from transplant, hematological parameters , rejection episodes or AZA dose. But the incidence of viral infections or cutaneous wart was higher in the high group (79% versus 27% $p = 0.015$) .In an other hand the children with cutaneous warts exhibited a higher E6TGN concentration (213 ± 34 vs 134 ± 18, $p = 0.039$).

These results suggest that E6TGN level could be very useful in transplantation : first to assess the AZA treatment compliance especially during the adolescent period , and second to evaluate the possible long term over imunosuppression and the carcinoma risk which is increased in these patients. Larger studies are necessary to confirm this last point.The bimodal distribution in cells could be explained by a difference of enzymatic activity with" low " and "high" metabolizer patients.

New Vitamin D analogues : Immunosuppressive Effects on skin allograft Survival in mice

Paule Veyron[1], Raymond Pamphile[2], Lise Binderup[3] and Jean Louis Touraine[1] - 1 : TRANSPLANTATION AND CLINICAL IMMUNOLOGY, PAVILLON P, HÔPITAL EDOUARD-HERRIOT, 69437 LYON, CEDEX 03. - 2 : LABORATORIES LEO S.A.78180 MONTIGNY, FRANCE. - 3 : LEO PHARMACEUTICAL PRODUCTS : DK-2750 BALLERUP, DENMARK.

Recent progress in the understanding of pathophysiological mechanisms of autoimmune diseases and the multiple therapies for organ or cell transplantation have expanded the use of immunosuppressive drugs. In this respect, 1,25-dihydroxyvitamin D_3, $(1,25(OH)_2D_3)$, the active form of vitamin D_3, has now attracted great interest. $1,25(OH)_2D_3$ is thought to exert its effects through binding to the vitamin D receptor (VDR). After binding of $1,25(OH)_2D_3$, the VDR mediates transcriptional activities through binding to specific DNA binding sites, in a manner analogous to classic steroid hormones, thyroxine and retinoic acid. Activated T lymphocyte proliferation is inhibited presumably by $1,25(OH)_2D_3$ interfering with cytokine mediated fonctions. The therapeutical use of $1,25(OH)_2D_3$ in the immunological field is limited by its potent effects on calcium metabolism, inducing hypercalcemia. New vitamin D_3 analogues have been developped in order to reduce the hypercalcemia effect. They are characterized by a modified stereochemistry at carbon 20 in the side chain of the molecule. Two of these analogues of $1,25(OH)_2D_3$, KH 1060 and CB 966, were tested on allogeneic skin graft in mice and were found to significantly delay the rejection of allogeneic skin from grafts in CBA recipient mice, transplanted with skin from C57Bl/6 donor mice. Graft survival was assessed in mice treated with KH 1060 or CB 966 (0.2 and 0.4 µg/kg/day i.p.) until the day of rejection, in comparison with the mice treated with vehicle, $1,25(OH)_2D_3$(0.2 and 0.4 µg/kg/day i.p.), or cyclosporine A (CsA) (20 mg/kg/day p.o). The following mean survival time in days was found : 16.6 ± 0.5 in CsA, 13.9 ± 0.6 and 15.5 ± 0.6 in $1,25(OH)_2D_3$, 14.3 ± 0.2 and 18.7 ± 0.5 in CB 966, and 13.5 ± 0.8, 15.9 ± 1.7, 19.6 ± 0.4 and 24.5 ± 0.5 in KH 1060 : 0.02, 0.1, 0.2 and 0.4 µg/kg/day, 10.9 ± 0.2 in controls. Combination of CsA with KH1060 (0.1 µg/kg/day i.p.) resulted in a synergistic effect : 23.4 ± 1.0 days compared to the 15.6 ± 1.7 days with KH1060 or CsA alone. KH 1060 was the most active, is effective at doses which marginally affect serum calcium levels. This association can therefore be regarded as a potent immunosuppressor in transplantation and can be used in combination with CsA. Actually novel vitamin D analogues are tested. This findings suggest that $1,25(OH)_2D_3$ and its analogues exert immunosuppressive effects different from those of CsA and thereby show synergistic effects during combined treatment and may lead to therapeutic regimens that combine low dosages of compounds and reduce the risk of unwanted side effects.

EFFECT OF INTRAOPERATIVE HIGH-DOSE SINGLE-BOLUS LYMPHOGLOBULIN PROPHYLAXIS ON THE OUTCOME OF RENAL TRANSPLANTATION

J. KADEN, G. MAY, P. MÖLLER, V. STROBELT, E. EGER, C. SCHÖNEMANN, J. GROTH

Friedrichshain Hospital, Kidney Transplant Centre and Division of Immunology, Berlin, Germany

In 19 cadaveric renal transplantations performed at the Kidney Transplant Centre Berlin-Friedrichshain during 8/1991 - 5/1992 we studied the influence of an intraoperative high-dose single-bolus equine anti-human thymocyte globulin prophylaxis (Lymphoglobulin, Institute Merieux, Lyon, France) on T-cell count, CD 4:8-ratio, hospital stay, incidence of rejection crises and CMV infections as well as on 1-year patient and graft survival. The results obtained were compared with those of historical control groups. The basic immunosuppression generally consisted of azathioprine, cyclosporine and low-dose prednisolone. In addition to this triple-drug therapy all recipients received intraoperatively 30 - 60 min after infusion of 500 mg methylprednisolone 1.5 ml Lymphoglobulin /kg b.w. just before the anastomoses were completed. This treatment protocol drastically reduced the peripheral T-cell count from preoperative $666 \pm 297/\mu l$ to $79 \pm 149/\mu l$ postoperative (flow cytometry). This T-lymphopenia lasted for three ($192 \pm 127/\mu l$) to five ($319 \pm 186/\mu l$) days. As an importand fact we found a much stronger initial effect on T helper cells, also indicated by a reduction of the preoperative CD 4:8-ratio from 1.3 ± 0.4 to 0.7 ± 0.4 postoperative. On the 3rd day after grafting this ratio was in the normal range again (1.2 ± 0.1). In comparison with the data of historical control groups this protocol did not shorten the hospital stay (43 ± 29 d) and not reduce the rate of rejection episodes (53 %). The CMV infection rate diagnosed by antigen as well as antibody detection was 63 % (12/19). From the clinical point of view it was very important to notice only but one light courses of CMV diseases (8/12). With respect to long-term results, both the 1-year graft survival (90 %) and patient survival (100 %) were pleasing good. Graft losses occurred only in two patients, one due to humoral rejection (detection of donor-reactive antibodies early after grafting) and one in connection with a severe CMV disease. Considering only the group of presensitized recipients (n = 15) with its high rate of 2nd and 3rd grafts (n = 7) the overall patient and graft survival after 12 month (100 % and 93 %, respectively) was excellent. Thus the high-dose single-bolus ATG prophylaxis in connection with triple-drug therapy seems to be an effective treatment protocol.
The rationale of this protocol is to produce maximal immunosuppression when the recipient is most likely to respond to the new organ.

A COMPARATIVE STUDY OF PROPHYLACTIC OKT3 VERSUS ANTILYMPHOGLOBULINS IN HIGLY SENSITIZED RENAL RECIPIENTS.

Vela C., Cristol J.P., Chong G., Okamba A., Lorho R., Mourad G., Mion C.
Service de Néphrologie , Lapeyronie,
34059 Montpellier Cedex. France.

Hyperimmunization remains a problem in kidney transplantation for its prolonged waiting time and higher risk of graft loss. Monoclonal antibodies were proposed as an effective prophylactic immunosuppressive treatment in such patients. In this study we compare the results obtained in our center in sensitized patients (SP) treated with OKT3 or antilymphoglobulins (ALG). Since January 1989 to January 1993, 38 transplantations were performed in patients with large Panel Reactive Antibodies (PRA > 50%), 22 women and 16 men, mean age 45 ± 2 (23-67) y. o., 10 second grafts, 2 third grafts. Peak PRA was $\geq 80\%$ in 24 SP, and 50-80% in 14 SP. All transplantations were performed with a current negative T-cell IgG cross-match; historical cross matches were negative in all sera in 30 SP and positive in one serum in 8 SP. Maximum HLA mismatches were 3. Patients were ramdomly assigned to either prophylactic OKT3 (5 mg/day, n=15) or ALG (5 ml/20kg/day; n=23). Oral cyclosporin A (10 mg/kg) was started at day 8 in OKT3 group and when serum creatinine level decreased to 200 µmol/l in ALG group. OKT3 was systematically withdrawn at day 10 but ALG was stopped only when total blood cyclosporin A concentration reached 150-200 ng/ml. The duration of ALG was 15 ± 1 (6-34) days. In both groups, azathioprine (150 mg/day) and prednisolone (20 mg/day) were given. During the first month, 6/15 gafts were lost in OKT3 group, (3 hyperacute rejections, 1 renal vein thrombosis, 1 steroid resistant rejection, 1 death); in ALG group 4/23 grafts were lost (1 hyperacute rejection, 2 steroid resistant rejections, 1 death). Incidence of rejection episodes was identical in ALG group and OKT3 group (48% and 53% respectively). However, OKT3 was associated with an increased rate of acute tubulopathy (53%) when compared to ALG treatment (22%). After 12 monthes of follow up, the graft survival was 71% (27/38) and did not significantly differ (Logrank test, ns) in OKT3 (60%; 9/15) versus ALG group (78%; 18/23).

We conclude that the use of the monoclonal antibody OKT3 as prophylactic agent in HSP does not improve the early graft survival when compared with prophylactic ALG. Polyclonal antibodies, which react with many epitopes and are much better tolerated seem to offer more powerfull strategy in this population.

MONITORING OF CD2 LYMPHOCYTES IN RENAL TRANSPLANT PATIENTS RECEIVING PROPHYLACTIC ANTITHYMOGLOBULINS

L. ROSTAING, J. TKACZUK, D. DURAND, M.H. CHABANNIER, J.J. LLOVERAS, E. OHAYON, J.M. SUC

CHU RANGUEIL, TOULOUSE

The aim of this study was to determine whether the monitoring of CD2 lymphocytes by cytofluorometry for renal transplant patients under antithymoglobulins (ATG) therapy would result a) in the use of a lower ATG dose/patient ; b) in fewer infectious complications ; c) in the same immunosuppressive effect.

In our center the immunosuppressive therapy include azathioprine (2 mg/kg/d), prednisone (1 mg/kg/d for two weeks, then progressively tapered to 0.2 mg/kg/d at day 90) and ATG (1.25 mg/kg/d) until serum creatinine (SCr) is below 200 μmol/l, then relayed by ciclosporine A -CyA- (6 mg/kg/d). We used to check the efficacy of ATG upon the absolute number of peripheral blood lymphocytes - PBL - (i.e. less than 100/mm3). Since August 1992 when a patient is under ATG therapy since five days we monitor three times a week the absolute number of CD2 lymphocytes by cytofluorometry . The goal to achieve is less than 50 CD2/mm3 ; when the CD2 number is less than 50/mm^3 the ATG daily dose is reduced by 50%; if the CD2 number is higher than 50/mm^3 the ATG daily dose is increased of 25 mg/day until next CD2 monitoring. From December 1991 to December 1992 51 adult renal transplants were performed in our department ; one patient received prophylactic OKT3 therapy (third graft) ; the others (50) received ATG ; 3 patients had early graft failure ; thus 47 patients could be evaluated with a follow-up of at least 4 months. They were divided in two groups ; group I included 28 patients with PBL monitoring ; group II included 19 patients with CD2 lymphocyte monitoring. The two groups were not different according to sex, patients'age and number of initial acute tubular necrosis.

	ATG (days/pt) (mean)	ATG (vial/pt) (mean)	Pt with rejection	CMV	Bacterial infections	SCr day 30 (μmol/l)	SCr day 90 (μmol/l)
Group I n = 28	8.8	24.4	9	5	4	120.7	133.5
Group II n = 19	8.8	20.4	8	1	7	122.1	134.5
p	NS	NS	NS	NS	NS	NS	NS

Even if the difference is not statistically significative, the monotoring of CD2 lymphocytes resulted in the use of less ATG/patient i.e. a mean of 4 vials/patient. Based upon 50 renal tranplants/year it will represent over one year $ 24464 savings. Furthermore the number of total rejections, the number of rejection/patient were not increased and SCr was at the same level as in group I. There were less CMV infections and more bacterial infections in groupe II but the difference was not significative. In conclusion CD2 lymphocyte monitoring by cytofluorometry under ATG therapy is useful since it allows to administer less ATG/patient with the same immunological efficacy. Nevertheless infections were not statistically diminished.

OKT3 TREATMENT FOR REJECTION IN RENAL TRANSPLANT PATIENTS AND OCCURENCE OF OKT3 BLOCKING ANTIBODIES.

L. ROSTAING, J. TKACZUK, M. ABBAL, O. FRITZ, D. DURAND, J.J. LLOVERAS,
A. MODESTO, E. OHAYON, J.M. SUC
CHU RANGUEIL, TOULOUSE - FRANCE

Since 01/01/88, 345 adult renal transplantations have been performed in our department. They all received the same sequential immunosuppression including azathioprine, steroids, antithymocyte globulins ; ciclosporine A -CsA- (6 mg/kg/d) was introduced as soon as serum creatinine was below 200 μmol/l. During this 5 year period 250 histological rejections were numbered ; most of them (184) were treated by methylprednisolone pulses (10 mg/kg/d for 3 days) ; the remainings (n= 66 i.e. 26.4 %) were treated by OKT3, 5 mg/day for 10 days ; CsA was stopped between day 0 and 8. Indications of OKT3 therapy included steroid-resistant rejections (n = 38 i.e. 58 %) and severe rejections with edema and/or fibrosis (n = 28 i.e. 42 %). Serum creatinine returned to baseline in 68 % of rejections whereas the improvement was partial in 14 cases (21 %) ; 7 rejections were not controlled by OKT3 (i.e. 11 %). Long term follow-up showed that in 36 cases (i.e. 54.5 %) renal function deteriorated ; 21 patients returned to haemodialysis in a mean time of 15 months (range : 2-53 months).

Under OKT3 treatment CD3 subsets were monitored at days 0, 5, 8 and 10 so as to maintain a CD3/total lymphocytes ratio below 0.1 . In 76 % of cases this was achieved at days 8 and 10. OKT3 blocking antibodies were assessed using cytofluorometric detection 1) 30 to 40 days after the begining of OKT3 therapy in 30 cases and 2) 6 months to one year after the end of OKT3 therapy in 14 cases. A positive response (i.e. presence of OKT3 blocking antibodies) was defined as an inhibition of fluorescence of blood bank donors' CD3 lymphocytes suspended with the patient's serum preincubated with FITC labelled OKT3. In 16/30 cases (53 %) we detected blocking antibodies that persisted in many cases 6 to 12 months later. There were no correlation between anti-OKT3 immunization and 1) the number of CD3 at the end of OKT3 therapy ; 2) subsequent acute rejection episode (s) ; 3) evolution to chronic rejection.

In conclusion OKT3 blocking antibodies developed in 53 % of patients treated by OKT3 and did not disappear in a one year follow-up thus precluding the reuse of OKT3.

Anti-mouse antibodies in OKT3 treated transplant recipients.

M.A. Rugo-Costa, E. Renoult, M.C. Béné, M. Kessler, G.C. Faure.

Nancy, France

OKT3 is amurine monoclonal antibody widely used in the prophylaxis or treatment of acute rejection in solid organ transplantation. Administration of these murine immunoglobulins could lead to an anti-isotypic or an anti-idiotypic immunisation in humans.

We investigated this possibility in 24/209 kidney recipients who received 1 (23 patients) or 2 (1 patient) course of OKT3 between 1989 and 1992. Fifteen men and 9 women were concerned (mean age: 37,9 years; 22-56). Twenty three episodes of rejection in 21 patients were treated with OKT3 and in 3 cases the monoclonal antibody was given in prophylaxis. In 6 cases, Cyclosporine was maintained during the treatment of rejection. Signs of intolerance were observed in 9 cases during the course of OKT3.

Eleven viral, 1 parasitologic and 2 bacterial infections were observed following treatment with OKT3.

We developed a sandwich ELISA assay to investigate the appearance of IgM and/or IgG anti-isotype and/or anti-idiotype in serum. One serum was considered as positive for a ratio OD patient/ OD negative serum ≥ 2.

No anti-idiotypic immunisation was observed but 3 patients developed anti-mouse IgG during the treatment. These IgG decreased in the following months.

This early immunisation, first observed in pediatric patients, evokes a secondary response directed against the Fc murine component and led us to propose investigation of anti-mouse immunoglobulins earlier during OKT3 course.

CD4 AND CD25 MONOCLONAL ANTIBODY COCKTAIL IN KIDNEY TRANSPLANT REJECTION PROPHYLAXIS. Clinical results of a pilot study.

Y. TANTER*, C. MOUSSON*, E. RACADOT**, J. WIJDENES**, P. HERVE**, G. RIFLE**.

* SERVICE DE NEPHROLOGIE-REANIMATION, CENTRE HOSPITALIER UNIVERSITAIRE, DIJON, FRANCE -**CRTS, BESANCON, FRANCE .

Among Monoclonal antibodies (mAbs), anti-IL2 receptor mAb gave interesting results in preventing transplant rejection. However, due to the murin origin of these mAbs, the patients are exposed to the risk of sensitization to the heterologous protein. More recently, it has been demonstrated that anti-CD4 mAb was able to induce donor specific unresponsiveness in rats. We report the results of a pilot study using simultaneously two mAbs: anti-CD4/B-F5 and anti-IL2R/B-B10 for kidney transplant rejection prophylaxis. The aim was to analyze the occurence of xenogenic antibodies and to evaluate the clinical impact of this treatment in terms of rejection episodes and infectious complications.

PATIENTS AND METHODS

Ten patients entered the study. They were 6 males and 4 females (age range 33-63 year, mean 47). All patients had received pre-transplant blood transfusions and 4 of them were immunized (between 20 % and 33 % towards a panel of 24 different donors). They all received a first cadaver kidney transplant and mean HLA A, B and DR mismatches was 2.6.

Anti-CD4/B-F5 and anti-IL2R/B-B10 are both mouse IgG1 produced in our laboratory. After dilution in 30ml of 4% diluted albumin, B-F5 mAb (20mg) was infused over 30mn before establishing revascularization; B-B10 (10mg) was infused over 30mn, 2 hours later. The following infusions were performed daily for 13 days at the same dose. Corticosteroids were administrated before the first B-F5 infusion and maintained at a dose of 1mg/kgBW/day until day 6, then progressively tapered to 15mg/day. Azathioprine (3 mg/kg/day) was started at day O, then progressively tapered to 1mg/kgBW/day on day 30. Cyclosporine was started at day 13 at oral dose of 4 mg/kgBW/day, then adjusted to blood levels (150-200ng/ml).

Xenoimmunization was analyzed by ELISA and immunofluorescence. Studies of lymphocyte subsets, cytokines and soluble receptors levels were performed, and will be reported separately.

RESULTS

All patients were alive. Three kidney grafts were lost, respectively from venous thrombosis (day 6) and arterial thrombosis (day 11 and day 12 respectively). Out of 7 evaluable patients, 1 presented 2 mild rejection episodes (day 40-day 180), 2 presented 1 mild rejection episode (day 19-day28). The remaining 4 patients did not present any rejection phenomenon. At the present time, the 7 patients have functionnal graft (mean creatinine clearance: 60 ml/mn) with a mean follow-up of 9.5 months (range: 6-21 months). mAb infusions were well tolerated, since only one transient cutaneous eruption occured. Infectious complications were neither severe, nor numerous: 3 mild CMV infections, 1 labial herpes, 1 bacteriemia (E.Coli). In addition, one patient experienced transient thrombopenia and hemolytic anemia of unknown origin on day 9, before starting Cyclosporine.

Xenogenic immunization occured in 4 patients (during mAb therapy only in 1 case).

CONCLUSION : The use of a mAbs cocktail CD4+CD25+ in kidney transplant rejection prophylaxis seems an interesting approach, without systemic side effects or severe infectious complications. However, the occurence of thrombosis in 3 patients, perhaps without any obvious connection with the use of mAbs, led us to evoke their possible responsability, as it has been described for OKT3 mAb. This hypothesis is under investigation.

OUTCOME OF LYMPHOCYTE SUBSETS AND CYTOKINES DURING COMBINED CD4/CD25 mAb THERAPY IN KIDNEY GRAFTING.

E. RACADOT*, C. MOUSSON**, Y. TANTER**, P. HERVE*, G. RIFLE**, J. WIJDENES***.
*CRTS *** Innothérapie BESANCON ** Service de Néphrologie-Réanimation DIJON FRANCE

An immunological follow-up was performed in 10 patients who received 2 monoclonal antibodies anti-CD4/B-F5 (20 mg) and anti-IL2R/B-B10 (10 mg) daily for 14 days for kidney transplant rejection prophylaxis.

Methods:

Lymphocyte subsets were analysed with mAbs: CD3, CD4, CD8, CD19, CD25 (Innotherapie), CD56, CD45RA (Coulter), CD11b, CD57, CD16 (Becton Dickinson) and flow cytometry (FACScan-Becton Dickinson). Cytokine and soluble receptor levels were evaluated by ELISA (IL6, sIL2R, sICAM, sTNF-R and sL-Selectin) or by IRMA (TNFα). In all patients the analysis were performed before the first CD4/B-F5 infusion, at day 6, at the end of the treatment (D14) and 15 days later (D30). In addition in 5 patients CD3, CD4, CD8, CD56, CD19, CD4/CD45RA+ cell enumeration and cytokine levels measurement were performed after the first B-F5 infusion, before and after the first B-B10 infusion and at day 1 before the second mAb infusion.

Circulating B-F5 and B-B10 were mesured by serial dilution in a double sandwich ELISA assay. Host antixenogenic Ig formation was determined by ELISA and screening for anti-idiotype antibodies was performed by flow cytometry.

Results:

As indicated in the table, B-F5 infusion induced a sharp decrease in CD4+ cells and in CD3+ cells. In the same time there was an increase in CD56+ cells. At the end of the treatment, a significant decrease in CD3 and CD4+ cell count was observed.

	Before treatment	After CD4/B-F5	Before anti-IL2R	after anti-IL2R	D6	D14	D30
lymphocytes	1477±1145	NT	NT	NT	966±271	921±528	863±383
CD3 %	68±10	32±12	34±11	34±9	58±12	53±11	59±8
CD4 %	41±8	10±8	11±5	12±7	30±10	28±9	28±5
CD8 %	29±8	37±9	37±11	33±19	27±8	28±10	32±2
CD19 %	7±3	11±7	9±5	11±5	19±12	16±10	8±3
CD56 %	23±9	52±16	55±14	51±14	24±4	27±16	31±14

Table: Evolution of lymphocyte subsets after CD4/B-F5 + CD25/B-B10 mAbs treatment

Two hours after the first CD4/B-F5 infusion, we observed an increase in IL6 and TNFα serum levels with a return to pretreatment values 24 hours later: 60±43 pg/ml after treatment versus 2±2 pg/ml before treatment for IL6 levels and 221±337 pg/ml after treatment versus 35±40 pg/ml before treatment for TNFα levels. There were no modifications in sIL2-R, sICAM1 and sL-selectin levels. Xenogenic immunization was observed in 4 patients post-treatment.

In conclusion: this mAb association did not induce major immune perturbations. However, the occurence of thrombosis in 3 patients led us to evoke the possible responsibility of mAbs by means of cytokine release as it has been described for OKT3.

Experience with monoclonal antibody against interleukin-2-receptor for treatment of acute interstitial renal transplant rejection

S.Carl, M.Wiesel, H.Reichel, G.Staehler. Depts. Urology and Nephrology, Transplant Centre, University of Heidelberg, Germany.

Monoclonal antibodies against interleukin-2 receptor (designated BT 563) have been used for prevention of acute rejection in liver, kidney and graft-versus-host-disease in bone marrow transplantation. Little experience exists with respect to the use of BT 563 in the treatment of acute interstitial rejection in renal transplant recipients. We, therefore retrospectively analyzed the efficacy of BT 563 in 8 patients (median age 39) with previously stable renal graft function (median 16 months after TPL; range 9-22), who had developed acute renal transplant rejection. The patients were on triple immunosuppressive therapy and received ß-methylprednisolone, azathioprine and ciclosporin. BT 563 was administered to patients with biopsy-proven acute interstitial rejection, which had been resistant to one course of corticosteroid bolus therapy (median cumulative steroid dose 850 mg). Serum creatinine concentrations before initiation of steroid therapy were 3.7 ± 0.6 mg/dl (mean$\pm$SD). There was no statistically significant difference in serum creatinine levels (3.6 ± 0.5) after completion of steroid therapy. Patients who had persistent acute interstitial rejection in re-biopsy after steroid therapy became eligible for BT 563. These patients received 10 mg/24 hr BT 563 as continuous infusion for 10 days. Side effects (e.g. fever, headache, seizures, clinically relevant infections) were not observed. After completion of BT 563 therapy, mean serum creatinine levels had significantly decreased to 2.0 ± 0.5 mg/dl ($p < 0.05$ vs pre-treatment levels). Re-biopsies after completion of BT 563 therapy showed resolution of acute rejection in renal grafts of all 8 patients. Follow-up of the patients for 12 months showed stable graft function in 6 of 8 patients (serum creatinine levels 2.2 ± 0.6). Two patients had progressive transplant failure and had become dependent on maintenance hemodialysis. One of these two patients had, in addition to acute interstitial rejection, signs of chronic vascular rejection. Our experience with a small number of patients suggests that BT 563 is, in the majority of patients, an effective and safe agent for treatment of acute interstitial renal transplant rejection, when steroid-bolus therapy had been ineffective.

Antithymocyte Globulins (ATG) contain antibodies against the b1 integrin molecule

Ticchioni M.*, G. Bernard-Pomier*, M. Deckert*, E. Cassuto-Viguier**, M. A. Rosenthal-Allieri*, J.R. Mondain**, J.C. Bendini**, L. Van Elslande** and A. Bernard*

From the *Laboratoire d'Immunologie, Hôpital de l'Archet, and the **Service de Néphrologie, Hôpital Pasteur, Nice, France.

Despite numerous progress in the management of kidney graft patients, Antithymocytes Globulins (ATG) are still widely used. Recently, it has been shown that Antilymphocyte Globulins (ALG) contain antibodies against the Lymphocyte Function Antigen-1 molecule (LFA-1, CD11a/CD18) which belongs to the b2 integrin subfamily. The b1 integrin molecule (CD29), expressed on T cells, plays an important role as a co-stimulatory molecule for T cell activation and mediates both cell-cell and cell-matrix interaction. In order to determine whether ATG contain also an activity against the b1 molecule, we used adherence assay. Thymi were obtained from children undergoing cardiac surgery. Thymocytes, labelled with a fluorescent product, BCECF, were incubated with ATG, Rabbit Immunoglobulins (RIG) or PBS, washed, and allowed to adhere to flat bottom wells coated with CD11a or CD29 mAb for various interval times at 37°C. Cells remaining after a final wash were quantified using the Cytofluor 2300 System (Millipore). Results showed that specific binding to both CD11a and CD29 was strongly inhibited by preincubation with ATG as compared to cells treated with RIG. Moreover, adhesion of thymocytes on plates coated with ATG was also weakly inhibited by preincubation with CD11a, CD29 and CD11a+CD29 mAb. Taken together, these data may suggest that antibodies against the b1 integrin are present in ATG.

ANTILYMPHOCYTE AND ANTITHYMOCYTE GLOBULINS (ALG/ATG) TRIGGER APOPTOSIS IN HUMAN B CELL LINES

L. Genestier, N. Bonnefoy-Bérard, M. Flacher, G. Lizard, N. Dedhin, M. Mutin,
G. Alberici and J.P. Revillard

Lab. Immunol. INSERM U. 80, Hôp. E. Herriot - 69437 Lyon Cedex 03

ALG and ATG are currently used as immunosuppressive agents in organ transplantation and for the treatment of acute graft-*versus*-host disease and aplastic anemia. Since any immunosuppressive treatment carries the risk of promoting B cell lymphoproliferative disorders, we investigated the *in vitro* effects of ALG/ATG on human B cells. We previously reported that, unlike all other T cell mitogens (including OKT3), ALG/ATG did not activate human B cells but blocked the proliferation of EBV-transformed lymphoblastoid cell lines and Burkitt's lymphoma (BL) cell lines (N.Bonnefoy-Bérard, M. Flacher, and J.P. Revillard, Blood 1992, **79**, 2164-2170). In this study we investigated the mechanisms of this proliferation inhibitory effect. Five different ALG/ATGs of horse or rabbit origin prepared by different manufacturers were found to induce apoptosis of a majority of human B cell lines, with the exception of BL70, an EBV-negative BL, while most myelomonocytic and T cell lines were resistant. Apoptosis was demonstrated : 1/ by nuclear condensation and/or fragmentation of cells stained with Hoechst 33342 ; 2/ by transmission electron microscopy showing the typical irregular chromatin condensation and disruption of the nucleus into discrete fragments with an undamaged cytoplasmic membrane ; and 3/ by the DNA breaks characteristic of apoptosis in DNA electrophoresis. Such apoptosis was achieved with F(ab')2 antibody fragments as well as with intact ALG/ATG, thus excluding a mechanism of reciprocal cell killing by antibody-dependent cell-mediated cytotoxicity. B cell apoptosis did not require *de novo* protein or RNA synthesis and occured in the absence of extracellular Ca^{2+}. Furthermore ALG/ATG did not induce a mobilization of intracellular Ca^{2+} in susceptible cell lines. Stimulation of protein kinase C activity by phorbol esters, which protects against apoptosis induced by Calcium ionophores or anti-Ig antibodies, did not antagonize the cytotoxic activity of ALG/ATG. The susceptibility of various B cell lines to ALG/ATG-induced apoptosis was not related to the level of Bcl-2 expression but grossly paralleled the reported expression of Apo-1. The cytotoxic activity of ATG/ALG was completely removed by absorption on susceptible but not on resistant cell lines, indicating that it was associated with specific antibodies against antigen(s) expressed on susceptible cell lines. A likely candidate is Apo-1, inasmuch as no such cytotoxicity was achieved by CD11a, CD18, CD19, CD21, CD24 and CD40 monoclonal antibodies, nor by antibodies to IgM or HLA-DR. Since this novel property of ALG/ATG might contribute to reduce the risk of B cell lymphoproliferative disorders *in vivo*, this activity (and possibly anti-Apo-1 antibody content) should be determined in ALG/ATG batches.

PART : D

INFECTIOUS COMPLICATIONS

EPSTEIN-BARR VIRUS-ASSOCIATED LYMPHOPROLIFERATIVE DISORDER CONFINED TO A RENAL ALLOGRAFT

R. CAHEN[1] , F. BERGER[2] , F. DIJOUD[2] , P. TROLLIET[1], J.P. MAGAUD[3], G. JEAN[1], H. DELECLUSE[2], M. DEVONEC[4], P. PERRIN [4],B. FRANCOIS[1]

[1] *Service de Néphrologie, Centre Hospitalier Lyon-Sud, 69495 Pierre Bénite Cédex*
[2] *Laboratoires d'Anatomie Pathologique, Hôpital E. Herriot et Hôpital Debrousse,Lyon*
[3] *Laboratoire d'Hématologie, Hôpital E. Herriot, Lyon*
[4] *Service d'Urologie, Hôpital de l'Antiquaille, Lyon, France*

The predilection of post-transplant lymphoproliferative disorders (PTLD) for extranodal sites and the tendency to infiltrate the allograft has been well recognized. However very few observations have been reported with an apparently isolated renal allograft involvement.

A 26 year-old woman with 50 % PRA received a kidney transplant on may 1989. The graft was matched for one HLA DR antigen. The recipient was seropositive to EBV and CMV prior to transplant. Immunosuppressive regimen consisted of ALG for 10 days, AZA, PRED and CsA started on day 8. Two acute cellular rejection episodes on post-operative days 15 and 60 were responsive to steroid pulse therapy. On march 1990, an allograft biopsy was performed because of increasing blood pressure and decreasing renal function, without graft ultrasound and arteriography abnormalities. It revealed a dense cellular proliferation compatible with the diagnosis of PTLD. Clinical status, blood cell count, liver function tests, serum immunoelectrophoresis, CT scans (brain, chest, abdomen) and bone marrow biopsy were unremarkable. There was no serological evidence of EBV reactivation: IgG VCA : 40 ; IgG EBNA : 20 ; IgG EA : < 5.

CsA was stopped with continuation of AZA and PRED. Blood pressure and creatinine serum level returned to previous values. ACYCLOVIR (10 mg/kg/d) was administered intravenously for 10 days. On november 1990 a solid mass was disclosed within the transplant by ultrasound examination and led to transplantectomy. Histopathological study showed a multifocal nodular infiltration limited to the graft , with large monomorphic B cells (CD 19+, CD 20+, CD 21+, CD 38+), without plasmacytic differenciation. Monoclonality was demonstrated by immunoglobulin gene rearrangement study. The EBV genome was detected within the lesion by in situ hybridization and Southern blot analysis. DNA fingerprinting using minisatellite probes demonstrated the tumor to be of recipient origin. Repeated extensive evaluation failed to document any other localization. Clinical status remained excellent 30 months after restarting dialysis.

As shown by this case, a PTLD may develop in the absence of clinical, biological or radiological abnormalities; it may be discovered on a transplant biopsy and apparently restricted to the renal allograft. It is suggested that the continued antigenic stimulation could facilitate the development in the allograft of EBV-associated PTLD.

EPSTEIN-BARR VIRUS-POSITIVE HUMAN B-CELL LYMPHOMAS IN SCID/HU MICE: MODEL FOR POST-TRANSPLANT LYMPHOMAS.

J.L. Garnier, J. Chargui, H. Plotnicky, J.L. Touraine.
Transplantation Unit, INSERM U80, Pav.P, Hôp. Ed. Herriot, Lyon, France.

Post-transplant B-cell lymphoproliferative diseases are associated with Epstein-Barr Virus (EBV) and represent an often fatal complication of immunosuppression. In order to progress in the understanding of the underlying mechanisms and to develop new therapeutic strategies, we have studied the development of human EBV-positive B-cell lymphomas in mice with severe combined immunodeficiency (Scid) which develop human lymphomas phenotypically and genotypically close to post-transplant lymphomas.

We have already reported that these lymphomas can be induced with human peripheral blood lymphocytes (PBL) injected intra-peritoneally; PBL from EBV-seropositive donors, PBL from seronegative donors infected in vivo with B95-8, or EBV lymphoblastoid cell lines (LCL) can be used. Lymphomas develop within 4-8 weeks after injection of human lymphocytes. A high level of human immunoglobulins in the mice is present at the time of the lymphomas. Tumor cells are different from LCL since they are able to progress in vivo towards late stages of B-cell differentiation. EBV is present in the tumor cells. Most tumors are oligoclonal. Cmyc or Bcl2 oncogenes are not present. IL-10 is a potent B-cell activator and is homologous to EBV-BCRF1 gene; we performed an assay to evaluate the secretion of this lymphokine in the serum of Scid mice with tumors; we found that IL-10 was present at the time of lymphomas.

In order to alter the progression of the lymphomas in the Scid mice, we used anti-B-cell monoclonal antibodies (mAb) and LAK cells. We used anti-CD23 mAb and anti-CD40 mAb (given by F. Rousset), injected at the same time than B95-8, and could not prevent the development of lymphomas in 3 different experiments. We used anti-CD38 mAb (given by G.T. Stevenson); in the first experiment, no mice treated with this antibody directed against a marker of late stages of B-cell differentiation developed a lymphoma; a second experiment is currently performed. LAK cells have been prepared from the PBL of the same donor than the cells which were used in the Scid mice: 5.10^6 have been injected between week 3 and week 4; mice in the control group and mice treated with LAK cells developed tumors between week 5 and week 6.

The development of non-immunosuppressive therapeutic protocols based on anti-B-cell mAb or anti-lymphokines mAb or their association, and cytotoxic cells will benefit of the model of the Scid mice; if their efficiency can be proven, they will be used in transplant patients without the need of stopping the immunosuppression which is for the moment the basis of the treatment.

INFLUENCE OF HBV AND HCV INFECTIONS ON THE SURVIVAL OF LONG-TERM FOLLOW-UP KIDNEY GRAFT RECIPIENTS

P.CHOSSEGROS, N.LEFRANCOIS, P.CHEVALLIER, F.GERARD, C.POUTEIL-NOBLE, JL GARNIER, G.COZON, JP.REVILLARD, C.TREPO, JL.TOURAINE - INSERM U271 Transplantation Unit, Institut Pasteur, Lyon, France

The influence of long term immunosupression on HBV and HCV chronic liver infections is unknown.

We have studied the 64 patients, with a functionnal graft 10 years after their transplantation, out of 256 kidney graft recipients transplanted in our center from 1966 to 1976. Overall median follow-up, after transplantation, was 17.9 years (range 11-25.5 years). Sera for retrospective sological analysis were available in 62 cases.

At the end of follow-up 40% were HBsAg+ (18% HBeAg+, 20% anti HBe+, none anti HDV), 40% were anti HBs and/or anti HBc+, 30% were anti HCV+ (12.5% HBs Ag and anti HCV+). HBe Ag/anti HBe (with a delayed HBV DNA clearance) and HBs Ag/anti HBs seroconversion occured, respectively, in 5 and 1 cases. Out of 21 patients with a known histology, a cirrhosiswas present in 11 cases (9 HBs Ag+ HBV DNA+, 4 anti HCV+, median 17 years).

Death occured in 10 cases (8 HBs Ag+, 3 anti HCV+, median 13.5 years). 5 died of liver failure (4 HBs Ag, HBV DNA+; 1 anti HBc, anti HCV, HBV DNA+). Death was related to the presence of HBs Ag ($p < 0.012$), but not of anti HCV.

Conclusion: In patients with long-term follow-up after kidney transplantation, survival is mainly related to a persitent HBV active replication. HBV DNA clearance is associated to a limited fibrosis whatever the HCV serological status.

COINFECTION WITH HCV DOES NOT INFLUENCE THE OUTCOME OF CHRONIC HEPATITIS B AFTER KIDNEY TRANSPLANTATION (KT)

P.CHOSSEGROS, C.POUTEIL-NOBLE P.CHEVALLIER, F.GERARD, N.LEFRANCOIS, JL GARNIER, C.TREPO, JL.TOURAINE INSERM U271 Transplantation Unit, Institut Pasteur, Lyon, France

To study the influence of HCV coinfection on chronic hepatitis B we have studied the evolution of liver histology in 115 HBsAg+ kidney graft recipients (no HDV coinfection): 246 liver biopsy (range 1 to 5) were performed a median of 75 months after transplantation. At the time of the latest biopsy Hbe Ag was present in 58% (87.5% HBV DNA+) of the cases and anti-HBe in 33% (28.6 HBV DNA+). Anti HCV detection in 37% of the cases was independent of HBe serology and HBV DNA distribution.

The prevalence of cirrhosis increased from 3.6% less than 5 years after transplantation to 31.7% after 20 years. At the end of follow-up HCA was present in 50.5% of the cases. If anti-HCV prevalence at all time and HBV DNA or HBe Ag detection, less than 20 years after KT, were identical in the patients with and without an evolution to cirrhosis, HBV DNA was detected in 78% of the patients with a cirrhosis (20% anti-HBe+) and 38.5% (50% anti-HBe+) of those without after 20 years of evolution (decrease of the prevalence of HBV DNA: 100% <5 years, 43% >20 years).

Conclusion : A spontaneous but delayed clearance of HBV DNA is possible after KT. It is related to an absence of progression of liver fibrosis. HCV coinfection does not influence the outcome of the chronic hepatitis B.

LIVER BIOPSY IN HEMODIALYSIS (HD) PATIENTS WITH CHRONIC HEPATITIS C VIRUS INFECTION. A PROSPECTIVE STUDY TO DETERMINE THE IMPACT OF LIVER INJURY SEVERITY ON PATIENTS OUTCOME.

Authors: Teresa Casanovas, Carmen Baliellas, Glòria Fernàndez Esparrach, Rosa Rota, Romi Casas, Carmen Benasco, Josep M. Griñó, Enric Andrés i Luis A. Casais.
Liver and Kidney Transplant Unit. Hospital de Bellvitge - Hospitalet de Llobregat (Barcelona - SPAIN).

The aim of this study is to evaluate the impact of histologic liver injury due to HCV chronic infection either of the group who remain on HD or patients who received a renal graft.

Patients and methods.- 32 patients were studied over 60 months. 14 patients were on HD awaiting a kidney transplant. 18 patients were already kidney transplant recipients; of those, 13 had a functioning transplant and in 5 the transplant failed and were again on HD when liver biopsy was done. All patients were positive for anti HCV by EIA2 (Abbot Lab. Chicago, Ill.).

Chronic Liver Disease (CLD) was arbitrarily defined as a sustained elevation of ALT (at least twice the normal value) over 6 months.

Patients with diabetes, heart disease, amyloidosis, previous alcoholism or treatment with Azathioprine were excluded. Also excluded were the HBsAg o HBcAb positive patients.

Histological features of the liver are reported following the classification and terminology of the International Group (1977).

Statistics.- Time of follow up is expressed as mean $\pm$ SD. Comparison between patients groups were made with Fisher's exact test. A p value less than 0.05 was considered significant.

Results.-

Pathological Features	H D Group	Mean* ALT	K T Group	Mean ALT
- Minimal Lesions (ML)	1	1,6	2	1,4
- Chronic Lobular Hepatitis (CLH)	3	4,3	3	3,4
- Chronic Persistent Hepatitis (CPH)	5	1,8	6	2,9
- Chronic Active Hepatitis (CAH)	5	2,4	2	2,7
- Chronic Active Hepatitis with bridging hepatitis necrosis (CAHB)	0		5**	4,2
	----	----	----	----
	14		18	

(*Normal values of ALT < 0,7 μkat./l. -   ** p < 0,05)

Clinical evolution.- - HD group: 14 patients. Follow up 27 $\pm$ 18.2 months. On the whole the biochemical abnormalities remained stable. 4 patients received a KT: 3 with CLH or CPH had improvement or normalization of ALT, 1 with CAH had increasing ALT.

- KT group: 18 patients. Follow up 37.9 $\pm$ 17 months. In 16 patients the ALT did not change or improved to normal values. In 2 patients the transplanted kidney failed and the liver lesion progressed. A combined L-K transplant was performed. 1 patient died; the cause was unrelated to liver disease. Both had CAHB in their initial biopsy.

Conclusions.- 1.- In our patients ALT changes do not reflect the severity of the pathological changes, and should not be used as a subrogate marker . Liver biopsy should be used to establish an accurate diagnosis and prognosis.

2.- We found CAHB only in the KT group (statisticaly significative p < 0.05).

3.- Liver biopsy in patients with chronic HCV infection awaiting kidney transplantation will permit:
- Better selection of patients.
- Better timing of the procedure.
- Assess the benefits of Interferon and/or antiviral therapy before transplantation.
- Assess the effects of post transplantations immunosuppression on the liver disease.

HCV-PCR AS A MARKER FOR LIVER DISEASE PROGRESSION OF HCV HEPATITIS IN RENAL TRANSPLANT RECIPIENTS ?

J.L. Garnier, P. Chossegros, O. Boillot, P. Chevallier, N. Lefrançois,
X. Martin, J.M. Dubernard, J.L. Touraine.
Transplantation Unit, Pav.P-Pav.V, Hôpital Ed. Herriot, Lyon, France.

Objective: The frequency of HCV infection in renal transplant recipients can be as high as 25%. In order to evaluate critical markers to follow the progression of liver disease in patients infected with HCV after renal transplantation (tr.), and to establish the basis for anti-viral therapeutic protocols, we sought to know the value of HCV-PCR besides standard parameters of chronic hepatitis.

Patients and Methods: Twenty patients who had received a kidney graft were included in the study. Three of them received a combined kidney + pancreas transplant. Ten patients received ciclosporine from the day of the tr.; 4 were converted from azathioprine to ciclosporine because of liver disease; 6 patients were under azathioprine therapy. HBV serology was performed in all patients; viral replication (DNA polymerase and HBV-DNA) was studied in HBV positive patients. HCV infection was detected by ELISA and RIBA for anti-HCV antibodies; PCR was performed using a nested PCR protocol.

Results: *Group 1: Seven patients had a HBV + HCV infection;* mean follow-up after tr. was 92 months (± 39); good graft function was present in 3 patients; 4 presented with impaired graft function due to chronic kidney rejection/portal hypertension. HCV-PCR was positive in 4 patients; HBV replication was positive in 4 patients. Chronic cytolysis was present in all patients starting at 21 months (± 11) after tr. Liver fibrosis/cirrhosis was noted in 6 patients at 72 months (± 28) . Two patients presented decompensated cirrhosis and one underwent liver transplantation. One patient was treated with Ganciclovir for HBV replication; cytolysis persisted in spite of negativation of HBV-DNA in his serum: Ribavirin therapy was started in this patient (follow-up at 2 months will be presented). *Group 2: Thirteen patients had HCV infection;* mean follow-up after tr. was 105 months (± 62); good graft function was present in 3; chronic rejection/glomerulonephritis was noted in 8; portal hypertension impaired kidney function in 2. HCV-PCR was positive in 12 patients. Chronic cytolysis was noted in 7 patients starting at 43 months (±70) after tr. Liver biopsy was performed in 8 patients; chronic hepatitis was present in all patients, with fibrosis in 4 (118 ± 63 months). Two patients presented with a decompensated fibrosis.

Conclusions: HCV-PCR was positive in almost all patients and did not seem to be a prognostic marker in group 1 or 2. Double HBV and HCV infection seemed associated with progression of liver disease. Anti-viral therapeutic criteria and protocols should be based on clinical, biological and pathological data.

RESPIRATORY VIRAL INFECTIONS IN LUNG TRANSPLANT RECIPIENTS

O. Jarry, J.F. Mornex, M. Bertocchi, F. Thevenet, F. Philit, J.P. Gamondes, M. Chuzel, O. Jegaden, G. Champsaur, O. Bastien, C. Girard, D. Thouvenot, S. Bosshard, A. Calvet, M. Celard. Hôpital Louis Pradel, et Laboratoire de virologie, Université Claude Bernard, Lyon, France.

As any individual, lung transplant recipients are exposed to person-to-person transmission of respiratory viral infections. These viruses are then able to infect the allograft, a unique situation in transplantation. In order to assess the incidence of respiratory viral infections, we prospectively monitored lung transplant recipients by serology and detection of viruses in bronchoalveolar lavage and nasal swab. Evidence of infection was demonstrated by a fourfold or greater increase in the antibody titer and/or virus isolation. Virus isolation was shown by monoclonal antibody staining of the cells in the biological sample or 2 to 3 days after inoculation to tissue culture. Among thirty three adult transplanted patients (heart lung: 12, single lung: 14, double lung: 7) followed for more than 3 month (i.e. 44 winter periods) 28 presented 1 or more viral infection. The viruses were: parainfluenza (23), respiratory syncytial virus (11), influenza A (2), adenovirus (2), coronavirus (2) and rhinovirus (1). Furthermore, despite the ability of these immunosuppressed patients to mount an antibody response, recurrent isolation of respiratory syncytial virus in 2 patients suggests persistance. Most of the patients presented, at the time of the infection, with upper respiratory tract symptoms and/or bronchitis. In 2 instances acute pneumonia was demonstrated by transbronchial biopsy with a cytopathic effect: parainfluenza 3 (1), respiratory syncytial virus (1). Most of these viruses are able to induce an inflammatory process and/or epithelial damage that may contribute to the degradation of the graft function. To support this hypothesis a deleterious effect of respiratory syncytial virus infection was demonstrated by a mean drop in FEV1 of 18% after infection and, in 2 cases, the initiation of a progressive obstructive disease (so-called obliterative bronchiolitis). Thus respiratory viral infections are frequent in lung transplant recipients leading to preventive (isolation of infected patients) and therapeutic (use of aeorosolised and intraveinous antiviral agents) decisions.

FUNGAL INFECTIONS ARE FREQUENT AFTER LUNG TRANPLANTATION

M. Bertocchi, J.F. Mornex, O. Jarry, O. Bastien, M. Rabonirina, F. Thevenet, J.P. Gamondes, M. Chuzel, M.A. Piens, M. Celard. Hôpital Louis Pradel, Lyon, France.

Infections are the major complication of lung transplantation. While, progressively a better control of infection by bacteria and cytomegalovirus have been achieved, other pathogens such as fungi are causing problems. In order to assess the incidence of fungal infection we retrospectively assesssed isolation from blood, bronchoalveolar lavage and bronchial aspiration in 50 adult transplanted patients surviving more than 1 week (heart lung: 19, single lung: 23, double lung: 8; bronchectasies were present in 8 of the total). Repeated isolations of fungal agents were obtained in 29 patients. *Aspergillus* sp. were observed in 7 (*A. fumigatus*, *A. niger*, *A. flavus*, *A. nidulans*, *A. clavatus*) and *Candida* sp. in 22 (*C albicans*, *C. tropicalis*). In 7 patients a coinfection by *Aspergillus* sp. and *Candida* sp. was observed. In addition, *Rhizopus* was isolated from a *post mortem* sample and *Torulopsis glabrata* from multiple *pre mortem* samples in a patient. In 13 of the cases the fungal infection was symptomatic. Fever, pneumonia and/or septicemia was associated with a *C. albicans* infection in 5 patients, furthermore in all of them antibodies and antigenemia were observed, they all survived this episode. Ulcerative invasive bronchitis due to *A. fumigatus* was succesfully treated during more than 6 month in a patient. More importantly 7 patients died in the context of a fungal infection by *C. albicans* in 5 (associated with *Aspergillus* sp. in 2, *Rhizopus* in 1), *A. fumigatus* in 1 and *T. glabrata* in 1. In all of them, both antibodies and circulating antigens were detected, in 3 the pathogen was demonstrated in autopsy specimens. These observations prompted us to use IV prophylactic amphotericin B during 3 weeeks after transplantation. Unfortunately, despite this prophylactic treatment, a patient died of pulmonary and systemic infection by *Pseudallerscheria boydii* known to be resistant to amphotericin. The source of fungal infection is unknown, it could be the recipient, the donor or the operating rooms. In conclusion, fungi are a cause of pulmonary and sytemic infections that can lead to death after lung transplantation.

PART : E

PRESERVATION, SURGERY, RADIOLOGY

AND GENERAL ASPECTS

ISCHEMIA-REPERFUSION INDUCED LIPOPEROXYDATION IN KIDNEY TRANSPLANT : PREVENTION IN VITRO BY ADDITION OF DEFEROXAMINE IN COLD STORAGE SOLUTION.

Cristol J.P., Fourcroy* S., Rebillard X., Iborra F., Bonne* C., Modat* G., Mourad G.
Department of Renal Transplantation, Lapeyronie Hospital, 34059 Montpellier.
* Laboratoire de Physiologie Cellulaire, Faculté de Pharmacie, Montpellier France.

Reactive oxygen species (ROS) generated in kidney transplant as a consequence of ischaemia/reperfusion are an important cause of tissular injury and are involved in acute transplant failure. In this study we determined the lipidperoxidation induced by cold hypoxia/warm reoxygenation in biopies from rabbit or human kidneys conserved in Eurocollins in presence or absence of deferoxamine, an iron chelator.

Renal cortical slices from rabbit kidneys were incubated in the cold storage solution, Eurocollins for 24 to 72 h at 4°C. Reoxygenation was then performed in vitro by incubating the kidney slides in M199 supplemented with 2% fetal calf serum, under normoxic conditions (95% air, 5% $CO2$) for 24h at 37°C. Amounts of thiobarbituric acid reactive substances (TBARS) in disrupted slices were used as an index of lipid membrane peroxidation. Cold hypoxia induced a time dependent increase in TBARS in rabbit biopsies which were furthermore significantly enhanced by reoxygenation. Addition of deferoxamine (10^{-3}) to Eurocollins reduced TBARS formation during cold hypoxia (max. $51.5 \pm 2.16\%$ after 72 h) and during the 24h of warm reoxygenation ($44.09 \pm 6.76\%$). Similar data were obtained with human kidney biopsies.

The present results suggest that addition of iron chelators or free radical scavengers in cold storage solutions would be usefull to preserve kidney transplants for longer periods and to prevent ischaemia / reperfusion -induced tissular injury.

HEART GRAFT REPERFUSION APPARATUS FOR XENOPERFUSION ASSESSMENT.

R. FERRERA[1], A. LARESE[2], J. GUIDOLLET[3], R. GALLETTI[4], G. DUREAU[1,3], D. RIGAL[2]

1- INSERM Unité 63 - 22 avenue du Doyen Lépine - 69675 BRON CEDEX
2- Centre Régional de Transfusion Sanguine de LYON
3- Hôpital Cardiologique de LYON BRON
4- Ecole Vétérinaire de Lyon

In order to investigate animal graft reaction submitted to human blood perfusion, we have set up an *ex-vivo* organ perfusion system. Animal hearts from three different species (Pig, Sheep, Calf) were harvested then reperfused during four hours with whole human blood. It was observed a different behaviour according to the species when xenogenic reperfusion. Pig hearts beatted without dysfunctionment whereas Sheep and Calf hearts stopped rapidly. These latters suggested from an hyperacute rejection symptoms (arythmy, cardiac function impaired, AMP catabolites production, myocardial injury). From these preliminary data we can draw 2 conclusions : (i) our *in vitro* reperfusion system allows a good way to assess the xenograft hyperacute rejection and (ii) Pig hearts tolerate very well the human blood.

KIDNEY GRAFT SALVAGE USING NEW RADIOLOGICAL INTERVENTIONAL PROCEDURES AFTER COMPLICATED BIOPSIES

C.NOEL, JM.COULLET, M.HAZZAN, FR.PRUVOT, L.LEMAITRE, G.LELIEVRE.
CHRU LILLE FRANCE

A Percutaneous needle biopsy of kidney graft is often required to distinguish between rejection and other causes of dysfunction, particularly since the use of cyclosporine A (CsA). The occurrence of arterioveinous fistula (AVF) is a well known complication. Between January 1986 and December 1992, 145 patients underwent a total of 172 percutaneous renal allograft biopsies in our department of transplantation. Three percent of these patients developed hematuria requiring hospitalisation and active treatment, but only 3 patients required embolisation. We report these 3 demonstrative cases where radiological interventional procedures permitted the rescue of the patients and the grafts.

The first one, a 26 year-old woman grafted 30 months ago with a cadaveric kidney, presented under CsA an isolated renal failure with serum creatinine increasing progressively (1.5 to 2.7 mg/dl). The second one, a 35 year-old woman grafted 36 months ago with a cadaveric kidney presented with heavy proteinuria without renal failure. The third one, a 29 year-old man, grafted 15 days ago with a cadaveric combined liver-kidney (oxalosis), presented with a delayed renal graft function.

To perform the graft biopsies, kidney localisation was determined by palpation in 2 cases and ultrasonography in 1 case. Kidneys were punctured three times with lower poleusing thinner-core biopsy needles (diameter 1.7 mm) equipped with an automatic spring system. In the 3 cases, immediately following the biopsies the patients presented abdominal pain and macroscopic hematuria with a marked drop in blood pressure and haemoglobin level. The renal ultrasonography revealed a large perirenal hematoma. The persistency of a gross hematuria with hemodynamic repercussion led us to perform a renal arteriography. It showed at least one free diameter AVF near the inferior third of the little calyx. Through the contolateral femoral artery, a set french guiding catheter was positioned in a peripheral arterial-branch, then micro catheter (Tracker* 2.7 french) was advanced coaxialy up to the 1 mm diameter feeding branch using a 0.14 steerable guiding wire (Seeker**) under digital mapping. Dye injection in this place showed both fistula and leaking of the dye around the thrombus of the calyx, in 2 cases. The AVF were occluded with injection of 1 or several 0.18 inch coil (diameter : 2 or 3 mm). In 2 cases, twenty-four hours later, the patients were anuric and ultrasonography revealed an hydronephrosis with large blood clots in the calyces. A percutaneous pyelostomy, passing through the superior calyx was performed under ultrasonic supervision. Renal cavities were washed with salt serum. Then, renal function rapidly improved and the pyelostomy catheters were removed on the 8th day. In the 3 cases renal function return toward normal.

AVF often closes spontaneously but, infrequently, profuse bleeding required surgical measures which often led to graft removal prior to the emergency. Each graft lost is catastrophic for the patient particularly when histology reveals the absence of serious lesions. So, these cases demonstrate that it is possible to save the graft by high technology derived from intracerebral embolisation.

UPPER POLE DEFECT INDUCED BY CAPTOPRIL ENHANCED SCINTIGRAPHY IN A RENAL TRANSPLANT

TRELUYER C., YATIM A., DAOUD S., PEYRIN J.O., TOURAINE J.L. (Lyon, France)

We report an hypertensive patient with a renal transplant who presented an upper pole renal defect induced by CAPTOPRIL premedication before renography.

He was 43 years old and has been transplanted recently because of a terminal renal insufficiency on a chronic glomerulonephritis which etiology was not known. Hypertention had appeared at the end of the first year of hemodialysis, three years ago. No historical or physical finding, except failure of antihypertensive therapy, was specific in the suspicion of renovascular hypertention. Several treatments with angiotensin converting enzyme inhibitors and calcium blockers were ineffective : blood pressure was noted at 180-110 mmHg. A concentric myocardic hypertrophy and a cardiac insufficiency progressively developed. Despite a nicotism, angiography just revealed an atherosclerotic plaque of 1 cm of length at the distal left iliac bifurcation and healthy coronary arteries. After injection of 1.5 MBq/kg of 99mTc-MAG3 data were acquired in 2 seconds frames for one minute (perfusion study) and in 20 seconds frames for 23 minutes.

Immediately post transplantation the patient underwent a renal perfusion study : the radionuclide renal scanns confirmed good renal transplant vascularisation. Because of still poorly managed hypertention (BP:180-110) and persistent high plasma creatinine level (220 µmol/l), a CAPTOPRIL renography was realized : while perfusion study was normal, baseline renogram was disturbed, particularly in the upper pole of transplant which showed impaired uptake and excretion with parenchymatous stasis. After administration of 50 mg CAPTOPRIL, a passage in acute renal failure was observed (a lost of the second segment of renogram whith a plateau pattern suggestif of renal function's worsening). Control renographies were performed 2 and 10 months later; the upper pole was not vascularized and not functional; the lower pole was visualized but presented impaired functional and kinetic's parameters. Pulsed and color doppler ultrasonographies just showed decreased vascularisation and increased resistive index in the upper area; it did not detect any vascular occlusion. Actually blood pressure is normalized with heavy treatment (calcium blocker and central antihypertensive therapy) and plasma creatinine level is stabilized at 250 µmol/l.

A rise of plasma creatinine level may occur after angiotensin converting enzyme inhibitors administration. It can be related to hemodynamical disturbance. An artery thrombosis or thrombosis on segmental branchies is a more uncommon occurrence, which should not be seen : in hypertensive patients, baseline study showing parenchymatous stasis, (particularly if it's located in one of the pole), with dissociated kinetic's parameters may be related to spontanously decompensated artery stenosis; these constatations should contra-indicate CAPTOPRIL administration.

Diagnosis of segmental branchies requires invasive methods. Angiography currently used in the detection of artery pathology is often contraindicated in the transplanted patients. Nuclear medicin methods due to their non invasive nature and capability to asses blood flow may be able to detect segmental artery thrombosis : they could be helpfull in these cases.

Laparoscopic treatment of lymphocele complicating renal transplantation.

G BURGARD*, N DIAB, C BROYET, C LAMBERT, F BERTHOUX
*General surgery, Nephrology dialysis and transplantation dpt,
Hopital Nord, CHRU St Etienne, 42055 St ETIENNE Cedex2

Pelvic lymphoceles occur in 0.6 to 18% of renal transplantation (RT). They may be responsible for graft dysfunction through ureteral or vascular compression requiring treatment. The best cure actually admitted is internal and permanent drainage by marsupialization. This procedure is usually preformed by laparotomy.

We report the cure of post-RT lymphoceles in two patients by laparoscopy:

A 65 years old polycystic man had impairement of graft function one month after transplantation due to compression of the uretere by a large (87x48mm) lymphocele. 3 external drainages had only transient effects. A 61 years old polycystic female had ureteral and vascular compression by a large lymphocele complicating a severe rejection, on day 83 of transplantation. Laparoscopic drainage under general anesthesia was followed by complete and permanant anatomical correction. A complete renal function recovery was observed in the first patient.

We concluded that laparoscopic marsupialization applicated for compressive post-renal transplantation lymphocele is a good procedure with minimal surgical trauma and rapid patient recovery.

HEMODIALYSIS AND RENAL TRANSPLANT PROGRAM IN IRAN

K.Rahbar, A.Nobakht, F.Proushani, A.Shafii, R.Abdi. Tehran, Iran

The widespread chronic hemodialysis (HD) was started in 1976 in Iran. Actually 4542 patients are hemodialyzed in 94 centers in Iran. Other forms of dialysis are not performed. Although the first renal transplant in Iran was performed in 1968, the transplant program was not started before 1985 This report presents the distribution and progression of dialysis and transplantation in Iran. Since 1985 to 1993, 2511 patients received renal transplant at 6 big and 11 small transplant centers in our country. Only one patient was transplanted by a local cadaveric kidney and the other patients received kidney from living related or unrelated donors. The geriatric population receiving maintenance HD are increasing regularly. This increase is due to our liberal patient selection policy that accepts all patients diagnosed, rather than the increase in life expectancy of general population. Despite the regular increase in the number of new elderly patients treated by HD, the number of transplants in geriatric population after a rapid increase from 1 in 1986 to 26 in 1989 reaches a plateau. This could be explained by the worse results of transplantation in this population, who are not accepted by most of the transplantation centers in Iran. Twenty percent and 9 oercent of hemodialyzed and transplanted patients respectively, had more than 50 years of age. The renal replacement therapy (RRT) is financed and is under the supervision of the Renal Replacement Therapy Office at the Ministry of health in Tehran. Further results and the demographic pattern of RRT in Iran will be presented at the congress.

CENTERS' EFFECT AND GRAFT SURVIVAL

Ph. ROMANO*, M. BUSSON*°, P. N'DOYE°

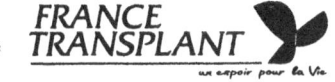

FRANCE TRANSPLANT   Hôpital Saint-Louis, PARIS

° INSERM U93

France-Transplant follow up for kidney graft is devided in two groups regarding years of the graft.

1979-1984 :   20 centers performed 3 665 grafts mean 183 (15 to 540)

1985-1991 :   38 centers performed 10 511 grafts mean 277 + - 208 (24 to 869)

RESULTS
*1979-1984

	M	1 year	5 years	10 years
< 183	12	67	48	31
> 183	8	77	57	42

*1985-1991

	M	1 year	5 years
< 277	20	85	67
> 277	18	84	66

*Comparative follow up for **14 centers**

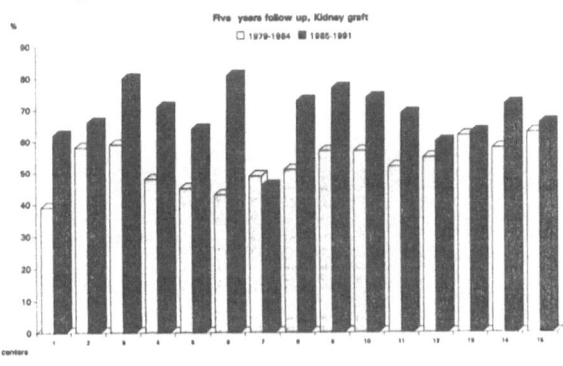

Discussion
Some years ago center's effect existed : high activity gave better results.
Since 1985 there is not yet center's effect.
If there is a difference it seems to be slightly in favour of not very important centers.

NAME INDEX